Pathophysiology of Blood

of

Third Edition

Allan J. Erslev, M.D.

Cardeza Research Professor of Medicine
Director, Cardeza Foundation for Hematologic Research
Department of Medicine
Thomas Jefferson University, Philadelphia

Thomas G. Gabuzda, M.D.

Professor of Medicine
Thomas Jefferson University
Chief, Division of Hematology
Lankenau Hospital, Philadelphia

1985

W. B. Saunders Company

Philadelphia □ London □ Toronto □ Mexico City
Rio de Janeiro □ Sydney □ Tokyo □ Hong Kong

W. B. Saunders Company: West Washington Square
Philadelphia, PA 19105

Library of Congress Cataloging in Publication Data

Erslev, Allan J.

Pathophysiology of blood.

Includes bibliographies and index.

1. Blood—Diseases.   2. Physiology, Pathological.
   I. Gabuzda, Thomas G.   II. Title.   [DNLM: 1. Blood—
   physiology.   2. Hematologic   Diseases—physiopathology.
   WH 100 E73p]

RB145.E75 1985   616.1′507   84–23612

ISBN 0–7216–1170–2

Listed here is the latest translated edition of this book together with the language of the translation and the publisher.

Spanish (*2nd Edition*)—Nueva Editorial Interamericana S. A. de C. V. Mexico 4 D. F., Mexico

Pathophysiology of Blood   ISBN   0–7216–1170–2

Last digit is the print number: 9   8   7   6   5   4   3   2   1

PREFACE

The first edition of *Pathophysiology of Blood* was published in 1975 to meet the need for a small readable and profusely illustrated paperback on the normal and abnormal physiology of blood cells and their supporting plasma components. Since then, the explosive development of cellular and molecular biology necessitated a second edition in 1979 and now a third edition. All of the chapters have been updated and rewritten to an extent that it is difficult to find remnants of what was thought to have been an up-to-date review in 1975. The overall structure has been simplified with fewer major chapters but with more subchapters followed by appropriate references. New illustrations have been added and old illustrations have been upgraded, and we have attempted to catch up with the rapidly changing concepts of hematologic physiology and the mechanism of disease.

Although hematology has evolved from static morphology to a dynamic metabolic science, we have striven to maintain and integrate light and EM morphology with biologic and biochemical observations. Thereby we hope that this monograph will be capable of preparing students for courses in hematology and oncology, residents and fellows for board examinations, and internists, pediatricians, and pathologists for postgraduate programs or recertification. However, it is also hoped that the monograph can be read generally by physicians as an enjoyable exposure to hematology and as a help in choosing therapy that is based increasingly on understanding of disease processes at the molecular level.

As in the previous edition, we would like to thank our medical artist, Andrew S. Likens, for his excellent illustrations and photomicrographs. In order to maintain a uniform style, all graphs are either original or redrawn, and all legends on the ordinate have been turned for more readable horizontal presentations. Our secretaries—Rosemarie Silvano, Doris Riso, and Rosemary McGlynn—have provided valiant support, our associates at the Cardeza Foundation, helpful criticism, and our wives, patient endurance. For all of this we are most grateful.

ALLAN J. ERSLEV, M.D.
THOMAS G. GABUZDA, M.D.

CONTENTS

Introduction

Hematology is traditionally defined as the study of the formed elements of blood. The combined mass of these elements constitutes an organ of considerable size and complexity. On the average, it measures 30 ml. per kg. body weight, or about the same as the liver. The inclusion of active bone marrow, spleen, lymph nodes, and mononuclear macrophage tissue further adds to the size of the hematologic system and to the importance of hematology. Hematology also has close ties with the fluid phase of blood and with the function and kinetics of other organ systems, and it has been increasingly difficult to establish its pathophysiologic limits. The erythrocytes need the cooperation of the heart, lungs, vessels, and kidneys in order to bring oxygen to the tissues; the granulocytes need a host of supporting plasma factors for their phagocytic mission; the lymphocytes produce and react with immunoglobulins; and the thrombocytes cannot be functionally separated from the coagulation factors. With this in mind, we will attempt here to correlate structure, function, and kinetics of the formed elements of blood with those of other organ systems and with overall human pathophysiology. This correlation and its documentation must of necessity be of an introductory nature, but it is hoped that the reader will be stimulated to seek more information from the monographs and key references listed.

1

Hemopoietic Tissues

Bone Marrow

With the exception of lymphocytes, blood cell formation in the normal adult is the exclusive prerogative of bone marrow. Even lymphocytes, however—both T and B cells—are derived from bone marrow, and multipotential stem cells in the marrow cavities are probably directly or indirectly responsible for all blood cell formation. Other areas can support hemopoiesis, but the bones appear to provide an optimal environment for differentiation and multiplication of blood cells. Before bone cavities form during the fifth fetal month, blood cell formation takes place first in the yolk sac and then in the liver and spleen (Fig. 1–1). During the brief yolk-sac phase, the erythrocytes produced are nucleated and contain embryonic hemoglobins, but the subsequent crops of fetal erythrocytes produced by the liver, spleen, and marrow are non-nucleated and contain primarily fetal hemoglobin with $\alpha_2\gamma_2$

polypeptide chains. Although the spleen in the human fetus plays only a brief role in hemopoiesis between the third and seventh months, the splenic microcirculation appears to be well suited for blood cell formation, and the spleen serves as the principal back-up organ for the marrow. At birth, the splenic and hepatic phases have ceased, the slow transformation from fetal to adult hemoglobin production is under way, and all bone cavities are actively involved in blood cell formation.

STRUCTURE

For the first few years of life, there is a precarious balance between the need for blood cells of a rapidly growing infant and the available bone marrow space, and reactivation of

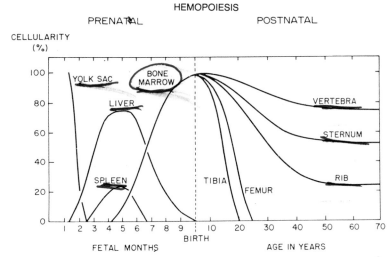

Figure 1–1 Expansion and regression of hemopoietic tissue during fetal and adult life.

hepatic and splenic hemopoiesis takes place whenever there is an increased demand for blood cell formation. At about the age of 4, the growth of bone cavities has outstripped the growth of the circulating blood cell mass, and fatty reserve bone marrow becomes noticeable. Fatty replacement occurs first in the diaphysis of the peripheral long bones, then slowly creeps centripetally until at the age of about 18, hemopoietically active bone marrow is found only in the vertebrae, ribs, pelvis, sternum, skull, and proximal epiphyses of the long bones. This obviously must mean that the available bone marrow space has continued to grow faster than the circulating blood cell mass, since the ratio between progenitor cells in the marrow and mature cells in the circula-tion is the same at all ages. In support of this assumption are measurements by Hudson that indicate that the volume of bone marrow cavities increases from about 1.5 percent of body weight at birth to about 4.5 percent of body weight in the adult, while the blood volume actually decreases from about 8 percent of body weight at birth to about 7 percent of body weight in the adult. During adult life the expansion of bone cavities continues, owing to bone resorption, and there is a gradual increase in the amount of fatty tissue present in all bone marrow areas. Because of the abundant bone marrow space, compensatory reactivation of extramedullary sites rarely takes place in later life, even during periods of accelerated hemopoietic activity. When pres-

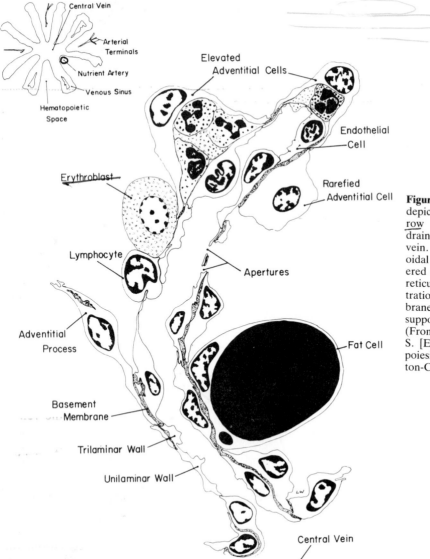

Figure 1–2 Sketch in upper left depicts cross section of bone marrow with spokelike sinusoids draining into a central longitudinal vein. Larger sketch depicts sinusoidal basement membrane covered on the outside by adventitial reticular cells guarding the fenestrations in the basement membrane and providing structural support for hemopoietic cells. (From Weiss, L.: *In* Gordon, A. S. [Ed.]: Regulation of Hematopoiesis. Vol. 1. New York, Appleton-Century-Crofts, 1970.)

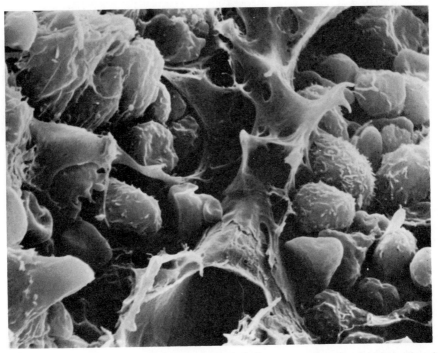

Figure 1–3 A venous sinus crossing the field with luminal endothelium exposed to the right but otherwise covered by adventitial reticular cells. The cytoplasm of these cells extends far into the hemopoietic compartment and provides structure and support for hemopoietic cells. (Courtesy of Weiss, L.: Anat. Rev., *186*:161, 1976.)

ent, extramedullary hemopoiesis often indicates inappropriate rather than compensatory blood formation.

Measurements of blood flow and hemopoietic activity have shown a close relationship between cellular production and blood supply, and some interesting experiments by Huggins suggest that this relationship goes in both directions and that induced vascularization is followed by increased hemopoietic activity. Huggins and coworkers implanted the tip of a rat's tail into the abdominal cavity or enclosed it in a heating chamber and found after some weeks that the inactive fatty marrow had become red and hemopoietically active. The conclusion from these experiments was initially that the low peripheral temperature in the long bones impairs blood cell formation and is responsible for the centripetal regression of active marrow in the adult. However, fatty marrow appears in the fingers even before birth, and active marrow is found in peripheral epiphyses when more proximal diaphyses are completely inactive. It seems more likely that temperature is merely one of many variables that control vascularization and that it is the vascular density of the bone marrow that determines hemopoietic activity. More recent studies by Crosby suggest that this vascular density is inherently lower in the peripheral areas of the body, rendering them particularly vulnerable to decreased temperature.

Structurally, the marrow is highly organized with a spokelike pattern of venous sinuses and cords of hemopoietic tissue (Fig. 1–2). The cords are percolated by arterial blood draining into the central venous sinuses through a basement membrane partly covered on the inside by endothelial cells and on the outside by reticular cells. Projections from the reticular cells subdivide the cords and provide support for hemopoietic cells (Fig. 1–3). They also control available hemopoietic space by gaining or losing lipid globules. Within the cords, the megakaryocytes lie close to the outside of the sinus wall and appear to reel off strings of cytoplasmic platelets directly into the sinus. The erythroblasts also lie close to the venous sinuses in distinctive clusters or islands. Each island consists of a central macrophage, or nurse cell, with maturing and dividing erythroblasts nestled in cytoplasmic pockets (Fig. 1–4). When mature enough for independent existence, the erythroblasts and reticulocytes as described by Chamberlain and Lichtman "bore" through the basement membrane and its endothelial coverage. During this passage through de novo apertures, pyknotic

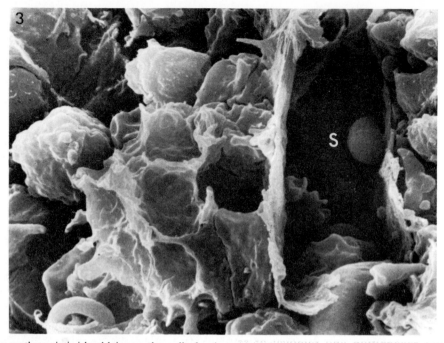

Figure 1–4 An erythropoietic island lying on the wall of a sinusoid (S) in rat bone marrow. The erythroblasts, nestled in the pockets of the island, were removed during the preparation of this scanning electron microscopic picture. (Courtesy of Weiss, L.: Anat. Rev., *186*:161, 1976.)

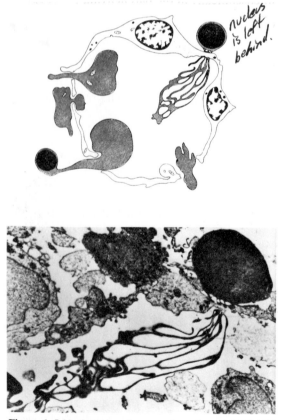

Figure 1–5 Nucleated and non-nucleated red blood cells "boring" through the basement membrane into a venous sinus. The nucleus is incapable of the necessary deformation and is snared off. (Courtesy of Bessis, M.: Life Cycle of the Erythrocyte. Sandoz Pharm., 1966.)

and nondeformable nuclei not lost previously to macrophages are expelled (Fig. 1–5). The maturing and dividing granulocytic precursors are situated deep in the hemopoietic cords and do not move toward and through the sinus wall until they reach a motile metamyelocytic stage.

The nervous supply to the marrow is quite extensive, as everyone having experienced a bone marrow aspiration can attest to. Some of the nerves are in close contact with the hemopoietic islands and may sense pressure changes caused by cellular proliferation. If such signals are transmitted to the nerves attached to the vessel walls, an autoregulatory system may well exist, adjusting the flood flow to permit undisturbed proliferation and maturation before the cells are released into the circulation.

The fatty tissue that in the adult fills about 50 percent of the bone cavities probably serves merely as a space-occupying material. It is preserved even during severe starvation, but so far it has not been found to play a significant role in marrow cell proliferation and maturation (Tavassoli, 1984).

FUNCTION

The marrow is one of the major mononuclear phagocyte organs and is involved in antigen processing, cellular and humoral immu-

HEMATOPOIESIS

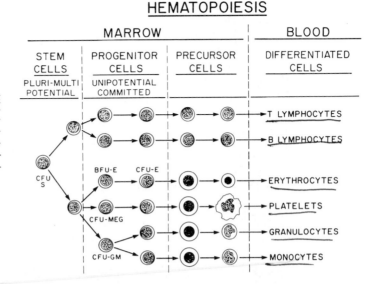

Figure 1–6 Outline of hematokinetics. CFU-S = colony-forming unit—spleen; CFU-GM = colony-forming unit—granulocyte, monocyte (also called CFU-C for culture); CFU-MEG = colony-forming unit—megakaryocyte; BFU-E = burst-forming unit—erythroid; CFU-E = colony-forming unit—erythroid.

nity, and the recognition and removal of senescent cells. Its main mission, however, is the production of differentiated blood cells (Fig. 1–6). These cells are derived from pools of morphologically similar but functionally dissimilar cells capable of both self-renewal and differentiation. The capacity for self-renewal diminishes slowly as the cells move from early stem cell pools to late progenitor pools and is finally lost when they become recognizable marrow precursor cells. The capacity for differentiation in many cellular directions diminishes similarly as the cells move from pluripotential stem cells via multipotential myelopoietic and lymphopoietic stem cells to unipotential progenitor cells committed to single cell lines. However, the proliferative activity increases steadily as the cells become more and more differentiated. (See 1983 review by Ogawa and coworkers.)

The pluri- and multipotential stem cells are rarely in cycle and are only moderately affected by tritiated thymidine given in doses high enough to cause radiation-induced "suicide" of cells incorporating thymidine for the synthesis of new DNA (Quesenberry and Levitt, 1979). These stem cells are believed to provide a dormant reserve first activated by marrow depletion or injury. Such activation into a regenerative and differentiating cell cycle was first described by Till and McCulloch in their classic observations of the spleens of irradiated mice, in which surviving or transplanted marrow attempts to replenish the hemopoietic tissues. Initially, the few available stem cells enter into intense proliferative activity and produce minute clonal colonies of un-

differentiated stem cells. After the fifth day, specific differentiation takes place, and discrete marrow colonies can be observed macroscopically on the surface of the spleen and microscopically in the parenchyma of the spleen and the marrow (Fig. 1–7). Since chromosomal studies have shown conclusively that each colony is derived from a single stem cell, it is possible to quantitate the number of multipotential stem cells (CFU-S [colony-forming units—spleen]) present initially. In the mouse, it has been estimated that there are about one

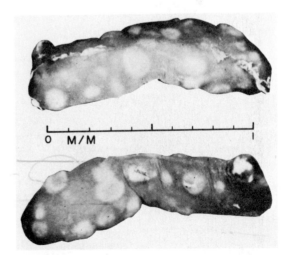

Figure 1–7 Each white raised plaque on the surface of these mouse spleens contains a colony of marrow cells. These colonies were found 7 days after total body radiation immediately followed by a transfusion of marrow cells obtained from an isogeneic donor. Each colony is derived from a single sequestered multipotential stem cell, which is designated as a CFU-S (colony-forming unit—spleen).

to three multipotential stem cells per 1000 nucleated marrow cells.

The dependence of a specific microenvironment for the capture and growth of CFU-S can also be demonstrated in cultures on semisolid media. In such media, short-term growth of marrow progenitor cells can be achieved, but sustained growth of multipotential stem cells can be accomplished only if the marrow cells are plated on a "hospitable stroma" consisting of endothelial cells, fat cells, macrophages, and other supporting marrow cells (Dexter et al., 1977). With this technique, it has been possible to isolate and identify CFU-S in human marrow. Barr and Whang-Peng have also identified human CFU-S in the lymphocyte fraction of blood. In this fraction, they could be separated from B and T lymphocytes

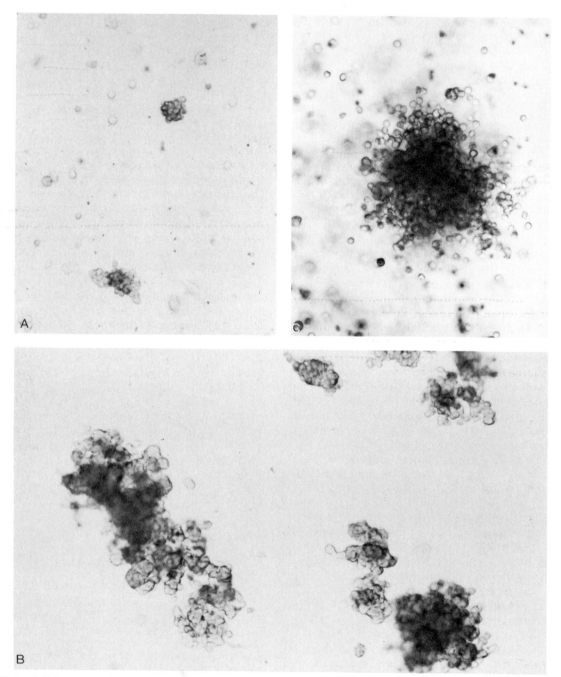

Figure 1–8 Stem cell cultures in semisolid media. *A*, Two CFU-E colonies. *B*, One BFU-E colony. *C*, One CFU-C (or GM) colony. (× 200)

but morphologically they were found to resemble small lymphocytes.

Studies on the distribution and composition of marrow colonies in the spleen have provided valuable information about the interrelationship between parenchymal structure and subsequent cellular differentiation. Each colony is made up of a mixture of hemopoietic cellular elements, usually with one cell type dominating. Although the specific differentiation probably is determined by humoral stimuli, it has been demonstrated by Trentin that the immediate cellular environment, or HIM (hemopoietic inductive microenvironment), modifies the effectiveness of the stimuli. Colonies derived from stem cells lodged on the surface of the spleen are primarily erythroid, whereas colonies from cells lodged in the center of the spleen or in the marrow are primarily granulocytic and megakaryocytic. This effect of the microenvironment on cellular differentiation is undoubtedly of major importance for normal hemopoiesis, but it is not known whether it is caused by a modification of the activities of progenitor cells or of precursor cells (see reviews by Tavassoli and Friedenstein, 1983 and by Dexter and coworkers, 1984).

The unipotential progenitor cells have been shown by the use of tritiated thymidine "suicide" techniques to be in active cell cycle. They are also capable of limited self-renewal, but in order to undergo blast transformation and further differentiation regardless of the microenvironment they need the stimulus of humoral "poietins." Erythropoietin is known to be the specific "poietin" for progenitor cells committed to erythropoiesis, but there is also evidence for the existence of leukopoietins and thrombopoietins needed for the differentiation of progenitor cells committed to granulopoiesis and thrombopoiesis.

In the presence of even small amounts of erythropoietin, bone marrow suspensions plated on fibrin clots or on methyl cellulose plates will form tiny erythroid colonies consisting of from 8 to 64 hemoglobin-containing erythroblasts (Fig. 1–8). The responsible cell has been identified by Clarke and Houseman as a small mononuclear lymphocyte-like cell. It has been designated as a CFU-E (colony-forming unit—erythroid) and it is probably identical with the unipotential, erythropoietin-responsive progenitor cell. In addition to these early occurring CFU-E, a second kind of colony begins to appear after 8 to 10 days of culture if the medium contains large amounts of erythropoietin. These colonies grow to macroscopic size and may contain thousands of erythroblasts. Because of their irregular outline with many CFU-E subcolonies they are called "bursts," and the responsible cell is called a "burst-forming unit—erythroid," or BFU-E (Fig. 1–8). BFU-E have been demonstrated in both peripheral blood and bone marrow, while CFU-E have been found only in the marrow.

Recent studies by Iscove have suggested that the primary stimulus of the BFU-E is a burst-promoting activity or factor (BPF) released by macrophages and T lymphocytes, but large amounts of erythropoietin appear to have enough BPF activity to initiate recruitment of CFU-E. A current hypothesis envisions BFU-E as early descendants of CFU-S (Fig. 1–9). They contain a few erythropoietin receptors enabling them to respond to large concentrations of erythropoietin with proliferation and maturation. According to Gregory and Eaves, the progeny will contain an increasing number of erythropoietin receptors until at a certain point of maturation the progenitor cells acquire the properties of CFU-E and undergo blast transformation to hemoglobin-producing erythroblasts. A problem with this hypothesis

ERYTHROPOIESIS

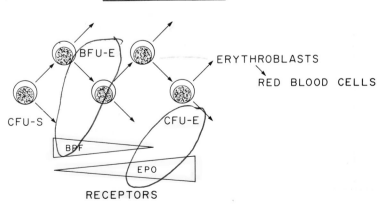

Figure 1–9 Kinetics of erythroid stem cells with hypothetical density of receptors for BPF (burst-producing factor) and EPO (erythropoietin). CFU-S = colony-forming unit—spleen; BFU-E = burst-forming unit—erythroid; CFU-E = colony-forming unit—erythroid.

Table 1–1 NORMAL MARROW KINETICS

Cell Type	Marrow		
	Number *(cells/kg)*	*Transit Time (days)*	*Production (cells/kg/day)*
I. Red cells			
Erythroblasts	5.3×10^9	5.0	3.0×10^9
Reticulocytes	8.2×10^9	2.8	3.0×10^9
II. Megakaryocytes	15×10^6	7	2.0×10^6
III. Granulocytes			
Proliferation pool	2.1×10^9	5.0	0.85×10^9
Postmitotic pool	5.6×10^9	6.6	0.85×10^9

(Courtesy of Finch C. A., et al., Blood, *50*:699, 1977.)

is that erythropoietin-responsive progenitor cells appear to be in active cell cycle even in the absence of erythropoietin. An explanation may be that these progenitor cells have a certain base line rate of proliferation with wastage and death of cells not exposed to erythropoietin. Studies summarized by Craddock and coworkers provide some support for this explanation by demonstrating the presence of short-lived mononuclear cells in the bone marrow.

Marrow plated on agar has also been shown to grow large colonies composed of granulocytes and monocytes when exposed to a colony-stimulating activity or factor, CSF (Fig. 1–8). These colonies have been designated CFU-C (C for culture) or CFU-GM (G for granulocytes and M for macrophages). The CSF originates from monocytes or macrophages and apparently is capable of transforming granulocyte-committed unipotential progenitor cells to myeloblasts and monoblasts (see review by Burgess and Metcalf). Although it acts as a leukopoietin in vitro, its physiologic significance, if any, for in vivo granulopoiesis is still moot. Megakaryocytic colonies (CFU-MEG) originating from bone marrow plated on fibrin plates and stimulated by various factors have been described by Nakeff and Daniels-McQueen, but their relationship to physiologic thrombopoiesis is also unknown.

The newly formed proerythroblasts and myeloblasts will subsequently undergo three to five mitotic divisions, resulting in an 8- to 32-fold multiplication (Fig. 1–6). The nucleus of the megakaryoblast will undergo the same number of endomitotic divisions, resulting in the formation of a few huge cells with multilobed nuclei. Concomitant with nuclear proliferation, the cytoplasm will undergo specific maturation, and 3 to 5 days after the initial differentiation the cells are almost completely mature and functional.

The maturing reticulocytes and the maturing granulocytes remain in the bone marrow for some days before they are released into the circulation. The length of this delay appears to be responsive to the immediate needs for circulating blood cells. However, because the circulating granulocyte mass is much smaller than the circulating red cell mass, a premature release of the marrow reserve of maturing cells is of importance only for the adjustment of the peripheral granulocyte count. After the release from the marrow, the erythrocytes are all in active use in circulating blood, while about 50 percent of the granulocytes and 30 percent of the thrombocytes are sequestered in the microvasculature or in the spleen as functional reserves. Figure 1–10 and Table 1–1 give a summary of the cellular morphology and composition of the hemopoietic tissue. The apparent discrepancy between the 2:1 ratio between erythroid and granulocytic cells and the 1:2 ratio found in marrow smears is caused by the fact that the marrow reticulocytes are included in the table but usually not in marrow differential counts.

Figure 1–10 The normal morphology of the hemopoietic cells.

References

Barr, R. D., and Whang-Peng, J.: Hemopoietic stem cells in human peripheral blood. Science, *190*:284, 1975.

Burgess, A. W., and Metcalf, D.: The nature and action of granulocyte-macrophage colony stimulating factors. Blood, *56*:947, 1980.

Chamberlain, J. K., and Lichtman, M. A.: Marrow cell egress: specificity of the site of penetration into the sinus. Blood, *52*:959, 1978.

Clarke, B. J., and Houseman, D.: Characterization of an erythroid cell of high proliferative capacity in normal human peripheral blood. Proc. Natl. Acad. Sci. USA, *74*:1105, 1977.

Craddock, C. G., Longmire, R., and McMillan, R.: Lymphocytes and the immune response. N. Engl. J. Med., *285*:324, 1972.

Crosby, W. H.: Experience with injured and implanted bone marrow: relation of function to structure. *In* Stohlman, F. Jr. (Ed.): Hematopoietic Cellular Proliferation. New York, Grune & Stratton, 1970, p. 87.

Dexter, T. M., Allen, T. D., and Lajtha, L. G.: Conditions controlling the proliferation of hemopoietic stem cells in vitro. J. Cell Physiol., *91*:335, 1977.

Dexter, T. M., et al.: The regulation of hemopoietic cell development by the stromal cell environment and diffusible regulatory molecules. *In* Young, et al. (Eds.): Aplastic Anemia. New York, Liss, Inc., 1984, p. 13.

Ebbe, S.: Thrombopoietin. Blood, *44*:605, 1974.

Erslev, A. J.: Feedback circuits in the control of stem cell differentiation. Am. J. Pathol., *65*:629, 1971.

Finch, C. A.: Pathophysiologic aspects of sickle cell anemia. Am. J. Med., *53*:1, 1972.

Finch, C. A., Harker, L. A., and Cook, J. D.: Kinetics of the formed elements of human blood. Blood, *50*:699, 1977.

Gregersen, M. I., and Rawson, R. A.: Blood volume. Physiol. Rev., *39*:307, 1959.

Gregory, C. J., and Eaves, A. C.: Human marrow cells capable of erythropoietic differentiation in vitro. Definition of three erythroid colony responses. Blood, *49*:855, 1977.

Hudson, G.: Bone marrow volume in the human foetus and newborn. Br. J. Haematol., *11*:446, 1965.

Huggins, L., and Blockson, B. H.: Changes in outlying bone marrow accompanying a local increase of temperature within physiologic limits. J. Exp. Med., *64*:253, 1956.

Iscove, N. N.: Erythropoietin-independent stimulation of early erythropoiesis. *In* Golde, D. W., et al. (Eds.): Hematopoietic Cell Differentiation. New York, Academic Press, 1978, p. 37.

Killmann, S. A., Cronkite, E. P., Fliedner, T. M., and Bond, V. P.: Mitotic indices of human bone marrow cells. III. Duration of some phases of erythrocyte and granulocytic proliferation computed from mitotic indices. Blood, *24*:267, 1964.

Nakeff, A., and Daniels-McQueen, S.: In vitro colony assay for a new class of megakaryocyte precursor: colony-forming unit megakaryocyte (CFU-M). Proc. Soc. Exp. Biol. Med., *151*:587, 1976.

Ogawa, M., Grush, O. C., O'Dell, R. F., Hara, H., and MacEachern, M. D.: Circulating erythropoietic precursors assessed in culture: characterization in normal men and patients with hemoglobinopathies. Blood, *50*:1081, 1977.

Ogawa, M., Porter, P. N., and Nakahata, T.: Renewal and commitment to differentiation of hemopoietic stem cells. Blood, *61*:823, 1983.

Quesenberry, P., and Levitt, L.: Hematopoietic stem cells. N. Engl. J. Med., *301*:755, 1979.

Reissmann, K. R., and Udupa, R. B.: Effect of erythropoietin on proliferation of erythropoietin-responsive cells. Cell Tissue Kinet., *5*:481, 1972.

Robinson, W. A., and Mangalik, A.: The kinetics and regulation of granulopoiesis. Semin. Hematol., *12*:7, 1975.

Tavassoli, M.: Marrow adipose cells and hemopoiesis: An interpretative review. Exp. Hematol., *12*:139, 1984.

Tavassoli, M., and Friedenstein, A.: Hemopoietic stromal microenvironment. Am. J. Hematol., *15*:195, 1983.

Till, J. E., and McCulloch, E. A.: A direct measurement of the radiation sensitivity of normal mouse bone marrow cells. Radiat. Res., *14*:213, 1961.

Trentin, J. J.: Determination of bone marrow stem cell differentiation by stromal hemopoietic inductive microenvironment (HIM). Am. J. Pathol., *65*:621, 1971.

Weiss, L.: The hemopoietic microenvironment of the bone marrow: an ultrastructural study of the stroma in rats. Anat. Rev., *186*:161, 1976.

Weiss. L., and Chen, L. T.: The organization of hematopoietic cords and vascular sinuses in bone marrow. Blood Cells, *1*:617, 1975.

Wu, A. M., Till, J. E., Siminovitch, L., and McCulloch, E. A.: A cytological study of the capacity for differentiation of normal hemopoietic colony-forming cells. J. Cell. Physiol., *69*:177, 1967.

Spleen

STRUCTURE

The normal spleen—no longer involved in hemopoiesis—is the largest of the lymphoid organs (Videbaek et al., 1982). Yet it is also a unique filtration bed for the circulating blood well equipped with macrophages to remove undesired particles from the circulation. The parenchyma, or "pulp," is partitioned by fibrous trabeculae, through which run the arteries, veins, and lymphatics. Arterioles run out from the trabeculae into the white pulp, branch at right angles into the marginal zone, and then terminate in the red pulp (Fig. 1–11). The venous drainage system originates in the sinus system of the red pulp. The blood then flows out through the trabecular veins and on into the portal system. The efferent lymphatic drainage runs into the thoracic duct.

In the white pulp, a sleeve of T lymphocytes—the "periarterial lymphatic sheath"—is wrapped around the central artery (Fig. 1–12). Nodular accumulations of lymphocytes, often at the sites of the right-angled vascular branches, form follicles along the course of the central arteriole. These contain germinal centers rich in B lymphocytes surrounded by mantle zones of T lymphocytes and macrophages. The cellular structure is held together by a network of fibrillar reticular cells.

The marginal zone is an ill-defined boundary between the white and red pulp. Into its interstices, also held together by fibrillar reticular cells, empty many arteriolar branches filling the spongy network with blood cells. Under provocative stimuli, macrophages readily migrate into this area.

Blood from the marginal zone as well as from central arterial terminals drains into the red pulp, either directly into venous sinuses and on out through the efferent veins or into the cords that lie between the sinuses (Fig. 1–13). The blood cells that enter the cords must pass through the fenestrated wall separating the cords from the sinuses before gaining access to the venous draining system. They are thus delayed to varying degrees in their transit. The fenestrations in the wall separating the cords and sinuses are about 3 μ in diameter, so small that erythrocytes must be squeezed through with effort. They pass through because their pliability and deformability are normally very great (Fig. 1–14). The sinus side of the wall is lined by reticular endothelial cells lying upon the fenestrated basement membrane. The cordal side of the wall is made up of the adventitial network of reticular cells and macrophages surrounding and separating the sinuses.

Blood flow through the spleen is both fast and slow. Rapid transit is achieved by the fraction that bypasses the cords and enters directly into the sinuses. The slow transit fraction is temporarily detained in the cords. Normally, this detention is not very great; the time required for complete mixing of blood within the spleen as measured with tagged erythrocytes is only about 2 minutes. When the spleen enlarges, however, the detention time of the "slow-flow" fraction may increase to as long as an hour, with potentially deleterious effects on the survival time of erythrocytes, particularly if they do not have their customary flexibility and become more easily entrapped in the splenic cords.

Plasma-skimming is another important aspect of the splenic circulation. Laminar flow in the central arteries directs leukocyte-rich plasma into the perpendicular branches feeding the germinal follicles and the marginal zone. This leaves behind more viscous high-hematocrit blood in the central artery to flow on into hemoconcentrated red pulp.

FUNCTIONS

Filtration

The spleen is the most discriminating filter of the circulating blood. The liver has a much larger filtration capacity because of its greater

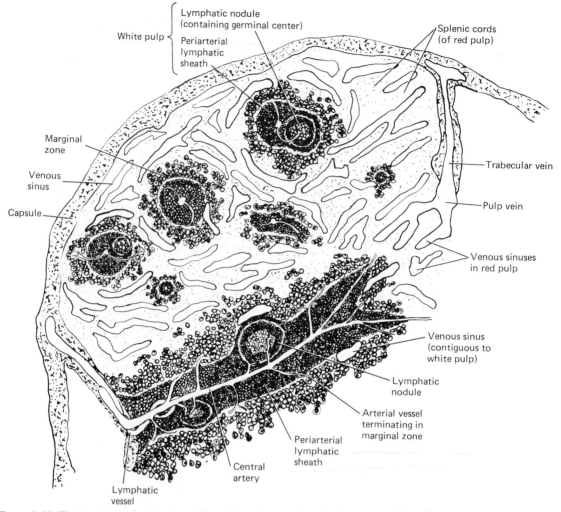

Figure 1–11 The structure of the spleen. The white pulp consists of the periarterial lymphatic sheath and lymphatic nodules with germinal centers. The red pulp contains the splenic cords and sinuses. The marginal zone is interposed between white and red pulp. The central artery sends branches out into the marginal zone and then terminates in the red pulp. Blood from the splenic cords passes through a fenestrated wall into the sinuses and is then collected into the splenic veins. (From Weiss, L., and Tavassoli, M.: Semin. Hematol., 7:372, 1970. Reprinted from Weiss, L., and Greep, R. O. [Eds.]: Histology. New York, McGraw-Hill Book Company. Copyright © 1977, McGraw-Hill Book Company.)

blood flow, but the spleen with its specialized network of cords and sinuses is able to select out for phagocytic clearance the more subtly altered particles. For example, Hosea and associates (1981) found that red blood cells and pneumococci that are only lightly coated with antibody are efficiently cleared from the circulation when the spleen is intact, but when it is absent a much denser antibody coating is required to achieve the same rate of clearance by the macrophages remaining in the liver and in other organs. Analogous principles apply to the autoimmune hemolytic anemias and thrombocytopenias. Red cells and platelets more lightly coated with autoimmune IgG are selected for destruction in the spleen, but in its absence they are not recognized by hepatic macrophages, past which they circulate too rapidly to be noticed. Hepatic uptake occurs when the antibody coating is more dense and especially when complement has been fixed to the surface of the circulating cells.

Cell Grooming

Erythrocytes undergo a certain degree of restructuring as they percolate through the splenic cords. Reticulocytes endure preferential splenic delay in transit, possibly because

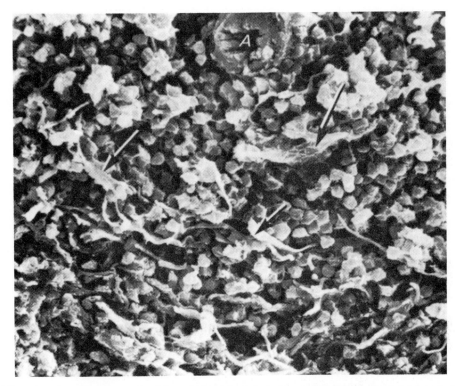

Figure 1–12 Scanning electron micrograph of the splenic white pulp in the region of the periarterial lymphatic sheath. A sea of lymphocytes is held together by reticular cells and their associated fibrils (shown by arrows). The central arteriole (A) is shown in cross section near the upper margin. (From Weiss, L.: Blood, *43*:665, 1974.)

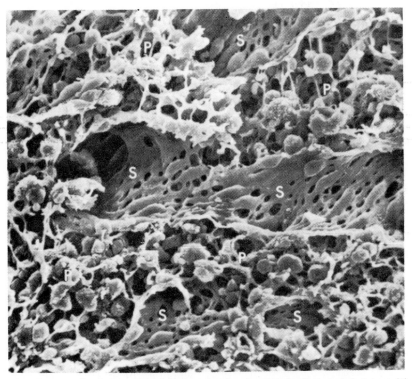

Figure 1–13 Scanning electron micrograph of the splenic red pulp, showing the fenestrated sinuses (S) and the spongy cords (P) that lie between the sinuses and consist of hematogenous cells enmeshed in an adventitial reticular network. (From Miyoshi, M., and Fujita, T.: Arch. Histol. Jpn., *33*:225, 1971.)

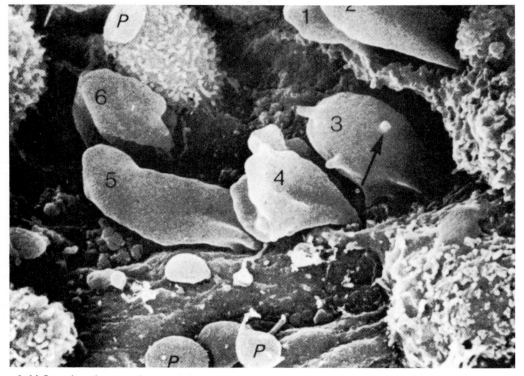

Figure 1–14 Scanning electron micrograph demonstrating erythrocytes (numbered 1 through 6) squeezing through the fenestrated wall in transit from the splenic cord to the sinus. The view shows the endothelial lining of the sinus wall, to which platelets (P) adhere, along with "hairy" white cells, probably macrophages. (From Weiss, L.: Blood, *43*:665, 1974.)

their transferrin coating makes them more "sticky" than mature erythrocytes. Intracytoplasmic inclusions left over after extrusion of the newly formed erythrocyte into the marrow sinusoid are plucked by splenic macrophages from the cell interior, usually without detriment to the integrity of the self-sealing red cell membrane. These inclusions consist of iron granules, hemoglobin precipitates, fragments of DNA, and even the entire erythroid cell nucleus. They are not numerous unless bone marrow function is hyperactive or abnormal, such as in Cooley's anemia or sickle cell anemia. In these conditions, the asplenic state is characterized by large numbers of circulating normoblasts and inclusion-containing erythrocytes. Loss of membrane surface along with membrane cholesterol accompanies the cellular grooming during splenic transit. The spleen, with the other organs of the mononuclear phagocyte system, removes senescent cells from the circulation.

Reservoir

In humans, the spleen is an important reservoir of platelets, as reported by Aster in 1966. About 30 percent of the body's platelets are sequestered there in slow transit and in dynamic equilibrium with the circulating pool. The splenic platelets are immediately moved into the circulation after stress or injection of epinephrine. The transitory platelet increase is accompanied by a parallel increase in Factor VIII level. Neither response is seen in the splenectomized individual. There is no significant storage pool of red or white cells in the human spleen, although in some animals, such as the dog, horse, and sheep, muscular contraction of the splenic capsule abruptly increases the peripheral hematocrit by means of "autotransfusion" of a reservoir of splenic blood.

Immunity

The spleen is a major station for lymphocyte traffic. It contains about 25 percent of the exchangeable pool of T lymphocytes and about 10 to 15 percent of that of the B lymphocytes. The T cells spend about 4 to 6 hours there, whereas the B cells linger somewhat longer. Opportunities are presented for cell-to-cell interactions, and then destination markers lure the T and B cells to their preferential sites of localization.

Because it is an efficient filter and is so well equipped with macrophages, the spleen is ideally suited for initiating the response to bloodborne antigen (Lockwood, 1983). It may also participate significantly in the immune response to antigen presented by other routes (e.g., specific antibody production in response to polyvalent pneumococcal vaccine given subcutaneously is impaired when it is absent). The spleen makes an especially important contribution to IgM production, and, in its absence, serum concentrations of IgM are significantly reduced.

Although filtration and antibody formation are the two functions most missed when the spleen is absent, deficient activities of the alternate complement pathway and of tuftsin, a tetrapeptide phagocytosis-promoting factor, have also been described.

In summation, the spleen, although not indispensable, is a most useful and occasionally vital component of the defense network of the body (Eichner, 1979).

PATHOPHYSIOLOGY

Asplenia

The asplenic state is usually the result of surgical removal. Splenectomy may be performed on hematologically normal individuals for traumatic rupture or incidentally during the course of surgery initiated for other reasons. Splenectomy is also done for hematologic indications, including hereditary spherocytosis, autoimmune hemolytic anemia or thrombocytopenia, staging laparotomy for Hodgkin's disease, Cooley's anemia, and any of a variety of causes of "hypersplenism." For some time, the spleen was considered dispensable because its absence did not seem to disturb vital functions. It has since been recognized that splenectomized individuals carry an increased risk of serious and often fatal infection, most often caused by encapsulated strains of *Streptococcus pneumoniae*, *Hemophilus influenzae*, and *Neisseria meningitidis* (Singer, 1973). The specific incidence depends on the age of the patient and on the presence of underlying disorders (Schwartz et al., 1982; Zarrabi and Rosner, 1984). Infants and small children are particularly susceptible, probably because of the immaturity of their immune system. Individuals

who were splenectomized because of lymphoma, Cooley's anemia, or other serious systemic disorders are also at an especially high risk. The overall incidence of serious infection is about 3 to 4 percent, with an associated mortality rate of about 50 percent.

In rare instances, the spleen is congenitally absent (Kevy et al., 1968). Atrophic spleens may occur as a result of splenic radiation or in association with malabsorption syndromes (Coleman et al., 1982; Wardrop et al., 1975). Extensive infiltration of the spleen (e.g., with amyloid) may cause an asplenic state (Hurd et al., 1980). Repeated splenic infarction in sickle cell anemia during childhood is a form of "autosplenectomy." Even before this transpires and when the spleen is still intact or even enlarged, youngsters with sickle cell anemia have a reversible "functional asplenia"; the state of chronic hemolysis causes a blockade of the mononuclear phagocyte system, including that present in the spleen. A similar blockade occurs in systemic lupus erythematosis because of high levels of circulating immune complexes that saturate phagocytic capacity and cause decreased splenic function (Dillon et al., 1982).

The removal of the spleen is followed by a rise in platelet and granulocyte counts, often reaching peaks after about 10 days of more than 1,000,000 and 30,000 per mm^3, respectively. The elevated counts gradually return to normal values in most cases. Late postsplenectomy effects include an absolute lymphocytosis, monocytosis, and the presence of occasional immature cells in the peripheral blood. Interaction between the spleen and bone marrow has been postulated to explain these changes, but experimental proof for this hypothesis has never come forth.

The asplenic state can usually be suspected by the presence of red cell inclusions, especially Howell-Jolly bodies, which otherwise are removed by the normal spleen (Fig. 1–15). In pathologic states, these may be very numerous. Significant numbers of target cells and spiculated erythrocytes, or "burr" cells, are also present, along with a parallel increase in erythrocyte membrane surface, membrane cholesterol content, and osmotic resistance. The erythrocyte mean corpuscular volume (MCV) is often high, the number of reticulocytes may be slightly increased, and a few giant platelets can be seen. Special microscopic techniques demonstrate erythrocyte vacuoles that give the cell surface a pitted appearance (Fig. 1–16).

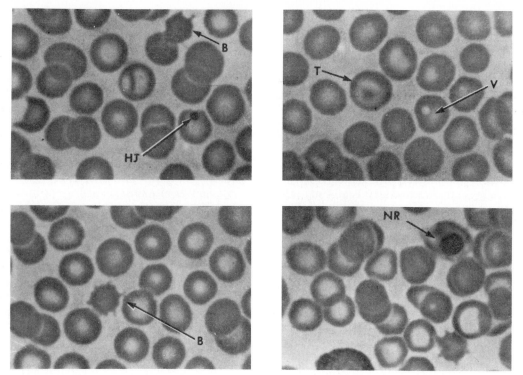

Figure 1–15 Morphologic signs in the peripheral blood of asplenia. HJ = Howell-Jolly body (fragment of DNA); T = target cell; V = vacuole; B = "burr" cell; NR = nucleated red cell. (From Holroyde, C. P. *In* Custer, R. P.: An Atlas of the Blood and Bone Marrow. Philadelphia, W. B. Saunders Co., 1974, p. 125.)

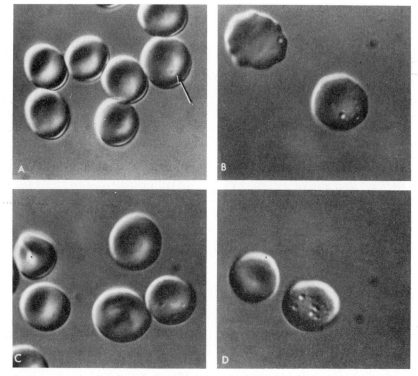

Figure 1–16 Interference contrast microscopy of erythrocytes. *A,* Cells of normal adult with intact spleen. Only 1 to 2 percent of the cells have vacuoles. *B,* Cells of normal adult after splenectomy performed because of ruptured spleen. About 50 percent of the cells contain vacuoles. Full-term infant *(C)* and premature infant *(D)* demonstrate an increased proportion of vacuole-containing cells, the latter to a more striking degree. (From Holroyde, C. P. *In* Custer, R. P.: An Atlas of the Blood and Bone Marrow. Philadelphia, W. B. Saunders Co., 1974, p. 134.)

2) Splenomegaly

Occasionally, splenic enlargement is caused by a disorder intrinsic to the spleen, such as a cyst, but more often it occurs as a feature of a systemic disease process (Table 1–2) (Eichner and Whitfield, 1981). A reactive response of the lymphoid white pulp is seen in infections, especially viral, whereas neoplastic proliferation is responsible for the splenomegaly of the lymphoproliferative disorders. The splenic pool of macrophages hypertrophies when subjected to a chronic work load (Bommer et al., 1981). This may be caused by bacterial infections, such as subacute bacterial endocarditis and miliary tuberculosis, or by the state of chronic hemolysis itself. Hypertrophy of the splenic pool of lipid-laden macrophages is responsible for the splenomegaly of the lipidoses.

The spleen may return to shades of its past developmental history and become swollen with hemopoietic myeloid tissue. Severe chronic hemolytic anemia is one stimulus for extramedullary hemopoiesis, especially in Cooley's anemia. Splenic infiltration with hematogenous elements also occurs as a common feature of the myeloproliferative syndromes. In temperate zones, some of the largest spleens

Table 1–2 CLASSIFICATION OF SPLENOMEGALY

Lymphatic Disorders
  Reactions to infections, especially viral (e.g., infectious mononucleosis)
  Reactions to connective tissue disorders (e.g., disseminated lupus erythematosus)
  Lymphoproliferative disorders (e.g., lymphatic leukemia, lymphoma)
Macrophage Disorders
  Reactions to infections (e.g., subacute bacterial endocarditis, miliary tuberculosis, tropical splenomegaly)
  "Work hypertrophy" secondary to chronic hemolytic anemia
  Lipidoses (e.g., Gaucher's disease)
  Proliferative disorders (e.g., histiocytic medullary reticulosis, Letterer-Siwe disease)
Infiltrative Disorders
  Myeloproliferative disorders
  Extramedullary hematopoiesis secondary to chronic hemolytic anemia (e.g., Cooley's anemia)
  Amyloidosis
Increased Splenic Vein Pressure (Congestive Splenomegaly)
  Splenic or portal vein thrombosis
  Liver cirrhosis
Miscellaneous
  Sarcoidosis
  Congenital cyst ("true," epithelial-lined, "primary")
  Post-traumatic cyst (not lined, "secondary")
  Rare tumors, primary and metastatic
  Nontropical idiopathic splenomegaly
  Abscess

occur in patients with myelofibrosis and myeloid metaplasia.

Vascular congestion—"congestive splenomegaly"—is seen most often as a consequence of portal hypertension secondary to hepatic cirrhosis, but obstructions of the portal and splenic veins are other etiologic considerations. Marked splenomegaly in patients living in tropical regions—"tropical splenomegaly"—apparently is caused by chronic malarial infestation or other infections endemic to the region. "Nontropical idiopathic splenomegaly" was so designated by Dacie and associates (1978) because of the nondiagnostic histology of the spleen after its removal in patients without evidence of other coexisting disease. A significant proportion of such patients subsequently develop lymphoma. Cysts, non-hemopoietic tumors, and abscesses are relatively infrequent causes of splenic enlargement (Chun et al., 1980).

3) Extra Spleens

Small accessory spleens are found in the splenic hilum, the mesentery, the region of the tail of the pancreas, or elsewhere in about 10 percent of normal individuals. They may enlarge after splenectomy and cause relapse of the hematologic condition for which the operation was originally done. This is, however, an unusual occurrence. "Splenosis" follows the seeding of multiple small implants of spleen tissue in the peritoneal cavity as a result of rupture of the splenic capsule. The spleen cells colonize and develop into nodules of spleen tissue studded on serosal surfaces.

Pearson and associates (1978) found that a large proportion of children splenectomized for traumatic rupture of the spleen had a partial return of spleen function because of splenosis. This observation may well explain why this group of splenectomized individuals has the lowest incidence of postsplenectomy infection.

The Spleen as a Trap

Hypersplenism is a term honored by both time and usage, but in the light of present concepts of the interactions of the hematogenous cells with the spleen, it lacks pathophysiologic precision. Hypersplenism is characterized by (1) reduction in erythrocytes, platelets, granulocytes, or any combination of these cellular elements in the peripheral blood; (2)

splenomegaly; (3) a cellular marrow implying adequate marrow compensation in response to the cytopenia; and (4) correction of the cytopenia by splenectomy (Pearson, 1980). Strictly speaking, the term should thus not be used until successful response to splenectomy has been documented.

The splenic blood volume, normally about 50 ml., may increase to such a degree in splenomegalic states that it contains as much as 25 percent of the total blood volume, and up to 90 percent or more of the total pool of platelets. However, the platelets, if otherwise untainted, withstand this altered distribution quite well. They easily escape from the splenic cords into the sinuses, where they are found temporarily adhering to the vascular wall, happily bathed by flowing blood with excellent preservation of their viability. Granulocytes, if otherwise normal, also seem to endure sequestration in the enlarged spleen without suffering undue damage. Red cells, dependent on glycolysis for energy, are susceptible to deterioration during repeated passages through the splenic cords. The depressed glucose concentration in the splenic red pulp (as low as one third the level in the blood) and the inhibitory action of the low pH (the result of lactic acid accumulation) severely limit glycolysis. Hemoconcentration and low Po_2 add insult to injury—especially in sickle cell disorders. The larger the spleen, the greater the likelihood of clinically significant sequestration phenomena, but precise correlation with the degree of splenomegaly is not always possible. Differences in the extent of cell entrapment in the splenic cords among patients with comparable degrees of splenomegaly may be explained by differences in the partition of splenic blood flow into rapid- and slow-transit streams.

The rigid inelastic cells of sickle hemoglobinopathy, homozygous hemoglobin C disease, and the Heinz body hemolytic anemias are more easily trapped and damaged in the spleen than normal erythrocytes. The erythrocyte in hereditary spherocytosis, by virtue of its high glycolytic requirement, is exquisitely sensitive to erythrostasis, and the stress of repeated passages through the splenic environment produces fragmentation at the membrane surface with sphering and, ultimately, entrapment and lysis. The state of chronic hemolysis provokes work hypertrophy of the spleen, which in turn may adversely reciprocate and worsen the hemolysis. In Cooley's anemia, the spleen may enlarge so massively that transfused erythrocytes do not survive sufficiently long to enable

the patient to maintain adequate hemoglobin levels. Splenectomy then becomes mandatory. If massive splenomegaly in the patient with myelofibrosis and myeloid metaplasia is responsible for intolerable transfusion requirements or for bleeding due to severe thrombocytopenia, splenectomy may be beneficial even in the face of marrow failure.

The Spleen and Autoantibodies

Erythrocytes and platelets coated with 7S antibody are selectively taken up and destroyed in the spleen. In autoimmune hemolytic anemia and thrombocytopenia, the antibody is of endogenous origin. During splenic transit, the antibodies on the cell surfaces cause adhesion to macrophages, the instruments of cell damage and destruction. When cells are more grossly affected with autoantibody and a phenomenon such as agglutination or complement-mediated membrane damage occurs in the circulation, cell destruction in extrasplenic sites predominates.

The observation that some patients achieve permanent remission after splenectomy with eventual disappearance of the autoantibody has led to the hypothesis that in these instances the spleen is the major or even the sole site of its synthesis. Indeed, experiments of Karpatkin and others (1983) have provided direct evidence that cells prepared from the excised spleens of patients with autoimmune idiopathic thrombocytopenic purpura do synthesize an antiplatelet antibody, leading to platelet destruction by the splenic macrophages.

The Spleen, Intravascular Volume, and Portal Hypertension

In patients with massive splenomegaly (Table 1–3), the blood flow through the organ increases from its normal value of 5 percent to

Table 1–3 SOME CAUSES OF CHRONIC MASSIVE SPLENOMEGALY

Myelofibrosis with myeloid metaplasia
Chronic granulocytic leukemia
"Hairy cell" leukemia
Chronic lymphocytic leukemia
Lymphosarcoma
Cooley's anemia
Gaucher's disease
Kala-azar
Malaria

as much as 50 percent of the cardiac output. The large volume of blood draining out through the splenic vein distends the portal vascular tree with two important consequences, "dilutional" anemia and portal hypertension.

Although anemia in the presence of massive splenomegaly may be primarily related to pooling of 25 percent or more of the red cell mass along with varying degrees of hemolysis, measurement of the total red cell mass may reveal that it is actually normal or even increased with an even greater expansion of total plasma volume and blood volume (i.e., there is a dilutional anemia). The mechanism of these changes in intravascular volume has been described by Hess and coworkers (1976). The portal vascular bed is expanded at the expense of the remainder of the intravascular space, including the renal circulation. Stimulation of the renin-angiotensin-aldosterone system causes retention of salt and water. Reduced colloid osmotic pressure then stimulates albumin synthesis. Normal albumin concentrations are restored, and the total albumin pool is expanded.

Massive splenomegaly is also associated with high cardiac output, hypermetabolism, and a wide pulse pressure. Decreased peripheral vascular resistance, necessary to meet the needs of heat dispersion, also compromises the renal circulation and stimulates renin secretion to expand intravascular volume.

If the spleen is surgically removed, the expanded blood volume only gradually returns to normal over a matter of several months. The reason for this slow reversal probably is the long time necessary for normal catabolic processes to dispose of the excess in the total body albumin pool.

Portal hypertension secondary to massive splenomegaly may be complicated by esophageal and gastric varices and risks of upper gastrointestinal hemorrhage. Varices may also form secondary to splenic vein thrombosis because of the increased blood flow from splenic accessory veins into the venous system of the greater curvature of the stomach and lower esophagus. When the spleen is the cause of serious portal hypertension, its removal may be the cure. However, outflow obstruction due to hepatic cirrhosis is by far the commonest cause of portal hypertension, for which splenectomy is almost never helpful, except perhaps when bleeding occurs in association with unusually severe thrombocytopenia.

References

Aster, R. H.: Pooling of platelets in the spleen. Role in the pathogenesis of "hypersplenic" thrombocytopenia. J. Clin. Invest., *45*:645, 1966.

Bommer, J., Ritz, E., and Waldherr, R.: Silicone-induced splenomegaly. Treatment of pancytopenia by splenectomy in a patient on hemodialysis. N. Engl. J. Med., *305*:1077, 1981.

Chun, C. H., Raff, M. J., Contreras, L., et al.: Splenic abscess. Medicine, *59*:50, 1980.

Coleman, C. N., McDougall, I. R., Dailey, M. O., et al.: Functional hyposplenia after splenic radiation for Hodgkin's disease. Ann. Int. Med., *96*:44, 1982.

Dacie, J. V., Galton, D. A. G., Gordon-Smith, E. C., and Harrison, C. V.: Non-tropical "idiopathic splenomegaly": a follow up study of 10 patients described in 1969. Br. J. Haematol., *38*:185, 1978.

Dillon, A. M., Stein, H. B., and English, R. A.: Splenic atrophy in systemic lupus erythematosis. Ann. Int. Med., *96*:40, 1982.

Eichner, E. R.: Splenic function: normal, too much, and too little. Am. J. Med., *66*:311, 1979.

Eichner, E. R., and Whitfield, C. L.: Splenomegaly. An algorithmic approach to diagnosis. J.A.M.A., *246*:2858, 1981.

Hess, C. E., Ayers, C. R., Sandusky, W. R., et al.: Mechanism of dilutional anemia in massive splenomegaly. Blood, *47*:629, 1976.

Hosea, S. W., Brown, E. J., Hamburger, M. I., and Frank, M. M.: Opsonic requirements for intravascular clearance after splenectomy. N. Engl. J. Med., *304*:245, 1981.

Hosea, S. W., Burch, C. G., Brown, E. J., et al.: Impaired immune response of splenectomized patients to polyvalent pneumococcal vaccine. Lancet, *1*:804, 1981.

Hurd, W. W., and Katholi, R. E.: Acquired functional asplenia. Association with spontaneous rupture of the spleen and fatal spontaneous rupture of the liver in amyloidosis. Arch. Int. Med., *140*:844, 1980.

Karpatkin, S.: The spleen and thrombocytopenia. Clin. Haematol., *12*:591, 1983.

Kevy, S. V., Tefft, M., Vawter, G. F., and Rosen, F. S.: Hereditary splenic hypoplasia. Pediatrics, *42*:752, 1968.

Lockwood, C. M.: Immunological functions of the spleen. Clin. Haematol., *12*:449, 1983.

Pearson, H. A.: Splenectomy: its risks and its roles. Hosp. Pract., *15*:85, 1980.

Pearson, H. A., Johnston, D., Smith, K. A., and Touloukian, R. J.: The born-again spleen. Return of splenic function after splenectomy for trauma. N. Engl. J. Med., *298*:1389, 1978.

Schwartz, P. E., Sterioff, S., Mucha, P., et al.: Postsplenectomy sepsis and mortality in adults. J.A.M.A., *248*:2279, 1982.

Singer, D. B.: Postsplenectomy sepsis. Perspect. Pediatr. Pathol., *1*:285, 1973.

Videbaek, A., Christensen, B. E., and Jonsson, V.: The spleen in health and disease. Chicago, Year Book Medical Publishers, 1982.

Wardrop, C. A. J., Lee, F. D., Dyet, J. F., et al.: Immunological abnormalities in splenic atrophy. Lancet, *2*:4, 1975.

Zarrabi, M. H., and Rosner, F.: Serious infections in adults following splenectomy for trauma. J.A.M.A., *144*:1421, 1984.

Lymphatic Tissues

STRUCTURE

The organs that give rise to lymphocytes and then foster their differentiation are called *primary lymphatic tissues*. These are the marrow, the thymus, and the sites of active hemopoiesis in the fetus. The *secondary lymphatic tissues* are the repositories of already differentiated lymphocytes. These include the lymph nodes, spleen, and visceral lymphocyte deposits such as those found in the subepithelial regions of the gastrointestinal tract (David, 1984).

The marrow and spleen have been described in previous sections. The structure of the other lymphatic tissues will be discussed here, along with the kinetics of lymphocyte production, circulation, and life span. Lymphocyte subsets will be covered more extensively along with pathophysiology in the section in Chapter 3 entitled Immunocytes.

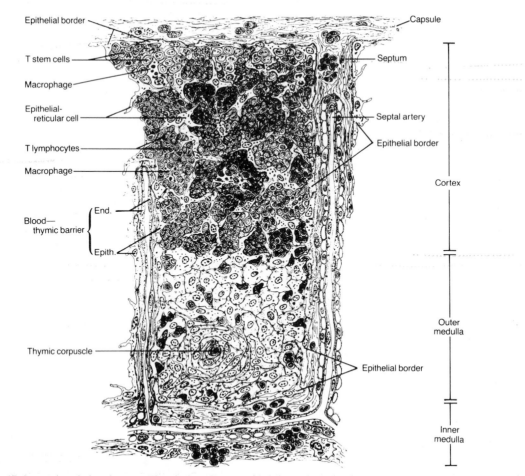

Figure 1–17 Structure of the thymus. Thymic lymphocytes (thymocytes) differentiate as they move from cortex to medulla. (From Weiss, L.: Textbook of Histology. 5th ed. New York, Elsevier North-Holland, Inc., 1983, p. 512.)

Thymus

The thymus gland is an epithelial organ that becomes densely invaded by lymphocytes newly derived from stem cells in the marrow or fetal hemopoietic organs. The thymic epithelium nurtures their differentiation into immunocompetent T cells (Scollay, 1983). In the absence of the thymus, T cell development does not occur; the T-dependent sites of the secondary lymphatic tissues are vacant, and the immune response is bereft of T cell–mediated functions.

The thymus arises at approximately the eighth week of gestation from the third and fourth branchial pouches. It is a bilobed structure located in the anterior mediastinum. Each lobe is subdivided into multiple lobules. It grows steadily until puberty, then it gradually involutes. In old age, it becomes atrophic. With aging, the secondary lymphatic tissues, already well populated with self-renewable immunocompetent T cells, become less dependent on the thymus.

The thymic lobules are separated by fibrous septa branching off from the organ capsule. In the lobular cortex, immigrant small and medium-sized lymphocytes ("thymocytes") predominate over the native epithelial cells, to which they seem to adhere. Macrophages are found, predominantly at the corticomedullary junction. The cellular arrangement is less compact in the medulla, where small lymphocytes and epithelial cells mingle with Hassall's corpuscles, characteristic small concentric whorls of squamoid epithelial cells, the function of which is unknown (Fig. 1–17).

Undifferentiated pre–T lymphocytes arrive in the cortex and, over several days, under the inductive influence of the thymic epithelium, differentiate into mature immunocompetent T cells as they migrate to the medulla. This maturation process is accompanied by changes in membrane surface markers ("differentiation antigens"). From the medulla, they enter the blood and then home into the T-dependent regions of the secondary lymphatic tissues.

Extracts of thymus have some activity in differentiating T cells, but the physiologic role of thymic hormones ("thymosin") is still uncertain (Ahmed et al., 1979).

Bursa Equivalent

In birds, a primary organ of epithelial origin induces the differentiation of B lymphocytes in a process analogous to the role of the thymus in T cell differentiation. The structure, called the *bursa of Fabricius,* is derived from the gut. In its absence, B cell development fails—lymphocytes are absent from B-dependent areas of the secondary lymphatic tissues, and humoral immunity is deficient. This organ is not present in mammals, and the term *bursa equivalent* is used to denote its functional counterpart, the site of which is thought to be the marrow (Goldschneider, 1982).

Lymphatics

The lymph nodes are strung out along a system of thin-walled channels called *lymphatics* (Fig. 1–18) (Mayerson, 1963). These conduct excess extravascular fluid back into the blood. Along the way, the lymph nodes add increasing numbers of lymphocytes, mostly T cells, also destined for return to the blood. The lymph nodes are anatomically grouped into a number of regions, some on the body exterior (submental, occipital, pre- and post-auricular, cervical, supraclavicular, axillary, epitrochlear, inguinal, and femoral) and some concealed in the interior (mediastinal, hilar, paraortic, iliac, mesenteric, and others).

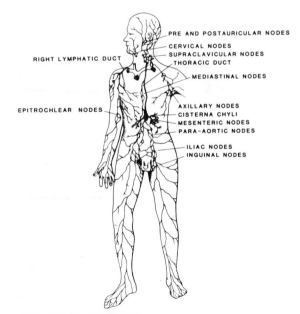

Figure 1–18 Lymphatics drain from distal to proximal sites in the body. Drainage from the lower portions of the body and the left arm, neck, and head is via the thoracic duct into the left subclavian vein. A minor drainage system from the right arm, neck, and head is via the right lymphatic duct into the right subclavian vein. (Adapted from Beck, W. S.: Human Design. Molecular, cellular and systematic physiology. Harcourt Brace Jovanovich, Inc. New York, 1971, p. 222.)

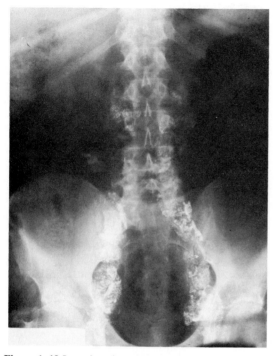

Figure 1–19 Lymphangiogram in a patient with Hodgkin's disease demonstrating enlarged abnormal iliac and retroperitoneal lymph nodes.

Lymph Nodes

Lymph nodes, distributed in large numbers throughout the body, bear a heavy responsibility for mounting immune responses (Fitch and Hunter, 1978). They contain lymphocytes, plasma cells, and macrophages along with vas-cular elements. An arrangement of the lymphocytes into follicles with germinal centers is a characteristic feature of the secondary lymphatic tissues. Germinal centers are not present in the marrow or thymus. Lymph nodes vary from 0.1 to 1.5 cm. in diameter. They may grow considerably larger in reactive or neoplastic conditions (Fig. 1–19).

The follicles are arranged in a row in the cortex of the lymph node just beneath the capsular sinus (Fig. 1–20). There are macrophages along with irregularly shaped large and medium-sized lymphocytes in the germinal centers. A mantle of small lymphocytes surrounds the germinal center. The outer pole of the mantle wears a cap of small lymphocytes. The deeper paracortex is a region of heavy lymphocyte traffic, also well endowed with macrophages. The medulla of the lymph node is arranged into parallel cords of small lymphocytes and plasma cells.

B and T lymphocytes settle in characteristic zones. B cells localize in the superficial cortex, the germinal centers, and the medullary cords. T cells home into the deep paracortex and into the periphery of the germinal follicles (Fig. 1–21).

The afferent lymphatic penetrates the capsule and enters the subcapsular sinuses, which dip into the nodal substance beside fibrous trabeculae. The sinuses combine in the medulla to emerge as an efferent lymphatic at the nodal hilum running along the artery and vein. Blood lymphocytes exit from the postcapillary venules in the deep paracortex. After some

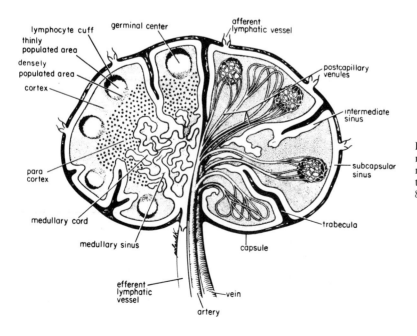

Figure 1–20 Structure of a lymph node. (From Samter, M. [Ed.]: Immunological Diseases. 3rd ed. Boston, Little, Brown & Co., 1978, p. 82.)

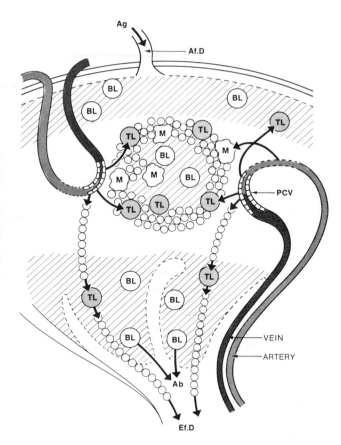

Figure 1–21 Localization of B and T cells in lymph node. TL = T lymphocyte; BL = B lymphocyte; M = macrophage; Ag = antigen; Ab = antibody; Af.d = afferent lymphatic duct; Ef.d = efferent lymphatic duct; PCV = postcapillary venule. The cross-hatched zones represent areas populated by B cells (superficial cortex, germinal centers, and medullary cords). Areas containing open circles represent T lymphocyte regions (deep paracortex, follicle periphery). T lymphocytes circulate in close proximity to both macrophages and B cells, allowing for cell–cell interactions. (From Craddock, C. G., et al.: N. Engl. J. Med., *285*:380, 1971.)

wandering, most of them enter the efferent flow of lymph, destined for return to the blood. The efferent lymph contains 50 times as many lymphocytes as the afferent flow.

KINETICS

Lymphopoiesis

Lymphocyte production in the primary lymphatic organs (marrow and thymus) proceeds continuously, independent of antigenic stimulation (Micklem, 1979). The production rate is far in excess of what is necessary; most of the lymphocytes appear to be destroyed in situ, and relatively few take up positions as differentiated cells in the secondary lymphatic tissues (Fig. 1–22).

In contrast, lymphocyte proliferation in the secondary lymphatic tissues proceeds appropriately and in response to antigenic stimulation, resulting in expansion of specific selected populations of lymphocytes specialized to take part in immune responses to particular antigens. The secondary tissues, although depend-

ent on marrow or fetal hemopoietic organs as their source of stem cells, maintain a capacity not only for proliferation but also for self-renewal.

Circulation

Most of the circulating lymphocytes, about 80 percent of them T cells, are mixed in the blood with other cell types. They selectively leave the blood at the postcapillary venules of the lymph nodes. They then enter the efferent lymphatic for a slower trip back to the blood via the main thoracic duct or the lesser right thoracic duct. The lymph is virtually a pure suspension of lymphocytes in extravascular fluid.

The T cells are more mobile than the B cells, most of which do not circulate. Most T cells recirculate, a fact amply demonstrated by the observation that depletion of the lymph by exterior drainage causes a fall in the blood lymphocyte count and desertion of the T-dependent zones of the secondary lymphatic tissues. T cells remain in the blood for about

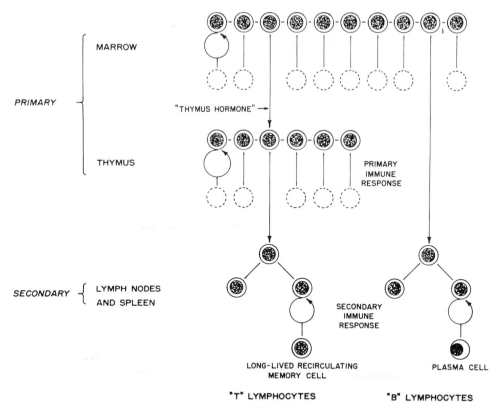

Figure 1–22 Lymphopoiesis. Interrupted circles represent effete cells. Proliferation takes place in both primary and secondary lymphatic tissue, and both have capacity for self-renewal. Augmentation of cell numbers in response to antigenic stimulation is characteristic of the secondary lymphatic tissue.

½ hour, in the spleen for about 6 hours, and in the lymph nodes for about 15 to 20 hours. Circulating B cells move somewhat more slowly. For example, they remain in the lymph node for about 30 hours.

Life Span

The life span of lymphocytes varies immensely from a few days to many months or even years. By means of DNA labeling or chromosomal markers, it has been shown that some small lymphocytes, presumably memory cells, survive for many years. However long-lived such cells may be, they still retain a viable nucleus with the ability to re-enter cell division upon appropriate antigenic stimulation. In this respect, lymphocytes differ from the red cells, platelets, and granulocytes of the blood, which all have finite life spans and can no longer divide. Plasma cells are end-stage

cells without a self-renewing capacity, and they appear to survive for only 2 or 3 days.

FUNCTION

Despite their simple morphology, immunocompetent lymphocytes are highly diversified and specialized. They have perfected a means of recognizing specific antigens, thereby directing defensive attacks on foreign invaders in close cooperation with phagocytic cells. With functional duties in such close accord, it is natural that these two families of cells should share common anatomic sites. Shared domiciles provide the proper setting for interactions of lymphocyte populations with each other and with macrophages.

Immune responses are classified as cell-mediated T-dependent and as humoral B-mediated. Although the two systems are distinct in functional development and in anatomic

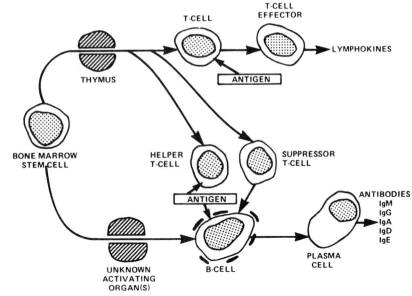

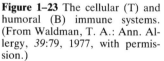

Figure 1–23 The cellular (T) and humoral (B) immune systems. (From Waldman, T. A.: Ann. Allergy, *39*:79, 1977, with permission.)

distribution, they must cooperate in an interdependent relationship (Fig. 1–23).

Cell-Mediated Immunity

The cell-mediated immune responses include delayed hypersensitivity; graft-versus-host reaction; defense against viral, fungal, and certain bacterial infections; and possibly even containment of neoplastic cells. After initial processing and recognition of specific antigen, T cells are programmed and become activated. They proliferate and secrete lymphokines. The latter are hormone-like substances that augment the immune response by a variety of actions, including the activation and proliferation of other T and B cells as well as of phagocytic macrophages. Activated T cells also serve as effector cells working with other effector cells—macrophages, mast cells, and mature granulocytes. Some of the activated T cells produce a population of small nondividing lymphocytes that bear a memory of the event, ready to resume immediate proliferation upon re-exposure to the antigen after prolonged periods of time, possibly even a lifetime.

Humoral Immunity

B cells must also be programmed with information about specific antigen. The formation of antigen-antibody complexes on their surfaces provokes activation, proliferation, and further differentiation into antibody-secreting plasma cells. The antibodies act as agglutinins, lysins, and opsonins. For many antigens, the B cell response requires the cooperation of T cells. In this respect, T cells exert important regulatory functions upon B cell activity. These are carried out by essentially separate T cell subsets, augmentation by the helper T cells and inhibition by the suppressor T cells (Fig. 1–23). The relatively immobile B cells also require the cooperation of the circulating T cells to spread the "message" quickly and thereby to achieve activation rapidly throughout the body. Like T cells, some long-lived B cells retain memory of specific antigenic encounters.

References

Ahmed, A., Wong, D. M., Thurman, G. B., et al.: T lymphocyte maturation: cell surface markers and immune function induced by T lymphocyte cell free products and thymosin polypeptides. Ann. N.Y. Acad. Sci., *332*:81, 1979.

David, J.: The organs and cells of the immune system. *In* Rubenstein, E., and Federman, D. D. (Eds.): Sci. Am. Med., New York. Sci. Am. Inc., 1984, p. 6:II:1.

Fitch, F. W., and Hunter, R. L., Jr.: Histology of immune responses. *In* Samter, M. (Ed.): Immunological Diseases. Boston, Little, Brown & Co., 1978, p. 81.

Goldschneider, I.: Heterogeneity of bone marrow "lymphocytes." Clin. Haematol., *11*:491, 1982.

Mayerson, H. S.: The lymphatic system. Sci. Am., *208*:80, 1963.

Micklem, H. S.: B lymphocytes, T lymphocytes and lymphopoiesis. Clin. Haematol., *8*:395, 1979.

Scollay, R.: Intrathymic events in the differentiation of T lymphocytes: a continuing enigma. Immun. Today, *4*:282, 1983.

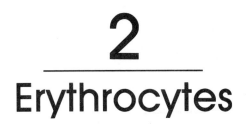

2

Erythrocytes

Structure and Function

MORPHOLOGY

The ultrastructure of the erythroid cell is increasingly being correlated with metabolic activities, and structure and function will be discussed together in this chapter. However, the morphology of blood cells stained with the Romanovsky dyes and the membrane topography deserve some separate remarks, since they are cornerstones in the clinical diagnosis and therapy of patients with hematologic disorders.

The earliest cell that can be recognized morphologically as a nucleated red blood cell is the proerythroblast. Preceding this precursor cell are several progenitor cells (CFU-E, BFU-E) that are committed but not yet triggered to enter the erythroid line (Fig. 1–9). These cells, like other progenitor or stem cells, morphologically resemble small to medium-sized lymphocytes. When exposed to erythropoietin they undergo transformation to proerythroblasts, large cells with diameters about 20 to 25 μ and nuclei that occupy about three fourths of the cells (Fig. 1–10). In a proerythroblast, the nuclear chromatin, stained dark violet with the usual Wright or Giemsa stain, is finely dispersed, and the nucleus with its one or several nucleoli is clearly separated from the deep-blue cytoplasm by a distinct membrane. The nucleus is usually perfectly round and the cytoplasm devoid of granules. The subsequent proliferation and maturation through the stages of basophilic, polychromatophilic, and orthochromatic erythroblasts are characterized by a stepwise reduction in cellular and nuclear size, by a condensation of the nuclear chromatin into well-defined chunks, and by a di-

lution of the blue-staining cytoplasmic ribosomes with newly synthesized hemoglobin. At the orthochromatic stage, the nucleus has become condensed into a small pyknotic mass and is extruded. Hemoglobin synthesis continues for a few more days until the nucleus-dependent synthetic machinery is exhausted. During this period, precipitation and condensation of the remaining basophilic ribosomes with oxidant dyes such as brilliant cresyl blue and methylene blue will result in the characteristic appearance of the reticulocyte on a blood smear. The final transformation of reticulocytes to mature cells is associated with a considerable loss in volume due to cytoplasmic dehydration and loss of cellular membrane.

The mature erythrocyte is a biconcave disk with an average diameter of about 8 μ and a central pallor occupying the middle third of the cell. Owing to a relative excess of surface over volume, the cell is soft and pliable, accounting for the ease with which it can pass through tissue capillaries and splenic fenestrations with diameters considerably less than its own. Its membrane has a remarkable self-healing capacity, and red cell injury may cause the production of viable fragments rather than intravascular hemoglobin leakage. As the cell grows older it becomes slightly more dense, but it maintains its normal pliable biconcave appearance until enzymatic failure leads to rigidity, macrophage trapping, and destruction.

Membrane Topography

The morphology of the mature red cell appears to depend almost exclusively on the

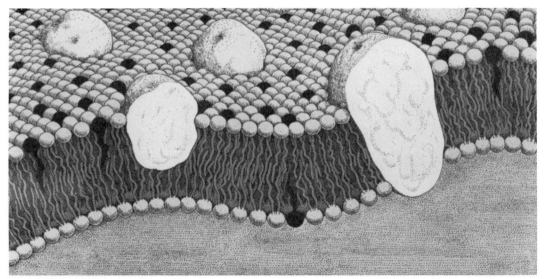

Figure 2–1 Floating iceberg model of cell membranes with globular proteins embedded in a bilayer of lipids (grey) and cholesterol (black). The proteins make up the membrane's "active sites." Some pass entirely through and may contain transport pores. (From Singer, S. J.: Hosp. Pract., 8:81, 1973.)

structure of the membrane. The spatial arrangement of hemoglobin and enzyme molecules in the cytoplasm is undoubtedly important, but this arrangement appears to be based on intermolecular forces rather than on the presence of a structural cytoskeleton.

The red cell membrane, like all cell membranes, consists of a viscous lipid matrix with protein globules in suspension (Fig. 2–1). As first proposed by Danielli and Dawson in 1935, the membrane is composed of a bilayer of tightly packed phospholipid molecules with their hydrophobic fatty acid tails intertwined in the center and their hydrophilic phosphoglycerol heads providing the intrinsic and extrinsic boundaries. Further dissection of the red cell membrane reveals that the choline phospholipids (phosphatidylcholine and sphingomyelin) predominate in the extrinsic layer, while the amino phospholipids (phosphatidylethanolamine and phosphatidylserine) are concentrated in the intrinsic layer. In addition, cholesterol molecules are interchelated between the phospholipids, contributing to the semiliquid consistency of the membrane at body temperature. The individual phospholipid and cholesterol molecules can move laterally within their respective layers, but due to polar forces, there is little, if any, opportunity for movements across the membrane.

In nucleated red cells, the lipid membrane can be renewed after injury or after loss from internalization during phagocytosis or pinocytosis. In non-nucleated red cells, limited membrane repair and remodeling are accomplished by a dynamic exchange of phosphatidylcholine and cholesterol in the extrinsic layer with phosphatidylcholine and unesterified cholesterol in plasma. In addition, there are enzymes that counteract the oxidation of phosphatidylcholine to the potentially dangerous lysophosphatidylcholine. However, lost membrane lipids cannot be replaced, and senescence of the red cells is associated with, or caused by, an irreparable loss of surface area.

Because the lipid bilayer acts as an almost impenetrable barrier, it appears that most transport across the membrane must be mediated by the protein globules, which, according to the Singer-Nicholson floating iceberg model, are suspended in the semifluid lipid matrix. These protein globules can be visualized directly by electron microscopy of freeze-cleaved red cell membranes (Fig. 2–2). It is assumed that they have a hydrophobic part deeply imbedded in the hydrophobic lipid center and a hydrophilic part emerging from the surface. Some proteins may even be banded like woolly bears with a hydrophobic center band embedded in the lipid center and the hydrophilic ends emerging from both interior and exterior surfaces. Such protein bridges would alone or in groups be well suited to mediate molecular transport across the membranes. In red cells, the transmembranous proteins are attached on the inner side to proteins that provide a biconcave scaffold for the lipid bilayer (Fig. 2–3). The predominant support-

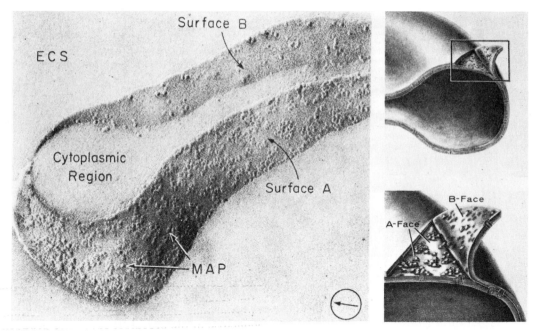

Figure 2–2 Artist's conception and actual electron microscopic view of a freeze-cleaved human red cell ghost membrane. Surface A is oriented toward the extracellular space (ECS) and is partly covered with clusters of 100 Å membrane-associated particles (MAP). Surface B has fewer particles and faces the cell's interior. (From Weinstein, R. S., and McNutt, N. S.: Semin. Hematol., 7:259, 1970.)

ing protein is spectrin, a molecular dimer composed of two nonidentical rod-shaped subunits. These dimers are linked together and attached to transmembranous proteins by a number of other proteins such as actins, ankyrins, and syndeins. The anchoring of membrane proteins to a submembranous structure explains why red cell proteins, when exposed to cross-link-

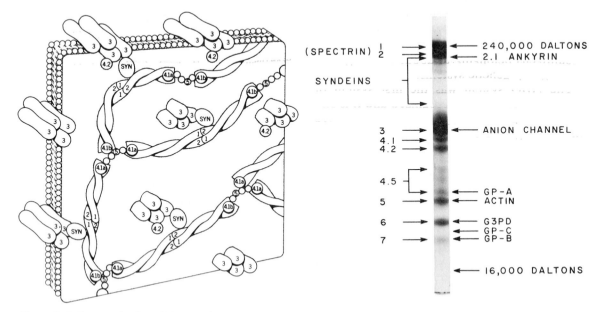

Figure 2–3 Characterization of the protein components of the red cell membrane and a hypothetical model of its protein and lipid structure. After solubilization of red cell membrane with sodium dodecyl sulfate, they are electrophoresed on a polyacrylamide gel and separated into a number of proteins numbered 1 to 7, ranging in molecular weight from 240,000 to 16,000 daltons. Component 3 provides an anion channel through the lipid bilayer and is attached to ankyrin, which in turn is attached to spectrin dimers 1 and 2. The spectrin dimers provide a scaffold for the membrane and are tied together by component 4.1 and by component 5, actin. Component 6 is glyceraldehyde-3 phosphate dehydrogenase. (Adapted from Goodman, S. R., and Shiffer, K.: Am. J. Physiol., 244:C121, 1983.)

Figure 2–4 Diagram of the red cell membrane with blood group antigens anchored on membrane proteins (band 3 and glycophorin A) and membrane lipids (ceramide). The sugars are designated by open and filled circles, and the amino acids are indicated by dots. The Rh antigen is depicted as an intramembranous particle of still unknown biochemical composition. (Adapted from Giblett, E. R. *In* Williams, W. J., et al. [Eds.]: Hematology. 3rd ed. New York, Mc-Graw-Hill Book Co., 1983, p. 1491.)

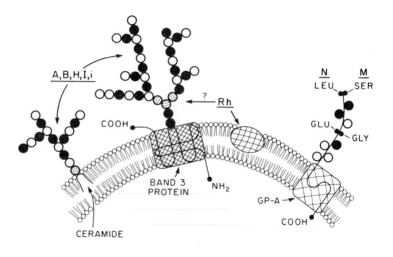

ing antibodies, do not gather together, or "cap," in one spot.

On the outside layer, protruding proteins serve a number of functions, such as receptors, cation pumps, and reducing enzymes. Furthermore, they act as anchors for the sugar and polypeptide chains that determine antigenic specificity. This specificity provides a "fingerprint" individuality to the membrane surface, apparently needed for the phagocytes to distinguish between self and non-self (Marcus, 1981).

During maturation from erythroid progenitor cell, the red cell membrane develops and loses a great number of such antigenic determinants until it is left with a few hundred alloantigens belonging to about 20 recognized blood group genetic systems.

The ABO system was the first system of surface markers to be recognized and it is still the most important. Its genetic locus is situated on the long arm of chromosome 9, and it is expressed on all cells of the body. Owing to its practical importance for blood transfusions, however, it has been identified with red blood cells.

The prime members of the ABO system, the A, B, and H antigens, are branching carbohydrate chains that extend above the membrane and are attached to the lipid membrane either directly by ceramide or indirectly by band 3 protein (Fig. 2–4). These sites begin to appear during the early maturation of nucleated red cells, and, at the time of release from the bone marrow, each red cell has about 1 million ABH sites. The ABH antigens, according to Watkins, are derived from a common precursor substance consisting of a chain of four sugars terminating in a galactose (Fig. 2–5). A genetic locus with the allelic genes H

and h determines the first step of differentiation (Fig. 2–6). The H gene codes for an enzyme that transfers fucose to the terminal galactose of the precursor substance producing the antigen H. Since this antigen is needed as substrate for the production of A and B anti-

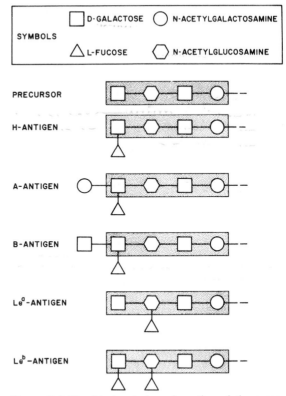

Figure 2–5 The biochemical configuration of the sugar chains in the closely linked group of ABH, Le^a, and Le^b antigens. They all have a common precursor skeleton, and the addition of sugar is accomplished through the activity of genetically determined transfer enzymes. (Adapted from Watkins, W.: Science, *162*:172, 1966.)

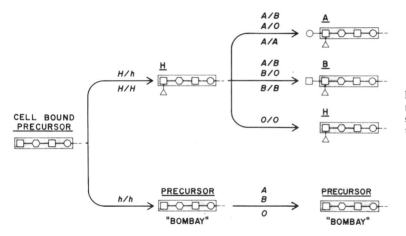

Figure 2–6 The enzymatic transformation of cell bound precursor substance for the ABO system. (See text.)

gens, individuals without the H gene (i.e., those homozygous for h) will not make any of the ABH antigens. People with this rare phenotype—called *Bombay*—will have all three isoantibodies, anti-A, anti-B, and anti-H, and the only compatible donors will be other individuals of the Bombay type.

After the production of H antigens, the final determination of the specific blood type is controlled by three allelic genes in the ABO chromosomal locus. The A gene codes for an enzyme that transfers acetylgalactosamine to the terminal galactose and changes the H antigen to an A antigen. The B gene codes for an enzyme that transfers galactose to the terminal galactose and changes the H antigen to a B antigen. The O gene dose not code for any recognized transferase, and the H antigen remains unchanged. (See recent review by Giblett.)

About 20 percent of individuals with A antigens belong to the clinically important subgroup A_2 (Table 2–1). The difference between this antigen and the common A antigen, so-called ":A_1," is, in part, quantitative rather than qualitative. The transferase, coded by the A_1 gene, transforms almost all the H substrate to A_1 antigen, while the transferase coded by A_2 is less active and leaves considerable

amounts of unchanged H on the surface. This explains why A_2 red cell agglutinates with both anti-A_1 and anti-H. The occasional but potentially dangerous presence of anti-A_1 antibodies in the plasma of A_2 individuals, however, cannot be explained merely by the low density of A_1 antigen on the cell surface, and it seems likely that there are additional subtle differences in transferases and substrates.

The same precursor substance attached to cell surfaces is also present in body fluids. In its soluble form, it is attached to a circulating lipoprotein and serves as a substrate for the ABO-determined transferases. The elaboration of soluble antigens, however, is more complex, since it involves the interaction of two closely related genetic loci—the "secretor" and the "Lewis" loci (Fig. 2–7).

About 20 percent of all individuals lack the secretor gene (Se) and are homozygous se/se. In these individuals, the soluble precursor substance cannot be altered by the transferase produced by the H, A, and B genes. They are so-called "nonsecretors" and have no ABH antigens in their saliva, regardless of their capacity to produce ABH antigens on cell surfaces. If they are also Lewis negative (le/le), they do not secrete Lewis blood groups either. However, if they are Lewis positive (Le/le or Le/Le), as is 90 percent of the population, the Lewis gene will code for a fucosyl transferase that transfers a fucose to the next to the last sugar molecule of the soluble precursor substance and changes it into a Lewis antigen—so-called "Le^a substance." This substance in turn will be passively absorbed to the membrane of circulating red cells, providing the cells with the phenotype Le$^{(a+b-)}$ (Table 2–2).

About 80 percent of all individuals possess the secretor gene (Se/Se or Se/se), and in these individuals, the transferases coded by the H,

Table 2–1 ABO SYSTEM

Subgroups	Antigens	Antibodies
0	H	Anti A + Anti A_1 + Anti B
A_1	A_1	Anti B
A_2	A_1 + H	(Anti A_1 in 1% of subjects)
B	B	Anti A + Anti A_1
A_1B	A_1 + B	None
A_2B	A_1 + B	(Anti A_1 in 25% of subjects)

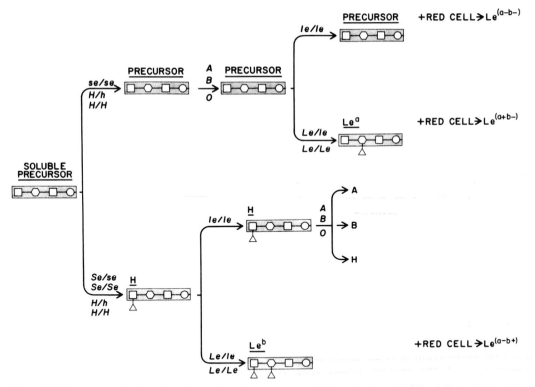

Figure 2–7 The enzymatic transformation of soluble precursor substance for the ABO Le system. (See text.)

A, and B genes can act on the soluble precursor substance and make specific soluble antigens parallel to their action on the precursor substance on the red cells. Ten percent of these individuals are Lewis negative, and no soluble Lewis substance will be produced or passed on to the red cells. In the 90 percent who have the Lewis gene, however, the precursor substance will be exposed to two fucosyl transferases, one coded by the Lewis gene and capable of transferring a fucose to the next to the last sugar molecule, and the other coded by the H gene and capable of transferring a fucose to the last sugar molecule. The result is the production of an Le^b substance that in turn will be absorbed to red cells and render them Le$^{(a-b+)}$ (Table 2–2).

Of the other blood group systems, the Ii system is closely related to the ABO and Lewis systems. The antigens of this system are carbohydrates; they are present in secretions as well as on cell membranes; they are present in close proximity to the ABH antigens on the red cell surface, and they are associated with naturally occurring isoantibodies. The phenotypic expression of the Ii system bears a resemblance to that of the fetal-adult hemoglobins. Antigen i is present during fetal development and is gradually replaced by antigen I at time of birth. In some individuals and in certain

Table 2–2 H-ABO-Se-Le SYSTEM

Genotype				Phenotype	
H (99.9%)*	ABO (100%)*	Se (80%)*	Le (90%)*	Soluble	Red cells
+	+	−	−	−	ABO
				−	Le$^{(a-b-)}$
+	+	−	+	−	ABO
				Le^a	Le$^{(a+b-)}$
+	+	+	−	ABO	ABO
				−	Le$^{(a-b-)}$
+	+	+	+	ABO	ABO
				Le^b	Le$^{(a-b+)}$

*Incidence of genes in population.

hematologic disorders, however, the antigen i reappears in a fashion analogous to that of fetal hemoglobin. Anti-I is a cold-reactive IgM antibody present in small amounts in all adults and in large amounts in patients with atypical (mycoplasma) pneumonia and in some patients with cold-reactive, acquired hemolytic anemia.

Naturally occurring isoantibodies may also be directed against antigens of the MN and P systems. These antigens are sialoglycopeptides anchored to glycoproteins A and B. In contrast to the antigens of the ABO system, their specificity is not determined by the sugars but by the amino acid sequence of their peptides (Fig. 2–4). The antigens in all systems with isoantibodies appear slowly during fetal maturation and are still not fully expressed at time of birth. The isoantibodies are usually not found until 3 to 6 months after birth, and if present earlier are acquired passively from the mother. The isoantibodies of the ABO system are primarily of the complement-binding IgM type. Even isoantibodies of the IgG type, however, will bind complement and cause hemolysis, presumably due to the great density of the ABH sites on the red cell surface.

Antibodies of the IgM type cause visible agglutination in vitro because their pentameric structure provides enough length to bridge the gap between cells. The IgG antibodies, however, usually cannot do so unless the negative repelling charge of red cells is decreased by trypsin or papain treatment or by coating with albumin. Albumin may also cause clustering of antigenic sites, thereby facilitating IgG-induced agglutination of cells sparsely covered by antigens. The addition of antibodies against IgG molecules or complement (Coombs serum) leads to visible agglutination of IgG-coated red cells. The immunologic origin of the naturally occurring isoantibodies is still unknown. They may be genetically determined, but it seems more likely that they are acquired during early infancy in response to AB-like exogenous antigens absorbed through the immature gastrointestinal mucosa.

In a number of blood group systems, such as Rh, Kell, and Duffy, naturally occurring antibodies are absent, and sensitization occurs first after repeated parenteral exposures to their antigens. Of these sytems, Rh is most important, since the strong antigenicity and early fetal emergence of the D antigen make it a frequent offender in transfusion reactions and in the development of erythroblastosis fetalis.

The Rh antigens are determined by genetic loci on the short arm of chromosome 1 and are present in a much smaller number on the red cell surface than the antigens of the ABO system. This low antigenic density, about 10,000 to 20,000 sites per cell, may explain the fact the IgG immune Rh antibodies rarely fix complement or cause intravascular hemolysis. The biochemical structure of the antigenic sites is poorly understood. They appear, however, to be integral parts of a surface protein, probably band 3, rather than elevated above it as is the case for the branching polysaccharide chain of the ABH sites. This conclusion is supported by the fact that in the absence of all Rh sites (as found in the rare genetic condition Rh null), the red cells are defective and short-lived, whereas in the absence of all ABH sites (as found in the Bombay type), the red cell surface is presumably normal, since the red cells survive normally in the circulation (Levine et al., 1973).

It has been proposed that the Rh sites in the surface layer of the membrane consist of three connected loci, with the first containing either C (rh′) or c (hr′), the second containing either E (rh″) or e (hr″), and the third containing either D (Rh$_o$) or no known antigen. Only the D is a strong antigen, and the antigenic behavior of the eight possible combinations (Table 2–3) is mostly determined by the presence or absence of D. Although the concept of three

Table 2–3 NOMENCLATURE AND FREQUENCY OF Rh-Hr SYSTEM

Separate Gene Hypothesis (Fisher-Race) Gene and Agglutinogen	Single Gene Hypothesis (Wiener) Gene		Frequency in Caucasians (Race and Sanger, 1962)
	Gene	Agglutinogen	
DCe	R′	Rh$_1$	41%
DcE	R^2	Rh$_2$	14%
Dce	R^0	Rh$_0$	3%
DCE	R^z	Rh$_z$	<1%
ce	r	rh	39%
Ce	r′	rh′	1%
cE	r″	rh″	1%
CE	r^y	rh$_z$	<1%

separate but connected loci (Fisher and Race) is attractive and easy to understand and remember, family studies indicate that each of the eight possible combinations behaves as the product of a single gene (Wiener), a finding justifying the use of the Rh terminology, at least by blood bankers. Since the blood type of each individual is determined by a pair of genes, 36 genotypes are possible, resulting in the production of 18 different phenotypes. This multitude of types is of great importance for genetic mapping, but for transfusion reaction and erythroblastosis, the presence or absence of the D (Rh$_o$) antigen is still the prime concern.

KINETICS

Self-Renewal and Differentiation

The earliest recognizable erythroid cell is the proerythroblast. However, since it is synthesizing and accumulating hemoglobin from the time of its appearance, it cannot renew itself merely through mitotic division but must be replenished from an earlier undifferentiated progenitor cell (Fig. 2–8). The morphologic identity of this cell has not as yet been firmly established, but it probably is a mononuclear lymphoid cell called CFU-E in accord with its cultural characteristics (Fig. 1–8). As described in the section on bone marrow, it is replenished

from an earlier erythroid committed progenitor cell called BFU-E, which in turn is replenished from a multipotential stem cell pool (CFU-S). The BFU-E is in active cell cycle, presumably maintained by a burst-promoting factor released by the microenvironment. As the cell matures to a CFU-E, it becomes increasingly responsive to erythropoietin until this hormone finally activates its potential as a hemoglobin–synthesizing cell and transforms it into a proerythroblast (Fig. 1–9).

The mechanism by which erythropoietin induces proliferation and blast transformation is still as obscure as was noted in a 1977 review by Nienhuis and Benz. It may directly cause a derepression of the production of a messenger RNA coded for a key enzyme in the synthesis of hemoglobin such as ALA synthetase. It is also possible that it acts indirectly on DNA transcription by activating a membrane adenyl cyclase, which in turn increases the production of cyclic AMP, a common second messenger for hormonal action. In either case, the activated cell appears to differentiate and proliferate according to a preformed program with only little additional stimulation by erythropoietin (Fig. 2–8).

Multiplication and Maturation

Following erythropoietin-induced blast transformation of the unipotential erythropoietin-sensitive progenitor cells, the emerging pro-

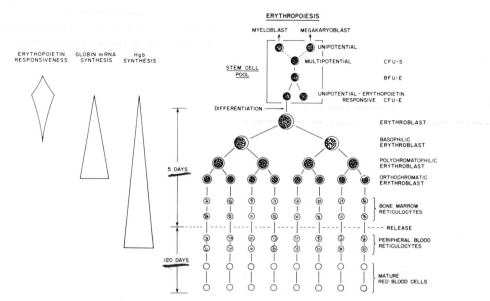

Figure 2–8 A pictorial model of the stem cell compartment and its differentiation by the action of erythropoietin to proliferating, maturing, and hemoglobin-producing erythroid cells.

erythroblasts immediately begin an integrated and controlled process of protoporphyrin production, globin-chain synthesis, iron uptake, and hemoglobin assembly. In the mitochondria, the newly formed ALA synthetase initiates synthesis of protoporphyrin by condensing activated glycine and succinic acid to ALA. The final step in this synthetic chain occurs again in the mitochondria and consists of the formation of heme from protoporphyrin and iron. Simultaneously, alpha and beta globin chains are produced in ribosomes strung together by mRNA. The synthesis of heme and globins is closely coordinated, and it appears that heme plays an essential role in this coordination. It exerts not only an end-product control on ALA synthetase activity but also a control on the transcription or processing of alpha and beta mRNA. The synthesis of other red cell proteins, such as membrane receptors, antigens, and glycolytic enzymes, are also closely integrated with the formation of heme and globins.

Iron necessary for the transformation of protoporphyrin to heme is provided from iron-charged transferrin, which becomes attached to specific receptors on the immature red cell membrane. The iron passes through the membrane while the iron-free transferrin, possibly after a brief sojourn inside the cell, is released and reused for shuttling iron from the macrophage system to erythroid cells. The intracellular iron is transported to the mitochondria for heme production or temporarily deposited as ferritin complexes in the cytoplasm. The fate of these so-called "siderotic granules" is not known. They may provide storage iron for further heme production, or they may be extruded and returned to the circulating iron pool.

Although transferrin-mediated delivery presumably provides adequate amounts of iron to the maturing cell, a second supply exists with iron provided by macrophages through direct cell-to-cell delivery. Since such an intercellular transport system also could facilitate removal or pitting of intracellular iron by the macrophages, the exact role played by these cells in cellular maturation is not clear. Nevertheless, it is known that erythroid development occurs in close physical proximity with macrophages (Fig. 2–9). This proximity is not always apparent on regular bone marrow smears, since the cells are torn apart from each other and from the thin, wide-flung cytoplasmic veil of the macrophages. However, biopsy sections and in vitro bone marrow cultures often show the presence of characteristic erythropoietic islands, each consisting of a macrophage and nucleated red cells at the same stage of maturation. As the cells mature and proliferate, the islands increase in size until they break up and release their finished cellular products.

Concurrently with the cytoplasmic maturation, the cell will undergo three to four mitotic divisions, causing a stepwise reduction in volume. Since all nucleated red cells are diploid, the reduction in nuclear size must be caused by a progressive condensation of nuclear protein, a condensation that eventually results in the appearance of a dense pyknotic nucleus incapable of further DNA synthesis. Occasionally in normal bone marrow and frequently in bone marrow from patients with accelerated red cell production, the last division may be incomplete, with the production of a cloverleaf nucleus or satellite nuclear pieces known as *Howell-Jolly bodies.* In most nonmammalian species, the condensed nucleus is carried as an inert inclusion by the mature circulating red blood cells. In mammals, however, it is extruded by a combination of intracellular demarcation and extracellular pressure. The cell is pitted when it forces its way into the circulation through narrow endothelial openings in the bone marrow sinusoids or when it passes a similar sievelike hazard in the spleen. The extruded nucleus is surrounded by a thin layer of hemoglobin, and in patients with accelerated red cell formation the breakdown of this hemoglobin may contribute significantly to the concentration of circulating bilirubin.

After the nucleus has been extruded, hemoglobin synthesis continues but at a gradually diminishing rate for another 3 to 4 days. The cells lose membrane receptors for transferrin-iron, the mitochondria diminish in number, and the polyribosomes disaggregate. When the ribosomes finally disappear, the cells no longer show the characteristic staining qualities of a reticulocyte, and they have become mature red blood cells. The cells also diminish in size, and the stickiness that characterizes immature red cells is lost. This stickiness may be caused by a coating of transferrin, and the diminishing number of iron receptors could be responsible in part for the loss of cellular cohesion and adhesion and could promote the release of cells into the circulating blood.

According to nuclear size and degree of cytoplasmic maturation, the developing bone marrow cell goes through five stages, designated respectively as *proerythroblasts, basophilic erythroblasts, polychromatic erythro-*

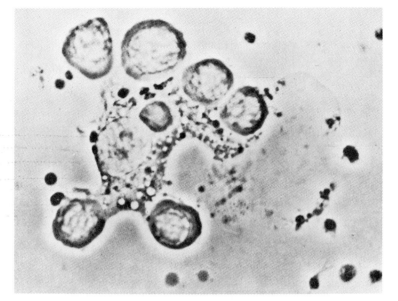

Figure 2–9 Phase contrast picture of a macrophage (nurse-cell) "servicing" attached erythroblasts. (From Bessis, M., Lessin, L. S., and Beutler, E. *In* Williams, W., et al. [Eds.]: Hematology. New York, McGraw-Hill Book Co., 1983, p. 259.)

blasts, orthochromatic erythroblasts, and bone marrow reticulocytes. Since each of the first three stages appears to be separated from the next by a mitotic division, it is possible to estimate their duration or generation time by enumerating mitotic figures. The fraction of cells in mitosis (mitotic index) depends on the duration of the mitosis (about 30 to 60 minutes) and on the generation time:

$$\text{Mitotic Index} = \frac{\text{Number of cells in mitosis}}{\text{Total number of cells}}$$

$$= \frac{\text{Mitotic time}}{\text{Generation time}}$$

The mitotic index has been measured to be about 2.5 percent for proerythroblasts, 5 percent for basophilic erythroblasts, and 6 percent for polychromatic erythroblasts, and the generation times have been calculated to be 30 hours, 15 hours, and 13 hours, respectively. Unfortunately, when generation times are measured by other techniques, the results have been somewhat different. The most popular alternate method has been based on the use of tritiated thymidine to label cells during their synthetic phase (lasting about 6 hours) and employment of radioautography to measure fraction of cells labeled, the so-called "labeling index" (see below).

The generation times calculated from such studies by Skårberg are 11 hours for proerythroblasts, 16 hours for basophilic erythroblasts, and 26 hours for polychromatic erythroblasts. In the absence of more consistent data, it seems permissible to use as a practical approximation 24 hours for each maturation phase. Since the orthochromatic erythroblasts and the bone marrow reticulocytes do not synthesize DNA or undergo mitotic divisions, the time spent in each of these stages is estimated from the turnover of appropriately labeled cells and is about 24 hours and 48 hours, respectively. Using a model based on these values (Fig. 2–8), one can estimate that the number of erythropoietic cells in the bone marrow is about 3 percent of the circulating red cells, or, if the red cell mass is 30 ml. per kg. body weight and the mean red cell count is 5 million per cu mm, about 5×10^9 cells per kg. body weight. More accurate methods for enumeration of erythropoietic bone marrow cells have disclosed higher values (Table 2–4), but a basic numerical agreement exists supporting the validity of the model presented in Figure 2–8.

Part of the transformation of nucleated red cells to mature red cells takes place in circulating blood, which contains about one third the reticulocyte pool. Under normal conditions, the reticulum persists for about 1 to 2

$$\text{Labeling Index} = \frac{\text{Number of cells in synthetic phase}}{\text{Total number of cells}}$$

$$= \frac{\text{Synthetic time}}{\text{Generation time}}$$

Table 2–4 ERYTHROID POOLS

Cell Types	Number of Cells in 10⁹ per kg. Body Weight
Proerythroblast	0.10
Basophilic erythroblast	0.48
Polychromatophilic erythroblast	1.47
Orthochromatic erythroblast	2.95
Marrow reticulocytes	8.20
Blood reticulocytes	3.10
Mature red blood cells	307.00
Daily production and destruction	3.00

(Adapted from Donohue D. M., et al.: J. Clin Invest., *37*:1571, 1958, and from Finch C. A., et al.: Blood, *50*:699, 1977.)

days, but in patients with accelerated red cell production, reticulocytes are released earlier and stay longer in the blood. As has been emphasized by Hillman and Finch, this must be taken into account when reticulocytes are used to estimate the rate of red cell production. The earlier release of reticulocytes is also reflected by the fact that these so-called "stress reticulocytes" are larger and more immature than normal circulating reticulocytes and that the bone marrow transit time is shortened. It has been suggested by Leblond and coworkers that the early release is caused by a direct action of erythropoietin on the bone marrow release mechanism. However, it could also be due to ecologic crowding of the bone marrow by new erythroid cells derived from an over-stimulated progenitor cell pool.

Regulation

Maturation and proliferation of nucleated red cells proceed at an integrated speed and rate. Changes in the speed of cellular maturation or in the rate of cellular proliferation could influence the total output of red cells from the bone marrow but cannot be solely responsible for the remarkable range of erythropoietic activity. A shortened maturation time or an early release of cells will augment the circulating red cell mass only slightly, and several extra mitotic divisions are needed in order to provide the bone marrow with its capacity to increase its rate of red cell production five- to tenfold. Since most studies indicate that an accelerated rate of red cell production is associated with a shortened transit time, it seems most unlikely that additional mitotic divisions can be squeezed in. Furthermore, direct measurements of cellular generation times have suggested that the maturation and

proliferation of immature red cells proceed at fairly fixed rates independent of the overall erythropoietic activity. Consequently, it seems more likely that the rate of red cell production depends on the number of operational erythropoietic units rather than on the activity within each unit. According to this widely accepted erythropoietic quantum theory, the rate of red cell production is controlled primarily, if not exclusively, by the rate at which progenitor cells differentiate to proerythroblasts and initiate the formation of an erythropoietic unit.

Under normal steady-state conditions, the rate of differentiation provides just enough red cells to replace the daily loss of cells. Maintenance of such a homeostatic balance demands the existence of a feedback system responsive to red cell loss and capable of inducing the necessary adjustment in the production of red cells. Occasionally, the reticulocyte count displays the oscillatory pattern that characterizes all feedback control systems (Fig. 2–10), but under normal conditions the system is usually too finely tuned to be visibly oscillatory. The triggering event in the activation of the adjustment must in some way be related to the physical or functional effect of red cell loss, and it has variously been suggested that red cell production is controlled by a device responsive to breakdown products of red cell destruction, to blood viscosity, to red cell volume, or to oxygen transport. Of these possibilities, a responsiveness to oxygen transport

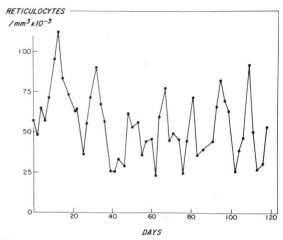

Figure 2–10 Absolute reticulocyte counts of a dog showing regularly spaced oscillations. The period is about 16 days, presumably twice the time from stem cell differentiation to reticulocyte maturation. (Redrawn from Morley, A., and Stohlman, F., Jr.: Science, *165*:1025, 1969. Copyright 1969 by the American Association for the Advancement of Science.)

is by far the most likely, since oxygen transport is the main function of the red cell mass. Furthermore, numerous studies have shown that a decreased supply of oxygen to the tissues almost invariably is associated with an increased rate of red cell production.

The existence of an erythropoietic feedback system responsive to the tissue tension of oxygen was first suspected by Dennis Jourdanet, a French physician who practiced medicine in the highlands of Mexico during the 1860s. He observed that the dark blood of his surgical patients was thick and flowed slowly, and he suggested that there was a connection between a low arterial content of oxygen and thick blood. Subsequent studies on the physiologic effect of low barometric pressure, conducted by the famous Parisian physiologist Paul Bert, led to the hypothesis that decreased arterial oxygen tension stimulates red cell production. Supporting evidence came from the fact that many patients with chronic pulmonary disorders or with right-to-left shunts were polycythemic. Since anemia, despite normal arterial oxygen tension, is also associated with increased red cell production, it was concluded that erythropoietic stimulation is caused by tissue hypoxia due to either a decreased oxygen tension or a decreased oxygen content of arterial blood.

Subsequent observations of the effect of an increased supply of oxygen to the tissues showed that the rate of red cell production is suppressed and that the tissue tension of oxygen apparently influences or controls the full range of red cell production. Direct confirmation of this hypothesis has been difficult to achieve because of our ignorance of the exact cellular location of the oxygen sensor. Measurements of the oxygen tension of subcutaneous tissue have disclosed an inverse relationship between oxygen tension and erythropoietic stimulation (Fig. 2–11). However, the oxygen sensor is probably not located in the subcutaneous tissue, and measurements of the oxygen tension in the kidney, a more likely site, have not been informative. This may be related to the fact that the oxygen sensor appears not to be responsive directly to the intercellular tissue tension of oxygen, but rather to a component of intracellular oxidative metabolism. Cobalt chloride administration, for example, causes an accelerated rate of red cell production despite an increase in the tissue tension of oxygen (Fig. 2–11), and the triggering event for the increase in both red cell production and tissue tension of oxygen appears to be impaired intracellular oxidative metabolism and oxygen utilization.

The mechanism that links the oxygen sensor to the bone marrow has been clarified and appears to consist of a feedback system mediated in one direction by red cell–bound oxygen and in the opposite direction by erythropoietin, a renal erythropoietic hormone.

The suggestion that tissue hypoxia causes the release of a humoral mediator was given its first solid experimental support in 1950

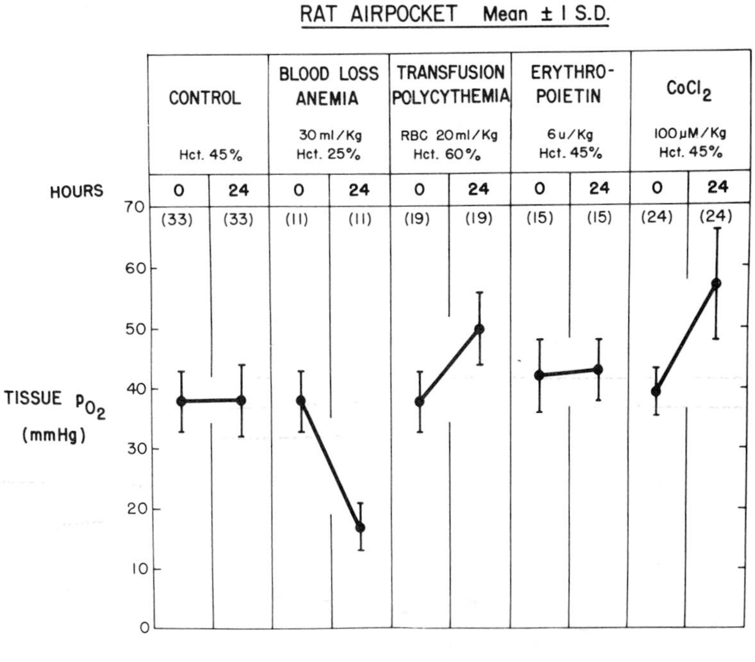

Figure 2–11 Oxygen tension of air pockets introduced subcutaneously in rats. The effects of bleeding, transfusion, erythropoietin, and cobalt on the oxygen tension are given. As expected, bleeding causes hypoxia, transfusion causes hyperoxia, and erythropoietin has no immediate effect. Cobalt causes tissue hyperoxia, presumably reflecting reduced oxygen utilization because of inhibited cellular oxidative metabolism.

RAT AIRPOCKET   Mean ± I S.D.

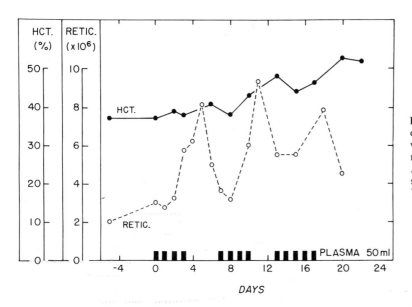

Figure 2–12 The erythropoietic effect of plasma from anemic donor rabbits when infused in large amounts to normal rabbits. (Redrawn from Erslev, A. J.: Blood, *8*:349, 1953, by permission of Grune & Stratton Inc., New York.)

when Reissmann demonstrated that hypoxia induced in one rat of a parabiotic pair causes increased red cell production in both partners. A few years later, Erslev found an erythropoietic factor in the serum of anemic rabbits (Fig. 2–12), and since then this factor, *erythropoietin,* has been isolated, purified, and partially characterized by Hiyahe and coworkers in Goldwasser's laboratory.

Erythropoietin is a glycoprotein with a molecular weight of about 35,000 and a sialic acid content of about 13 percent. It is present in both the plasma and urine of all mammals tested, and similar substances have been described in birds and fish. In humans, it has a biologic half-life of about 4 to 6 hours, but its renal clearance is quite low (about 0.5 ml. per minute). Attempts to characterize erythropoietin and to elucidate its site of production have been impeded by crude and cumbersome assay techniques. Direct measurement of biologic activity is provided by the in vivo bioassay. This assay is usually carried out in mice in which endogenous erythropoietin production has been abolished by transfusion or by hypoxia-induced erythrocytosis. The erythropoietin content of an unknown sample is estimated by the effect of the sample on the rate of red cell production as measured by the reticulocyte count or by the incorporation of radioactive iron into circulating red cells. Unfortunately, this technique is not sensitive enough to detect erythropoietin in normal sera because the lower level of sensitivity is 50 mU per sample, far above the normal serum concentration. However, erythropoietin is quite thermoresistant, and it is possible to deproteinize serum by boiling without losing more than 50 percent of its erythropoietin content. Such deproteinized sera can be concentrated and when assayed will provide discrimination down to 3 mU per sample. Using concentration techniques for sera from normals and direct assay for sera from patients with anemia, researchers have found that the erythropoietin titers correlate inversely with the hematocrit, establishing a range for normal serum from 3 to 17 mU per ml. (Fig. 2–13). In vitro bioassays measuring the effect of an unknown sample on iron incorporation or colony formation of erythroid cells in adult marrow or fetal livers have provided comparable data. More recently, pure erythropoietin has become available and with antierythropoietin antibodies has formed the basis for the development of a radioimmunoassay. So far, this assay has confirmed the results obtained by bioassay and has shown that biologic and immunologic activities of serum erythropoietin go in tandem. Due to simplicity and reproducibility, radioimmunoassays will in the future undoubtedly replace other assays and provide better data on the physiologic and pharmacologic roles of erythropoietin in erythropoiesis.

Based on the observations by Jacobson and coworkers that the production of erythropoietin ceases after bilateral nephrectomy, it has generally been accepted that erythropoietin has a renal origin. Support for this hypothesis has come from the observation that kidneys obtained from hypoxic animals and perfused in vitro will synthesize erythropoietin.

In order for the kidney to adjust its production of erythropoietin to oxygen needs, the

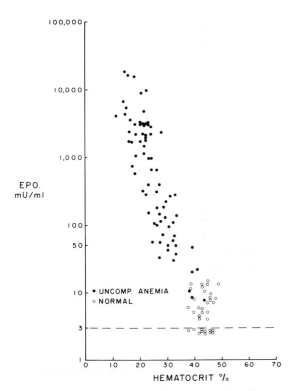

Figure 2–13 Plasma erythropoietin measured in mU per ml related to hematocrit percentage. Data obtained from normal individuals and from uncomplicated anemias (i.e., anemias not caused by renal failure or chronic disease).

rate of production must be controlled by an oxygen-sensitive device. The exact site of this device is still unknown, but since isolated normal kidneys perfused at a low oxygen tension will initiate erythropoietin production, it must be located in the kidney. In the kidney, this oxygen-sensitive device may communicate with the erythropoietin-producing cells by short-range signals, but it is more likely an integral component of these cells.

The glomeruli have been suggested as the site for this cellular interaction between oxygen tension and erythropoietin synthesis because fluorescence-tagged antibodies to erythropoietin are attached to the glomerular tufts. Juxtaglomerular cells are also contenders because renin production and erythropoietin production occur together in some, although not all, conditions. Finally, tubular cells have been considered because renal cysts and hypernephromas, which occasionally are the source of erythropoietin, are derived from the tubules. Actually, direct assay of kidney tissue separated into its components reveals four to five times as much erythropoietin in the tubules as in the glomeruli. Since mRNA coded for eryth-

ropoietin has been isolated from renal tissue, it seems almost certain that we shall know shortly from which renal fraction this mRNA is derived and in turn which cells are responsible for erythropoietin synthesis.

Studies of anephric animals and humans have disclosed that extrarenal erythropoietin production occurs. It amounts to approximately 10 to 15 percent of total production, and extrarenal erythropoietin is biologically and immunologically similar to renal erythropoietin. The site of production appears to be the liver and/or the mononuclear macrophage system. Since the production is enhanced by severe anemia and hypoxia, the extrarenal site, like the kidney, must be linked to an oxygen sensor. Extrarenal erythropoietin production has been described in association with various neoplasms, particularly cerebellar hemangiomas and hepatomas, but the relationship between this inappropriate secretion by neoplastic cells and the slight but appropriate secretion found in anephric mammals is unknown.

The action of erythropoietin on red cell precursors is better understood, although the exact target cells have not been morphologically identified or isolated. As outlined in Figure 2–8, the target cells are primarily the unipotential progenitor cells committed to erythroid development. Stimulating effects on the proliferation of early differentiated erythroblasts have also been described. Changes in granulocyte and thrombocyte counts are frequently observed under conditions of increased erythropoietin release. However, these changes are temporary and may depend on a secondary activation of multipotential cells with either an increased rate of differentiation in all directions or a possible competition among the unipotential progenitor cell pools for the attention of the multipotent cell compartment. Since an erythropoietin-stimulated bone marrow regularly displays a shortened erythroid transit time with an early release of large immature reticulocytes, a direct effect of erythropoietin on red cell maturation and release has been postulated. However, this effect could also be caused by the rapid growth of the early erythroid cells stressing the physical capacity of bone marrow to provide room for maturing erythroid cells.

Although the capacity of renal hypoxia to generate erythropoietin and in turn to accelerate red cell production explains most clinical and experimental observations on the control of red cell production, the existence of addi-

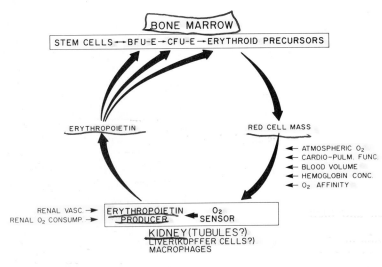

Figure 2–14 Current version of the feedback circuit.

tional regulatory mechanisms has been proposed. The pituitary, hypothalamus, and carotid bodies have all been claimed to be involved in the physiologic regulation of red cell production, but the experimental support for such neuroendocrine control is not convincing. More impressive are reports suggesting that hemolyzed red cells may exert an end-product feedback stimulation on red cell production. Because of the high reticulocyte count in hemolytic anemias, it has usually been assumed that these anemias exert a more powerful stimulation on red cell production than similar anemias caused by blood loss. However, the difference in the rate of red cell production between the two kinds of anemia

may actually not be as pronounced as suggested by the reticulocyte counts, since hemolysis often causes a selective destruction of old red cells, leaving relatively more reticulocytes in the circulation. Nevertheless, hemolyzed red cells do appear to have some effect on red cell production, mediated either by their iron content or by a "stimulatory" effect on the erythropoietin-producing cells in the kidney or elsewhere.

In summary, it appears that the main feedback system regulating red cell production is based on the capacity of the kidneys to sense tissue hypoxia and translate this information into production of erythropoietin. Figure 2–14 shows a feedback model that incorporates cur-

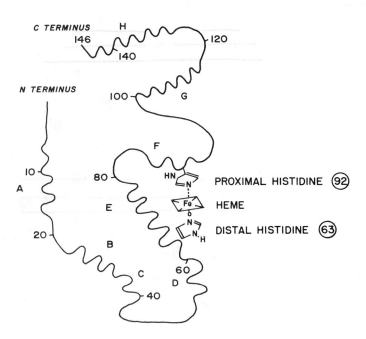

Figure 2–15 Diagram of the β polypeptide chain of hemoglobin with its eight helices (A to H) and the histidine-enclosed heme group. (Adapted from Giblett, E. R.: Genetic Markers in Human Blood. Oxford, Blackwell Scientific Publications, 1969, p. 349.)

rent concepts of oxygen transport and erythropoietin production and action.

Oxygen and Carbon Dioxide Transport

The red blood cells are usually considered functionally quite unsophisticated, since their only obligations appear to be the transport and protection of the oxygen-carrying pigment, hemoglobin. Nevertheless, the survival of cells containing neither nuclei nor mitochondria for about 4 months in a high-oxygen and high-sodium environment demands the presence of efficient metabolic defenses and long-lived enzymes. The cargo of enzymes provided during the nucleated phase of development must provide sufficient energy to maintain hemoglobin iron in its active ferrous state; to power the cation pump needed to maintain intracellular sodium and potassium concentrations despite the presence of unfavorable concentration gradients; to keep the sulfhydryl groups of globins, enzymes, and membranes in an active reduced state; and to preserve the integrity of the membrane. The metabolic pathways responsible for maintaining structure and function of the red cells will be described in the section dealing with the pathophysiology of red cell survival.

As mentioned earlier, the raison d'être for erythroid tissue and circulating red blood cells is the synthesis, transport, and protection of hemoglobin molecules. The importance of these molecules for oxygen transport has been known since 1862, when Hoppe-Seyler first isolated hemoglobin and demonstrated its affinity for oxygen. However, the molecular structure making a reversible oxygen-binding possible has been clarified only recently. The hemoglobin molecule is a tetramer consisting of two α and two β polypeptide chains, each with an attached heme group. The sequential mapping of the 141 amino acids of the α chain and 146 amino acids of the β chain has been of great importance for our identification of abnormal hemoglobins with specific amino acid substitutions. However, normal function of the hemoglobin molecules and the functional impact of such amino acid substitutions were not comprehended until the spatial positioning of the chains and of the individual amino acids had been established. Studies initiated by the classic x-ray crystallographic observation made by Perutz and coworkers have

shown that each of the four chains coils into eight helices (Fig. 2–15), forming an eggshaped molecule with a central cavity (Fig. 2–16). The polar, hydrophilic amino acid residues cover the surfaces, whereas hydrophobic residues line four superficial pockets, each containing a heme group with its iron positioned between two histidine radicals. The proximal histidine is firmly bound to the ferrous atom, whereas the distal histidine provides a protective and reversible link for deoxygenated iron. In our sequential nomenclature, these histidine radicals are far apart (histidine 58 and 87 for α chains and histidine 63 and 92 for β chains) (Fig. 2–15), but spatially they are close together in the wells of the heme pockets.

The uptake and delivery of oxygen by the

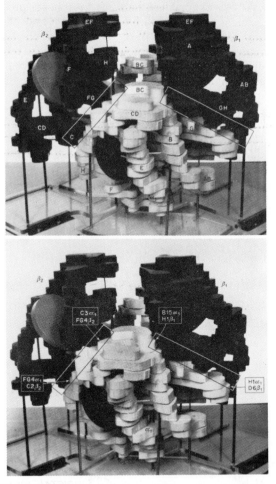

Figure 2–16 Model of the hemoglobin molecule depicting the α–β contact areas and the sliding motions that occur in the transformation from a deoxygenated form with a large central cavity *(top)* to an oxygenated form with a small cavity *(bottom)*. (From Muirhead, H., et al.: J. Molec. Biol., *13*:646, 1965.)

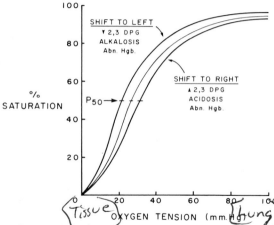

Figure 2–17 Oxygen dissociation curve of normal human blood showing that a shift to the right with an increase in P_{50} (the oxygen tension at which 50 percent of hemoglobin is deoxygenated) is found under conditions of acidosis or increased 2,3 DPG or with certain abnormal hemoglobins, whereas a shift to the left with a decrease in P_{50} is found under conditions of alkalosis or decreased 2,3 DPG or with other abnormal hemoglobins.

hemoglobin molecules are associated with considerable spatial rearrangement of the hemoglobin molecule, and, as Perutz has pointed out, the well-known oxygen dissociation curve can best be explained on the basis of such rearrangement (Fig. 2–17). The oxygen affinity of deoxygenated hemoglobin is low, and it takes a relatively large increase in oxygen

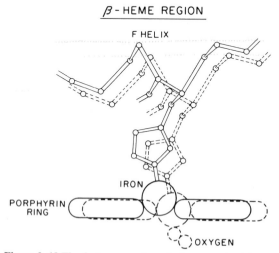

Figure 2–18 The first oxygenation of a heme pocket causes widespread molecular rearrangement with helix F changing configuration so that iron in all heme pockets moves down into the plane of the porphyrin ring, thereby facilitating its binding to an oxygen molecule. (Adapted from Perutz, M. F.: Sci. Am., 239:92, 1978.)

tension to attach an oxygen molecule to the first heme group. However, the oxygenation of this heme group causes a widespread molecular displacement "pushing" iron from its deoxygenated position above the plane of the porphyrin ring to a position permitting easy access and binding of an oxygen molecule (Fig. 2–18). The resulting molecular reorientation turns the relatively rigid α-β dimers at their $\alpha_1\beta_2$ interface, shrinks the central cavity between the β chains so it no longer can contain a stabilizing 2,3 DPG molecule, and widens the other heme pockets. In other words, the affinity for oxygen increases progressively as the hemoglobin molecule becomes oxygenated, and fully oxygenated hemoglobin has an oxygen affinity almost 100 times higher than that of deoxyhemoglobin. Concomitant release of protons accounts for oxyhemoglobin's having a greater acidity than deoxyhemoglobin.

The sequential changes in oxygen affinity are reflected in the sigmoid shape of the oxygen dissociation curve and are responsible for the ease with which hemoglobin can be loaded with oxygen in the lungs and unloaded in the tissues. Hemoglobin variants with amino acid substitution in a heme pocket or in the α_1-β_2 contact area often have altered oxygen dissociation curves. If these substitutions cause a shift to the left in the curve, the oxygen affinity is increased, the tissues become hypoxic, and a compensatory polycythemia ensues (Fig. 2–17). If the substitution causes a shift to the right, the oxygen affinity is decreased, and the tissues can be provided with adequate amounts of oxygen at low hemoglobin concentrations. Obviously, if the amino acid substitutions involve the proximal or distal histidine in the heme pockets, much more severe changes will occur, with loss of the oxygen-carrying capacity of the heme pockets involved. The oxygen dissociation curve for hemoglobins composed of like chains such as β^4 in hemoglobin H and γ^4 in Bart's hemoglobin are not sigmoid but are shifted far to the left, making these hemoglobin variants useless as oxygen carriers.

It has been known for many years that the shape of the oxygen dissociation curve is dependent on the pH (Fig. 2–17). Free protons apparently affect the charge of the histidines in the heme pocket, and the resulting displacement of attached amino acids decreases oxygen affinity. This so-called "Bohr effect" is responsible for the fact that the curve is shifted to the right in the acid microenvironment of hypoxic tissues, causing an enhanced capacity to release oxygen where it is most needed.

In addition to the Bohr effect, the oxygen dissociation curve is also responsive to the intracellular concentration of certain organic phosphates. This discovery explains the fact that oxygen affinity is reduced in conditions characterized by a decreased oxygen supply, such as at high altitudes, or an impaired oxygen supply system, such as in anemia. In both these conditions, there is an alkalosis: respiratory hyperventilation alkalosis at high altitude and intracellular alkalosis due to accumulation of the more alkaline reduced hemoglobin in anemia. Since alkalosis stimulates glycolysis, there is an increase in the intracellular concentration of 2,3-diphosphoglycerate (2,3-DPG). Furthermore, the binding of increased quantities of 2,3-DPG to deoxyhemoglobin depletes the unbound pool and thus also stimulates the increased synthesis of the low molecular weight phosphate. This phosphate fits into the expanded central cavity of deoxygenated hemoglobin and impedes the transformation of deoxyhemoglobin with a low oxygen affinity to oxyhemoglobin with a high oxygen affinity. The result is that the oxygen dissociation curve shifts to the right, permitting more oxygen to be released at a given tissue tension of oxygen. The opposite of such a facilitated oxygen unloading occurs in conditions in which the 2,3-DPG concentration is decreased, such as in stored bank blood. Here the shift of the curve is to the left, and the tissues may become hypoxic despite a normal oxygen-carrying capacity of the perfusing blood.

The respiratory function of hemoglobin also includes support for carbon dioxide transport from the tissues to the lungs. Carbon dioxide diffuses into the red cells and, catalyzed by carbonic anhydrase, becomes transformed into carbonic acid.

$$CO_2 + H_2O \rightarrow HCO_3^- + H^+$$

The hydrogen ions of carbonic acid are buffered by the relatively alkaline deoxyhemoglobin, and the bicarbonate ion diffuses back into plasma. In the pulmonary capillary, the same process in reverse will liberate carbon dioxide for pulmonary elimination. In addition to this Bohr effect on carbon dioxide transport, the amino groups of globin form reversible carbamino groups with carbon dioxide and are responsible for about 10 percent of carbon dioxide transport and excretion.

References

Bert, P.: La pression barométrique. Masson, Paris, 1878.

Danielli, J. F., and Dawson, H.: A contribution to the theory of permeability of thin films. J. Cell. Comp. Physiol., 5:495, 1935.

Erslev, A. J.: Humoral regulation of red cell production. Blood, 8:349, 1953.

Giblett, E. R.: Erythrocyte antigens and antibodies. In Williams, W. J., et al. (Eds.): Hematology. 3rd ed. New York, McGraw-Hill Book Company, 1983, p. 1491.

Hillman, R. S., and Finch, C. A.: Erythropoiesis: normal and abnormal. Semin. Hematol., 4:327, 1967.

Hiyahe, T., Kung, C. K.-H., and Goldwasser, E.: Purification of human erythropoietin. J. Biol. Chem., 252:558, 1977.

Jacobson, L. O., Goldwasser, E., Fried, W., and Plzak, L.: Role of the kidney in erythropoiesis. Nature (London), 179:633, 1957.

Jourdanet, D.: De l'anémie des altitudes et de l'anémie en général dans ses rapports avec la pression de l'atmosphère. Braillere, Paris, 1863.

Leblond, P. F., Chamberlain, J. K., and Weed, R. J.: Scanning electron microscopy of erythropoietin–stimulated bone marrow. Blood Cells, 1:639, 1975.

Levine, P., et al.: Hemolytic anemia associated with Rh null but not with Bombay blood. Vox. Sang., 24:417, 1973.

Marchesi, V. T.: The red cell membrane skeleton. Recent progress. Blood, 61:1, 1983.

Marcus, D. M.: Guest editor of issue devoted to blood group antigens. Semin. Hematol., 18:1, 1981.

Nienhuis, A. W., and Benz, E. J., Jr.: Regulation of hemoglobin synthesis during the development of the red cell. N. Engl. J. Med., 297:1318, 1977.

Palek, J.: Guest editor of issue on red cell membrane skeleton. Semin. Hematol., 20:139, 1983.

Perutz, M.F.: Hemoglobin structure and respiratory transport. Sci. Am., 239:92, 1978.

Reissmann, K. R.: Studies on the mechanism of erythropoietic stimulation in parabiotic rats during hypoxia. Blood, 5:372, 1950.

Skårberg, K. O.: Cellularity and cell proliferation rates in human bone marrow. II. Studies on generation times and radiothymidine uptake of human red cell precursors. Acta Med. Scand., 195:301, 1974.

Watkins, W. M.: Blood group substances. Science, 162:172, 1966.

Pathophysiology

DEFINITION AND CLASSIFICATION OF POLYCYTHEMIAS AND ANEMIAS

The polycythemias and anemias are defined as hematologic disorders with either too many or too few red cells in the circulation. Functionally, the polycythemias are better characterized by an increased hematocrit (more than 53 percent in males and 51 percent in females), since their clinical manifestations are not caused by a change in oxygen delivery but rather by hypervolemia and hyperviscosity, both consequences of a high hematocrit. The anemias, on the other hand, are functionally better characterized by a reduced hemoglobin concentration (less than 12 gm. percent in males and 11 gm. percent in females), since the clinical manifestations depend on the oxygen-carrying capacity of blood.

Based on the size of the red cell mass, both polycythemias and anemias can be classified as either relative, caused by changes in the plasma volume, or absolute, caused by changes in the red cell mass. Strictly speaking, the relative polycythemias or anemias are not primary hematologic disorders. However, from a differential diagnostic point of view, they play a considerable role in hematology.

The absolute polycythemias traditionally are subdivided into primary and secondary polycythemias, whereas the absolute anemias can be classified further into anemias caused by

Table 2–5 CLASSIFICATION OF ERYTHROCYTE DISORDERS

Stem Cell Disorders
Multipotential
  Polycythemia vera
  Aplastic anemia
Unipotential
  Secondary polycythemia
  Anemia of renal disease
  Anemia of chronic disease
  Anemia of endocrine disorders
  Pure red cell aplasia
DNA Disorders
Vitamin B_{12} deficiency
Folate deficiency
Refractory megaloblastic anemias
Antimetabolite therapy (methotrexate,
  6-mercaptopurine)
Heme and Globin Disorders
Porphyrias
  Hereditary porphyrias
  Acquired porphyrias (lead poisoning)
Iron
  Iron-deficiency anemia
  Iron-loading anemias
Globin
  Structural abnormality
    Hemoglobinopathies (sickle cell anemia)
  Quantitative abnormality
    Thalassemias

Survival Disorders
Intrinsic
  Hereditary spherocytosis
  Hereditary elliptocytosis
  Paroxysmal nocturnal hemoglobinuria
  Enzymopathies (G-6-PD, P.K.)
  Hemoglobinopathies
Extrinsic
  Toxic Factors
    Thermal burn
    Chemical damage
    Infection (malaria)
    Hyperoxia (hyperbaric conditions)
    Oxidative hemolysis due to drugs (sulfonamides)
  Hypersplenism
  Mechanical Factors
    March hemoglobinuria
    Traumatic cardiac hemolysis
    Microangiopathic hemolytic anemia
  Plasma Lipid Abnormality
    Spur cell anemia of cirrhosis
    Hereditary acanthocytosis
  Immune Hemolysis
    Isoimmune
      Transfusion reaction
      Erythroblastosis fetalis
    Autoimmune
      Cold type
      Warm type
  Blood Loss
    Acute blood loss anemia

decreased red cell production or decreased red cell survival.

From a pathophysiologic point of view, however, the erythrocyte disorders are best characterized by pathogenesis. Table 2–5 classifies these disorders according to one of four recognized causes: (1) disorders of stem cell function, (2) disorders of DNA synthesis, (3) disorders of heme and globin synthesis, and (4) disorders of red cell survival. In many instances, the pathogenesis involves a mixture of several of these causes, but this classification serves to direct attention to pathogenesis rather than to manifestations.

General Effects of Polycythemia

The pathophysiologic manifestations of polycythemia or, more correctly, of erythrocytosis are caused by hyperviscosity and hypervolemia associated with an increase in the red cell mass. Under normal conditions, the red cell mass is maintained carefully at about 30 ml. per kg. body weight, a value that presumably must be considered optimal. The reason for not maintaining a higher red cell mass does not reside in any bone marrow limitation, since a mere doubling of the rate of red cell production would sustain a red cell mass twice normal size. The reason seems to be that an increased red cell mass will be associated with a high viscosity and sluggish flow of circulating blood.

Such sluggish blood flow is responsible in part for the tendency to thrombosis found in patients with polycythemia, and would, if not compensated for, result in decreased oxygen flow to the tissues (Fig. 2–19) and obviate any benefits derived from the development of secondary polycythemia. Fortunately, the high hematocrit and high viscosity are associated with an increase in blood volume (Fig. 2–20), and the resulting vasodilatation will enhance the tissue perfusion with blood and oxygen. Using measurement for cardiac output and tissue oxygen tension, it can be shown directly that oxygen transport at a given hematocrit is greater in hypervolemic than in normovolemic animals (Fig. 2–21).

Nevertheless, there is still considerable doubt about the benefits derived from secondary polycythemia. The trade-offs in terms of increased viscosity and cardiac work seem to be too high, and the most telling argument against polycythemia as an adaptive device of high altitudes is that the llama and the bar-

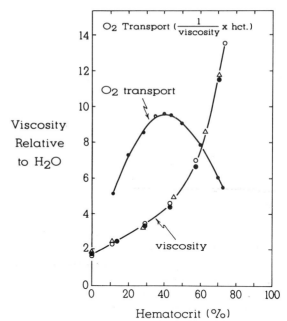

Figure 2–19 Oxygen transport as calculated from blood oxygen-carrying capacity (hematocrit) and blood flow (reciprocal of viscosity).

headed goose, both superbly adapted to hypoxia, are not polycythemic (Eaton, 1981).

The high blood volume in polycythemia is tolerated quite well, although symptoms such as headache, tinnitus, and dizziness and signs such as nose-bleeding and ruddy cyanosis probably are caused by the vascular dilatation needed to accommodate the blood volume.

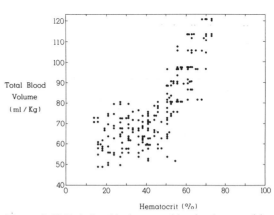

Figure 2–20 Relationship between blood volume and hematocrit. A reduction in hematocrit to about 15 percent does not cause a significant change in blood volume, but an increase in hematocrit above 50 percent appears to cause hypervolemia. (Data from Metcalfe, J., et al.: Circ. Res., *25*:47, 1969, by permission of The American Heart Association, Inc.)

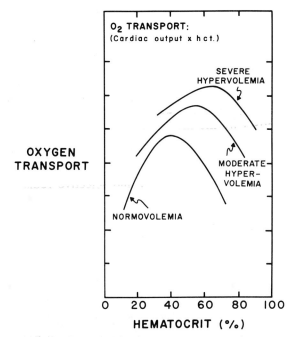

Figure 2–21 Calculated in vivo oxygen transport in normovolemic and hypervolemic conditions. As can be seen, the oxygen transport in hypervolemia is better than in normovolemic states, even at higher hematocrits. The curves also indicate that the optimal value for oxygen transport is higher at higher blood volumes. (From Murray, J. F., et al.: J. Clin. Invest., *42*:1150, 1963, and Thorling, E. B., and Erslev, A. J.: Blood, *31*:332, 1968, by permission of Grune & Stratton, Inc., New York.)

Since the increase in red cell production needed to sustain an erythrocytosis is quite moderate, clinical or laboratory signs of bone marrow hyperactivity are usually absent. However, a slight increase in uric acid and lactic dehydrogenase levels may occur, reflecting an increase in the number of red cells destroyed daily.

General Effects of Anemia

The pathophysiologic effects of a reduced oxygen-carrying capacity of blood are all related to tissue hypoxia and to the compensatory mechanisms mobilized to alleviate this hypoxia. Tissue hypoxia occurs when the pressure head of oxygen in the capillaries is too low to provide distant cells with enough oxygen for their metabolic needs. This may happen despite the presence of several times the needed oxygen in the circulating blood. Using approximate figures for a normal adult, the red cell mass has to provide the tissues with about 250 ml. of oxygen per minute to support life. Since the oxygen-carrying capacity of normal blood is 1.34 ml. per gram hemoglobin, or about 20 ml. per 100 ml. of normal blood, and the cardiac output is about 5000 ml. per minute, 1000 ml. of oxygen per minute is made available at the tissue level. The extraction of one fourth of this amount will reduce the oxygen tension of 100 mm. Hg in the arterial end of the capillary to 40 mm. Hg in the venous end (Fig. 2–17). This partial extraction will maintain a diffusion pressure throughout the capillaries sufficient to provide all cells within a truncated cone segment with enough oxygen for their metabolism (Fig. 2–22). In anemia, the extraction of the same amount of oxygen would lead to greater hemoglobin desaturation and a lower oxygen tension at the venous end of the capillary. Since this would result in destructive cellular hypoxia or anoxia in the immediate vicinity, compensatory and frequently symptomatic adjustment in the supply of blood and oxygen must be mobilized in order to keep the oxygen gradient almost unchanged. (See 1972 review by Finch and Lenfant.)

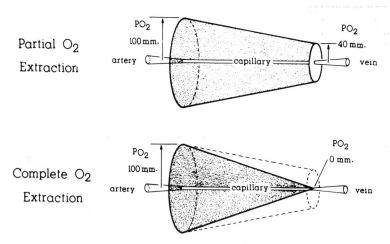

Figure 2–22 A hypothetical model of the tissue cone provided by oxygen when the blood is partially or completely extracted of oxygen.

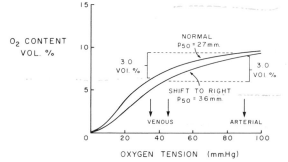

Figure 2–23 This figure depicts the effect on venous oxygen tension when 3.0 volume percent of oxygen is extracted from normal hemoglobin in an anemic individual. A shift to the right will permit this extraction of 3 volume percent with less reduction in venous oxygen tension and therefore an enhanced tissue oxygenation.

Decreased Oxygen Affinity. One of the earliest and least traumatic adjustments is a shift in the oxygen dissociation curve to the right, permitting the extraction of increased amounts of oxygen without a decrease in oxygen pressure. As mentioned before, the position of the oxygen dissociation curve is in part dependent on the intracellular pH. At an acid pH, as experienced in tissues in which anemic hypoxia has led to anaerobic metabolism and lactic acid accumulation, the curve will be shifted to the right, the so-called Bohr effect (Fig. 2–17). More important, however, is a stimulation of the production of 2,3 diphosphoglycerate. The reason for this stimulation in anemia is not clear, but it has been suggested that the binding of free 2,3-DPG to deoxygenated hemoglobin, present in increased amounts in anemia, will result in a compensatory increase in glycolysis and 2,3-DPG production. Alternately, deoxygenated hemoglobin may cause enough intracellular alkalosis to stimulate glycolysis and 2,3-DPG production. The binding of 2,3-DPG to reduced hemoglobin stabilizes the molecule in its low-affinity state and facilitates the unloading of oxygen in the tissues. According to Torrance and colleagues, this change in oxygen affinity plays a substantial role in reducing the arteriovenous oxygen pressure gradient and in minimizing cellular hypoxia (Fig. 2–23).

Increased Tissue Perfusion. Redistribution of blood from tissues with fairly low oxygen requirements and high blood supply such as skin and kidneys to oxygen-dependent tissues such as brain and myocardium provides an early and efficient protection of these vital tissues. The metabolic price for maintaining a high oxygen tension in some selective organs or tissues appears reasonable. Subcutaneous

vasoconstriction and oxygen deprivation are tolerated well, since dermal blood supply is geared more toward temperature regulation than toward oxygen delivery. The same is true for the kidney, in which the blood supply is far in excess of the oxygen requirement. The effect on renal excretory function is relatively minor, since the decrease in blood supply is offset by the increase in "plasma crit" of the perfusing anemic blood.

Increased Cardiac Output. In mild to moderate anemia, the combined effects of decreased oxygen affinity and selective redistribution of blood maintain oxygen pressure at close to normal levels, and these anemias are usually quite asymptomatic. However, with more severe anemias it becomes necessary to increase cardiac output in order to provide the tissues with enough oxygen. Although the low viscosity of anemic blood and the peripheral vasodilatation reduce the workload on the heart, the metabolic cost and the wear and tear on the moving parts of the cardiac pump make an increase in cardiac output an undesirable device for long-term compensation.

The clinical manifestations of severe anemia are to a great extent caused by the compensatory cardiac overactivity. Pallor is due primarily to dermal vasoconstriction and blood redistribution, but tachycardia and symptoms of decreased cardiac reserve are related to cardiac stress. The characteristic shortness of breath associated with severe anemia may be a sign of incipient cardiopulmonary failure rather than a manifestation of ventilatory compensation to the anemia. Owing to the almost complete saturation of anemic blood with oxygen in the lungs, a pulmonary compensation would actually be of little practical importance.

Increased Red Cell Production. The most appropriate but also the slowest compensatory device in anemia is an increase in the rate of red cell production. Tissue hypoxia will lead to increased erythropoietin production within a few hours, but owing to the time lag from stem cell differentiation to the release of reticulocytes from the bone marrow, a compensatory increase in the number of circulating red cells does not begin until 4 to 5 days later. Increased erythropoietin titers in serum (Fig. 2–14) causing increased bone marrow activity may be associated with sternal pain or tenderness and the presence of large immature reticulocytes on the blood smear.

These compensatory mechanisms are all designed to keep the capillary oxygen pressure up and the oxygen delivery adequate for the cellular needs. However, a complete rectification of tissue hypoxia cannot occur until the hemoglobin concentration has been restored to normal. Some degree of tissue hypoxia is needed in order to provide a driving force for the various compensatory devices. The symptomatology of such remaining hypoxia is difficult to separate from that of the compensatory mechanisms, but leg cramps, angina pectoris, and light-headedness appear to be caused directly by tissue hypoxia.

Relative Polycythemia

A relative erythrocytosis with a hematocrit of more than 53 percent can be found after severe fluid loss, and the hematocrit may serve as a useful gauge of dehydration. A relative erythrocytosis has also been observed in otherwise healthy individuals with no apparent fluid volume deficit. Careful measurements by Brown and coworkers of red cell mass and fluid volume in such patients have suggested that the increase in hematocrit is spurious and caused merely by the combination of a borderline high red cell mass and a borderline low plasma volume. Since many patients with such spurious erythrocytosis are tense, chain-smoking individuals, the condition has been called "stress polycythemia." However, tobacco by itself produces carbon monoxide hemoglobin, leading to a compensatory increase in the red cell mass, and nicotine may have a diuretic, plasma volume–lowering effect. Consequently, "stress polycythemia," as pointed out by Smith and Landow, probably should be called "tobacco polycythemia" and designated as a secondary rather than a relative polycythemia.

Relative Anemia

An expansion of plasma volume causing a dilution of the red cell mass with consequent reduction in the number of erythrocytes per cu. mm. is seen during the third trimester of pregnancy. This physiologic anemia of pregnancy is fortunately not associated with a decreased oxygen transport to mother or fetus, since the hypervolemia will compensate for the decrease in oxygen-carrying capacity (Fig. 2–21).

Macroglobulinemia and multiple myeloma may also cause an inappropriate increase in plasma volume, resulting in a dilution anemia. Because of the hypervolemic increase in oxygen transport, this anemia is not associated with hypoxemic symptoms. Determination of the absolute red cell mass in patients with dysgammaglobulinemia and anemia is advised to distinguish dilution anemia from anemia due to bone marrow replacement.

References

Brown, S. M., Gilbert, H. S., Krauss, S., and Wasserman, L. R.: Relative polycythemia: a non-existent disease. Am. J. Med., *50*:200, 1971.

Eaton, J. W.: Low altitude hominids at high altitude. Blood Cells, 7:509, 1981.

Erslev, A. J., and Caro, J.: Pathophysiology and classification of polycythaemia. Scand. J. Hematol., *31*:287, 1983.

Finch, C. A., and Lenfant, C.: Oxygen transport in man. N. Engl. J. Med., *286*:407, 1972.

Smith, J. R., and Landaw, S. A.: Smokers' polycythemia. N. Engl. J. Med., *298*:6, 1978.

Torrance, J., Jacobs, P., Restrepo, A., et al.: Intraerythrocytic adaptation to anemia. N. Engl. J. Med., *283*:165, 1970.

Stem Cell Disorders

Under physiologic conditions, the red cell mass is maintained at an optimal size by appropriate adjustments in the rate of transformation of stem cells and progenitor cells to nucleated red blood cells. These adjustments are accomplished by feedback systems, and a disruption at any point in the circuits of these systems will lead to disordered stem cell function and polycythemia or anemia. A disordered function of the multipotential stem cells such as observed in patients with polycythemia vera or aplastic anemia is usually believed to be caused by an intrinsic defect of the stem cells themselves. However, very little is known of their regulation, and it is possible that cellular dysfunction is secondary to defective feedback signals from the immediate microenvironment.

The feedback system regulating the unipotential erythropoietin-sensitive progenitor cells is much better understood, and it is now possible to relate various secondary polycythemias and aregenerative anemias to defects in specific key stations in this circuit. The major distinction between disorders of the multipotential stem cells and the unipotential progenitor cells is that multipotential stem cell disorders are characterized by pancytosis or pancytopenia, and unipotential progenitor cell disorders are identified by erythrocytosis or erythrocytopenia.

DISORDERS OF MULTIPOTENTIAL STEM CELLS

Polycythemia Vera

Polycythemia vera is a "myeloproliferative" disorder characterized by an uncontrolled proliferation of erythroid, myeloid, and megakaryocytic bone marrow elements. The proliferation is predominantly erythroid, and the circulating red cell mass is increased during the early part of the disease. The concomitant increase in granulocytes and platelets has led to the assumption that polycythemia vera is caused by an inappropriate activation of multipotential stem cells. However, the unipotential committed progenitor cells must also be involved in the disease process, since the erythropoietin-sensitive progenitor cells undergo differentiation despite the fact that the production of erythropoietin is almost completely suppressed.

Studies by Adamson and coworkers have shown that polycythemia vera is a clonal disorder caused by autonomous overactivity of a single abnormal multipotential stem cell. These authors studied two polycythemic women who were heterozygous for the X-linked A and B glucose-6-phosphate dehydrogenase isoenzymes (Fig. 2–24). Not only skin but also bone marrow fibroblasts showed a mosaicism of cells with A and B isoenzymes. However, all red cells, granulocytes, and platelets contained the same isoenzymes, type A, presumably derived from a single, type A, multipotential stem cell. Bone marrow from these patients cultured in the absence of erythropoietin grew out erythroid colonies, all with the same type A isoenzyme. When erythro-

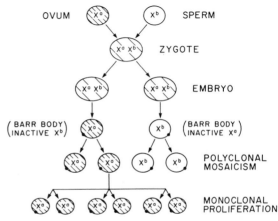

Figure 2–24 X-chromosomal inactivation in women heterozygous for the glucose-6-dehydrogenase genes a and b.

poietin was added, the number of type A colonies increased, but, in addition, colonies with type B isoenzyme appeared. These findings suggest firstly that the hemopoietic tissue represents a neoplastic, clonal hyperplasia, whereas the fibroblastic tissue, so characteristic of late polycythemia vera, represents a reactive, non-neoplastic hyperplasia. Secondly, that the autonomous clones of polycythemia vera are responsive to the stimulating effect of erythropoietin and that the bone marrow from patients with polycythemia vera in addition contains a number of normal erythropoietin-dependent clones.

The cause of this autonomous overactivity of the stem cell pool is unknown, but the existence of a virus-induced polycythemia in mice has raised the possibility that the human disorder also is virus-related. However, as is the case for most neoplastic proliferative disorders, firm evidence for a viral etiology is not available.

The increased rate of red cell production causes a steady rise in red cell blood count and hematocrit. The plasma volume remains unchanged or increases slightly, and the erythrocytosis becomes characterized by an increase in both the red cell mass and the blood volume. This process may be quite slow and may be accomplished by a slight but sustained excess of red cell production over red cell destruction. For example, a mere doubling of the rate of red cell production for a period of 4 months will result in a doubling of the size of the red cell mass. Since the establishment of a clinically recognizable polycythemia may take much longer, it is not surprising that a routine bone marrow examination may not show evidence of much erythroid hyperactivity.

Ferrokinetic studies, measuring total bone marrow activity, are more apt to demonstrate the presence of a slight increase in erythroid bone marrow mass. Such studies also show that the red cell production in patients with polycythemia vera is effective with the release of normal, long-lived red blood cells. Because of the increase in the number of erythroid cells in the bone marrow and circulating blood, a greater than normal amount of iron is "trapped" in the hemoglobin of these cells, and the tissue iron stores may become depleted. This trend is aggravated by the frequent therapeutic use of phlebotomy, by spontaneous nose and gastric bleedings, and by the lack of an "anemic stimulus" to intestinal iron absorption, and it leads to an iron-deficient erythropoiesis. Fortunately, the production of

microcytic and hypochromic cells may be of considerable symptomatic benefit, since the hematocrit and in turn the viscosity will become disproportionately lower than the red cell count.

Most symptoms are related to hypervolemia and hyperviscosity and are alleviated by phlebotomy. They frequently consist merely of nonspecific headaches, dizziness, blurred vision, and a feeling of "fullness in the head." Engorgement of thin-walled vessels may cause nose and gastric bleedings, serving as convenient means for spontaneous bloodletting. However, more serious symptoms may occur if the hyperviscosity causes venous stagnation, thrombosis, and embolization. Such events can cause fatal vascular accidents when they occur in cerebral, coronary, hepatic, or intestinal veins.

The characteristic splenomegaly found in polycythemia vera may be caused in part by vascular engorgement and in part by extramedullary hemopoiesis. However, it is probably caused primarily by fibrous tissue, an early manifestation of fibroblastic stimulation induced by the abnormal hemopoietic cells. The granulocyte count in polycythemia vera is regularly increased, although it rarely exceeds 30,000 cells per cu. mm. The resulting increase in granulocyte turnover is often reflected by an increase in serum and urine muramidase levels and in the concentration of B_{12} and B_{12} binders in serum. The granulocytes are usually mature and normally functioning, but more immature granulocytic elements may be present. The leukocyte alkaline phosphatase is either normal or high, a finding of uncertain functional significance but of use in distinguishing the granulocytosis of polycythemia vera from the granulocytosis of chronic myeloid leukemia. The granulocytes of polycythemia vera reportedly contain an increased amount of histidine decarboxylase, an enzyme involved in the production of histamine from histidine. Excessive histamine may be responsible for the common complaint of itching, especially following warm baths or showers.

The platelet count is regularly increased, but frequently not as much as would be expected from examining bone marrow specimens. These often reveal sheets of megakaryocytes, a finding that may justify bone marrow aspiration as a differential diagnostic test in the polycythemias. The characteristic tendency of patients with polycythemia vera to develop thrombotic complications is frequently related to the increased platelet count. However, mor-

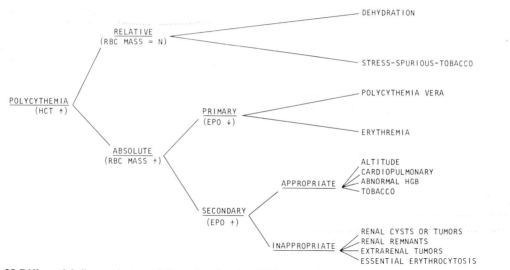

Figure 2–25 Differential diagnostic tree of the polycythemias. EPO = erythropoietin. (From Erslev, A. J., and Caro, J.: Am. J. Med., 76:57, 1984.)

phologic and functional studies of platelets indicate that their adhesiveness is reduced and that despite their increased numbers they may not be responsible for these complications. Actually, studies by Spaet and coworkers on the coagulation process in this disease suggest the presence of impaired hemostasis with poor clot formation rather than hypercoagulability. In evaluating the results from such studies, one must realize that the plasma volume is relatively decreased in polycythemic blood and that the amount of available coagulation factors may not be adequate for the establishment of a firm red cell clot. (See 1984 review by Schafer.)

It is usually not difficult to make a diagnosis of polycythemia vera in patients with full-blown pancytosis and splenomegaly (Fig. 2–25). However, early in the course, polycythemia vera may be more difficult to recognize. Table 2–6 gives some of the findings of value in the differential diagnosis of various polycythemias. The two diagnostic findings that most closely reflect the pathogenesis of polycythemia vera are the low to absent erythropoietin titer and the growth of erythroid colonies in vitro in the absence of erythropoietin. Unfortunately, they are also the most difficult to establish. As the disease progresses, patients with polycythemia vera develop specific and characteristic complications not seen in the other polycythemias. The paradoxic occurrence of both thromboses and hemorrhages occurs quite frequently, and cerebral, coronary, mesenteric, or portal thrombosis may cause life-threatening situations in a patient

who displays nasal, gastric, or dermal hemorrhages. In a considerable number of patients, the disease slowly changes in character, with myelofibrosis and myeloid metaplasia becoming predominant features. These features are the results of excessive fibroblastic activity, probably in response to growth promoting factors released by the abnormal hemopoietic clones. The reduction in available bone marrow space and the increase in splenic size will lead first to anemia and eventually to pancytopenia.

Acute myelogenous leukemia develops ultimately in about 10 to 15 percent of patients with polycythemia vera. The occurrence of this dreaded complication was believed initially to be related to the therapeutic use of radioactive

Table 2–6 DIFFERENTIAL DIAGNOSIS OF POLYCYTHEMIAS

	Relative Polycythemia	Polycythemia Vera	Secondary Polycythemia
Hematocrit	Increased	Increased	Increased
Red blood cell mass	Normal	Increased	Increased
Erythropoietin	Normal	Absent	Increased
Spontaneous erythroid colonies	Absent	Present	Absent
White blood count	Normal	Increased	Normal
Platelet count	Normal	Increased	Normal
Bone marrow	Normal	Hyperplastic	Erythroid hyperplasia
Spleen	Normal	Enlarged	Normal
Arterial oxygen saturation	Normal	Normal	Decreased or normal
Serum iron	Normal	Decreased	Normal
Serum B_{12}	Normal	Increased	Normal
Leukocyte alkaline phosphatase	Normal	Increased	Normal
Muramidase	Normal	Increased	Normal

phosphorus. Recent reports, however, suggest that the use of so-called "radiomimetic agents" such as chlorambucil and busulfan also may be followed by the development of acute myelogenous leukemia (Berk et al., 1981). Polycythemia vera was the first "neoplastic" disease with a long enough survival to make possible prolonged follow-up studies after the use of myelosuppressive agents. The more recent successes in the treatment of Hodgkin's disease, ovarian cancer, multiple myeloma, and transplantation rejection have permitted similar prolonged follow-ups after the use of other forms of radiation or radiomimetic drugs, and it has become clear that the development of acute myelogenous leukemia is an appreciable therapeutic hazard. So far, the therapeutic results have been well worth the risk, but obviously these agents should be used with reluctance and caution.

Primary erythrocytosis, with low or absent erythropoietin titers in plasma and with spontaneous growth of erythroid colonies, has also been described in a few patients who had no evidence of granulocyte or platelet hyperplasia. In some this condition represents early polycythemia vera, but in others the erythrocytosis remains pure. It has been named *erythremia* and presumably represents a clonal overgrowth of erythroid progenitor cells.

Aplastic Anemia

Aplastic anemia is a bone marrow disorder characterized by a reduction in the number or function of multipotential stem cells. This reduction leads in turn to a decrease in the volume of active blood-cell–producing bone marrow and to a pancytopenia. The remaining marrow becomes confined to small, often intensely active islands surrounded by fatty tissue. This fatty replacement is the sine qua non of true aplastic anemia.

The clinical manifestations are all directly related to the pancytopenia. The anemia may cause weakness, fatigue, and pallor; the granulocytopenia may cause fever and infections; and the thrombocytopenia may cause hemorrhages, hematomas, and petechiae. Hepatomegaly and splenomegaly are unusual findings in the early phase of the disease, and their presence should lead to re-evaluation of the diagnosis. However, after prolonged illness, recurrent infections may produce a reactive macrophage hyperplasia of the spleen, and transfusion hemosiderosis may lead to hepatomegaly and congestive splenomegaly.

The anemia is often macrocytic, and the reticulocytes are few in number but relatively immature. These findings reflect an accelerated bone marrow transit time and release, possibly caused by a high level of erythropoietin or by the crowded environment in the remaining bone marrow islands. Ferrokinetic studies reveal a reduced plasma iron turnover, but this reduction may be difficult to appreciate, since the normal baseline value is quite low.

Of greater importance for the demonstration of a reduced rate of red cell production are the iron clearance time and the red cell utilization of iron. The reduced bone marrow mass can clear iron from plasma only slowly, giving extramedullary tissues such as liver or spleen extra time in which to compete with the marrow for circulating radioactive iron. The result is a prolonged iron clearance time and a low red cell iron utilization. This combination is characteristic for all anemias caused by a reduction in erythropoietic tissue and distinguishes them from anemias caused by ineffective red cell production. In the latter anemias, intramedullary destruction of nucleated red cells will also cause a low utilization of radioactive iron, but the iron clearance is short because of an abundance of erythropoietic bone marrow (Fig. 2–26). This distinction is of particular importance in establishing whether pancytopenia is caused by bone marrow hypoplasia or by ineffective cellular production. This latter condition has been called "aplastic anemia with a hyperplastic bone marrow," a confusing term for a condition that often is preleukemic and may be pathogenetically quite different from aplastic anemia.

Both plasma iron and erythropoietin concentrations are high in aplastic anemia, possibly reflecting decreased utilization by a reduced bone marrow mass. The high plasma iron concentration may cause excessive tissue incorporation of iron and eventually hemosiderosis. Bone marrow preparations disclose many siderotic granules in the macrophages, but since maturation of the individual nucleated red cell is normal, siderotic granules in these cells are seen only rarely. The high erythropoietin titer in plasma and urine has made patients with aplastic anemia useful sources for the preparation of erythropoietin concentrates.

In some patients with aplastic anemia, particularly children, there may be a substantial increase in the production of fetal hemoglobin. This finding may merely reflect a rapid transit from early erythroid progenitors (BFU-E) to early erythroid precursor cells permitting fetal

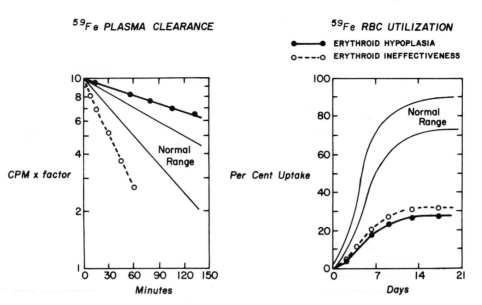

Figure 2–26 Plasma clearance and red cell utilization of radioactive iron in normals, patients with erythroid hypoplasia, and patients with ineffective red cell production. The clearance rate of ^{59}Fe injected intravenously at time 0 was determined by serial measurements of the radioactivity (CPM) over a 3-hour period. The subsequent utilization of the ^{59}Fe for hemoglobin synthesis was estimated by measuring the total radioactivity in circulating red cells (red cell mass × CPM) and relating it in percent to the total amount of ^{59}Fe injected. Although the utilization of ^{59}Fe is equally reduced in patients with erythroid hypoplasia or with erythroid ineffectiveness, the plasma clearance rate readily separates them from each other.

BFU-E potentials, usually lost in the adult during slow transit, to be expressed. Macrocytosis, fetal hemoglobin, and the persistence of a fetal surface protein, little i, have been suggested by Alter to be characteristic of "stress" erythrocytes rather than indicative of stem cell dysfunction.

Absolute granulocytopenia is always present in aplastic anemia, and its severity will determine to a great extent the immediate prognosis. As a rough guide, an absolute granulocyte count of less than 200 cells per cu. mm. suggests imminent danger of infectious complications and demands some kind of a sheltered environment. In addition to an absolute granulocytopenia, there is often a reduction in the total number of lymphocytes. The reason for and functional significance of this reduction is not known but immunoglobulin synthesis and delayed sensitivity reactions are usually intact.

Thrombocytopenia with its dramatic and visible hemorrhagic manifestations is also always part of the clinical picture of advanced aplastic anemia. Because of the insidious onset of this disease, it is difficult to assess the sequence by which the various cytopenias appear. However, during the recovery phase, thrombocytopoiesis is often the last bone marrow function to recover and many patients may have thrombocytopenia for years after the other cytopenias have been corrected.

Etiology and Pathogenesis (Table 2–7). Numerous drugs, illnesses, and physical agents have the capacity to alter stem cell function, presumably by interfering with intracellular metabolism. However, these agents could also alter the stem cell microenvironment, and the

---

Table 2–7 ETIOLOGIC CLASSIFICATION OF APLASTIC ANEMIA

I. Idiopathic
  A. *Constitutional* (Fanconi's anemia)
  B. *Acquired*
II. Secondary
  A. *Chemical and physical agents*
      Drugs
      Nonpharmacologic chemicals
      Radiation
  B. *Infectious*
      Viral (hepatitis)
      Bacterial (miliary TB)
  C. *Metabolic*
      Pancreatitis
      Pregnancy
  D. *Immunologic*
      Antibody
      Graft-vs.-host
  E. *Neoplastic*
      Myelophthisic anemia
  F. *Paroxysmal nocturnal hemoglobinuria*

relative importance of "seed" and "soil" in the pathogenesis of aplastic anemia is still not resolved. Although statistical and clinical cause-effect relationships between a specific agent or event and the development of aplastic anemia can be quite impressive, aplastic anemia is a disease in which the etiology can be only suspected, not established. No in vitro test system is capable of duplicating the in vitro events, and in vivo tests in patients are too potentially dangerous to be justified. This makes the designation of an etiologic agent a question of judgment and clinical experience, hallowed but quite vulnerable criteria. In patients without exposure to a suggestive etiologic agent, the term *idiopathic* is used to conceal our ignorance. Obviously, even in these cases an etiologic agent must exist and may be present among the host of environmental toxins that have become part of our civilized existence.

Drugs and Chemicals. The drugs suspected of being potentially toxic for the hemopoietic stem cells have been listed in booklets published by the American Medical Association in the 1960s and include about 329 items. The inclusion of all these drugs diluted the responsibility, since every medication from aspirin and penicillin to phenylbutazone and chloramphenicol was equally tainted. However, subsequent, more discriminating studies have emphasized incidence. Alter and coworkers, in a thorough study of 2109 cases, have produced a more meaningful list of potential marrow toxins (Table 2–8). This list emphasizes the etiologic importance of chloramphenicol and explains why this drug now is used sparingly, making chloramphenicol-induced aplastic anemia a rarity today.

Many attempts have been made to relate potential toxicity to the presence of a benzene

Table 2–8 SUSPECTED ETIOLOGIC AGENTS IN 2109 CASES OF APLASTIC ANEMIA REPORTED IN THE LITERATURE BETWEEN 1950 AND 1977

Idiopathic	44%
Chloramphenicol	26%
Benzene	2%
Sulfonamides	2%
Insecticides	3%
Anticonvulsants	2%
Phenylbutazone	4%
Solvents	1%
Gold	< 1%
Infections	2%
Hepatitis	1%
Other	14%

(From Alter B. P., et al.: Clin. Haematol., 7:431, 1978.)

or nitrobenzene radical in the chemical structure of suspected drugs. Benzene itself is a major bone marrow toxin capable of inducing both aplastic anemia and leukemia, and, in addition to chloramphenicol, many benzene-related chemicals such as trinitrotoluene, toluene, and the insecticides lindane and DDT have been strongly suspected of inducing aplastic anemia. However, many drugs without the benzene radical also appear to be toxic to stem cells, and the common denominator may reside in an intermediate metabolic product rather than in the parent molecule.

Because of the high incidence of aplastic anemia in patients receiving chloramphenicol, special efforts have been made to clarify the mechanism of the toxic action of this drug on the bone marrow. Although we talk about "high" incidence, it must be emphasized that only one of 10,000 to 20,000 treated patients develop aplastic anemia and that prospective metabolic studies are almost impossible. However, mild, reversible bone marrow suppression is observed in most treated patients, a suppression related to drug dosage and length of treatment. Clinically, it can easily be recognized by a decrease in reticulocyte counts and an increase in serum iron concentration. Bone marrow examination reveals vacuolization of erythroid cells. After prolonged treatment, vacuolization can be observed in other cellular elements as well, and granulocytopenia and thrombocytopenia may ensue. These effects were initially thought to be related to a suppressive action on the ribosomal protein synthesis similar to the action of chloramphenicol on the bacterial cells. However, in vitro studies of bone marrow suspensions by Yunis and coworkers have suggested that in the mammalian cell chloramphenicol inhibits mitochondrial protein synthesis. Since many consider the mitochondria to be intracellular inclusions of plant origin with independent mechanisms for replication and metabolism, this finding could provide a link between the bacteriostatic and the bone marrow suppressive actions of chloramphenicol.

It is tempting to consider the suppressive action of the bone marrow as an early, still reversible manifestation of a stem cell injury that eventually leads to irreversible aplastic anemia. However, it seems more likely that patients who develop aplastic anemia have an abnormal response to the bone marrow suppressive effect of chloramphenicol. Not only is the regularly occurring suppression readily reversible even after prolonged treatment with large amounts of chloramphenicol, but many patients who develop aplastic anemia do so weeks or months after exposure to relatively small amounts of this drug. It has been proposed that the few unfortunate victims have an underlying genetic or acquired hypersensitivity to chloramphenicol. This could reside in the rate or extent of detoxification of the drug or in a specific stem cell abnormality. Some in vitro studies of bone marrow taken from patients who have recovered from aplastic anemia or obtained from their immediate relatives have suggested a greater than normal susceptibility to the suppressive action of chloramphenicol. Other studies, however, have not supported such a genetic hypersusceptibility but have suggested that previously damaged stem cells, as in busulfan-treated mice, are excessively vulnerable to the toxic effect of chloramphenicol. We obviously are still far from having established the pathogenetic mode of action of chloramphenicol or from having learned how to predict individual hypersensitivity to this or to other potentially toxic drugs.

Radiation. Bone marrow supression is a well-recognized side effect of the diagnostic and therapeutic use of radiation. Radiation energy, whether mediated by a direct hit of waves or particles or by the production of highly reactive free radicals, is capable of breaking molecular bonds in critical intracellular macromolecules. Although all cells can be injured by radiation energy, organ systems dependent on a rapid cellular turnover of nucleic acids are particularly vulnerable. These systems can be ranked, according to Cronkite and Bond, with regard to radiosensitivity as follows: (1) germinal cells of the testes, (2) hemopoietic cells, (3) intestinal cells, and (4) epidermal basal cells.

Brief exposure to radiation of high energy as in reactor accidents leads to extensive destruction of the bone marrow and intestine, and death is usually caused by acute granulocytopenia and thrombocytopenia and by intestinal ulcerations. If the patient should survive the acute effects, the recovery is usually almost complete, since the dormant multipotential stem cells will have sustained very little radiation injury and are capable of bone marrow repopulation. In the aftermath of the atomic attacks on Nagasaki, for example, Kirschbaum and his Japanese coworkers found that aplastic anemia was observed in only a very small number of survivors.

Prolonged exposure to more moderate doses of radiation may cause chronic bone marrow failure and aplastic anemia. This has been described in patients intermittently treated with external or internal total body radiation or in Martland's classic report on watch-dial painters who accidentally ingested paint containing radium with a long biologic half-life. It has also been suspected as a pathogenetic mechanism in aplastic anemia occurring in physicians and radiologists exposed to minimal amounts of radiation for many years. However, as is the case for exposure to drugs and chemicals, a definite cause-effect relationship can never be firmly established. The reasons for defective bone marrow repopulation after chronic radiation exposure may be that multipotential stem cells are activated and then share in the radiation injury. An alternative explanation for the development of aplastic anemia after chronic radiation has been provided by Knospe and coworkers—namely, that radiation-induced damage to endothelial stem cells will change the structural microenvironment of the bone marrow and prevent bone marrow regeneration.

Immunologic Rejection. Aplastic anemia has been associated with a variety of seemingly unrelated diseases. Miliary tuberculosis has always been listed prominently among such disorders, but a critical evaluation of reported cases indicates that this association is rare indeed. Hepatitis with its many immunologic manifestations looms much larger as a possible etiologic event, and Camitta and coworkers, after reviewing many cases, have concluded that post-hepatitis aplastic anemia is especially malignant and should be treated with marrow transplantation promptly. Aplastic anemia associated with complement-sensitive red cells and nocturnal hemoglobinuria has been described so frequently by Lewis and Dacie in England and by Vincent and de Gruchy in Australia that this combination ought to contain some clue to etiology or pathogenesis.

The most reasonable explanation is that an immunologic mechanism underlies the development of aplastic anemia. In support of this hypothesis, aplastic anemia has been observed to develop after the transfusion of whole blood or bone marrow into immunologically deficient children. Miller has suggested that the disease in these unfortunate patients reflects a graft-versus-host immunologic rejection of either hemopoietic or structural stem cells. In vitro studies have furthermore demonstrated the presence of an increased number of suppressor or killer lymphocytes in some patients with aplastic anemia. The therapeutic implication of these findings would be to use immunosuppressive drugs, a most difficult decision to make because of the inherent bone marrow suppressive effect of currently used drugs. However, the effect of antithymocyte globulin has been very impressive. It has been used primarily in older patients and in younger patients without HLA-compatible donors, and its use has been associated with about 50 percent complete or partial remissions as compared with a 20 to 25 percent spontaneous recovery. The effect of prednisone has been too erratic to justify its use, although high-dose "bolus" prednisolone has been claimed to be beneficial.

Constitutional. Fanconi's anemia is a form of aplastic anemia that occurs as an inborn defect associated with other congenital abnormalities such as skin pigmentations, renal hypoplasia, absent thumb or radius, and microcephaly. Multiple abnormalities of the chromosomal pattern of lymphocytes and bone marrow cells have been described, but whether or not the basic disorder resides in the hemopoietic or the structural stem cells is no better known here than in the acquired cases. Fanconi's anemia is believed to be a recessive autosomal disorder with an estimated incidence of heterozygotes of 1 to 300 to 400 in the population. This appreciable incidence has led to the speculation that some with aplastic anemia due to idiopathic hypersensitivity are actually carriers of a Fanconi stem cell defect. Of more immediate interest, however, has been the demonstration by Shahidi and Diamond that the hypoplastic bone marrow in Fanconi's anemia appears to be quite responsive to the myelostimulatory effect of androgens. Many patients have been kept alive and well on a maintenance regimen of androgens, and these results have led to a revival of the therapeutic use of androgens in all cases of aplastic anemia. Androgens do enhance erythropoietin release, but this cannot explain their occasional effect on granulocyte and thrombocyte production, and, as emphasized by Gardner and coworkers, they must have some direct or indirect action on the hemopoietic or the structural bone marrow stem cells.

The conclusion from these etiologic and pathogenetic considerations appears to be that aplastic anemia is not one but many diseases. However, they all have one feature in common, a defect in the capacity of stem cells to restore a depleted multipotential stem cell compartment. Sustained blood cell production takes place in small and large islands in the

Table 2–9 POSSIBLE PATHOGENETIC MECHANISMS IN APLASTIC ANEMIA

Defective stem cell microenvironment
Depleted stem cells
Abnormal stem cells
Rejected stem cells

otherwise fatty marrow, indicating that stem cells can differentiate as well as replace their own number. But they cannot multiply and reseed the aplastic marrow. The reason for proliferative inhibition is not clear, but Table 2–9 lists some pathogenetic possibilities, explored in detail by Appelbaum and Fefer in 1981, by Camitta and coworkers in 1982, and by the contributors to a monograph edited by Young and coworkers in 1984.

The presence of a defective microenvironment is a possibility difficult to accept now in view of the therapeutic effectiveness of marrow transplantation. It has been suggested, however, that this procedure restores normal marrow function by transplanting both hemopoietic and structural stem cells. Although possible, it seems unlikely because fibroblasts of a post-transplantation marrow were found by Wilson and colleagues to be of recipient origin.

Depletion of normal multipotential stem cells can be envisioned as a primary pathogenetic mechanism only if the capacity to restore normal stem cell numbers after injury is finite. This would mean that proliferation without differentiation is the prerogative of very early stem cells and can be carried out only a limited number of times before the stem cells settle in a steady state condition during which each differentiation is associated with a single stem cell renewal. Support for this hypothesis comes primarily from the observation by Hellman and Mauch that during successive marrow transplantations in inbred mice stem cell pool restoration diminishes gradually until it fails altogether.

Dysfunction of the multipotential stem cells with reduced capacity for proliferation but preserved capacity for differentiation is another mechanism that would lead to marrow aplasia. Such dysfunction would presumably have to be clonal, and one has to assume that these clones—despite their limited proliferative capacity—have a survival advantage over normal clones. This could be accomplished by the release of suppressors of normal stem cell function, but if so it is difficult to explain the successful direct engraftment of stem cells from an identical twin.

Rejection, either humoral or cellular, of normal stem cells is a pathogenetic mechanism that has received considerable support. The identification in some patients of stem cell antibodies, the demonstration in marrow co-cultures of suppressive T lymphocytes directed against stem cells, the sporadic but impressive therapeutic benefit of antithymocyte globulin (Champlin et al., 1983), and the dependence on immunosuppression for successful marrow transplantation—even among some identical twin pairs—all have directed attention to immunologic rejection as a likely pathogenetic mechanism. The therapeutic implications are not clear. At present, marrow transplantation in children and young adults with HLA-compatible siblings seems to be the treatment of choice (Storb et al., 1984). However, various therapeutic regimens directed at humoral or cellular suppression are being tested and may provide a less traumatic treatment in the future.

DISORDERS OF UNIPOTENTIAL PROGENITOR CELLS

Secondary Polycythemia

Secondary polycythemia, or, more correctly, secondary erythrocytosis, is a condition characterized by an enhanced, erythropoietin-mediated stimulation of red cell production and an increased red cell mass. In most cases, the erythropoietin release is an appropriate response to tissue hypoxia, but in some the release is inappropriate, and the resulting erythrocytosis presumably serves no useful function (Fig. 2–25).

Appropriate Secondary Erythrocytosis

High Altitude. The erythrocytosis experienced by high-altitude dwellers is probably the most common of the secondary polycythemias, and it must be considered an appropriate physiologic adaptation rather than a pathologic disorder. However, sustained physiologic adaptations are usually achieved at a certain biologic cost, and individuals at high altitude pay for an enhanced oxygen transport by problems related to hypervolemia, hyperviscosity, and hyperventilation.

Many field studies of high-altitude erythrocytosis have been conducted in the small town

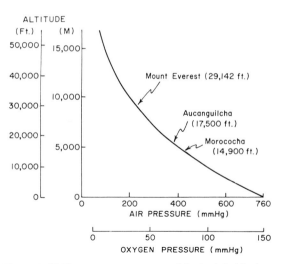

Figure 2–27 The oxygen pressure at altitudes inhabited or visited by humans.

of Morococha at 15,000 feet in the Peruvian Andes. Only a few precarious settlements exist above this altitude, with the highest permanent settlement probably being Aucanguilcha in the Chilean Andes at 17,500 feet. At this level, the atmospheric oxygen pressure is not much higher than the mean capillary oxygen pressure at sea level, making it very difficult to provide a downhill gradient for oxygen from air to cells. Above 17,500 feet, only short-term sojourns are possible, and only a few single-minded, superbly conditioned mountain climbers have managed to reach the top of the world, Mt. Everest—at 29,000 feet—without being sustained by supplemental oxygen (Fig. 2–27).

The ability of the inhabitants of the mining town of Morococha to live active, strenuous lives at 15,000 feet is directly related to their adaptable oxygen transport system (Erslev, 1981). The tissue requirements for oxygen are the same as or higher than at sea level, but increased pulmonary function, increased oxygen-carrying capacity of blood, and increased blood volume succeed in reducing the oxygen gradient needed to bring oxygen from the air to the tissues (Fig. 2–28). Such a reduction will ensure that the oxygen molecules in the capillaries are under enough pressure for their subsequent diffusion into the tissues.

Sustained hyperventilation causes a reduction in the oxygen gradient between ambient and alveolar air. Because of the inherent effect of dead space and water vapors, this part of the gradient can be only reduced moderately. However, hyperventilation causes a pulmonary "stretch" with enlargement of the alveolar

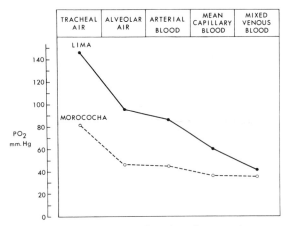

Figure 2–28 The oxygen gradient from lungs to tissues at sea level (Lima) or at 15,000 feet (Morococha). (Redrawn from Hurtado, A. *In* Weihe, W. H. [Ed.]: Physiological Effects of High Altitude. New York, Pergamon Press, 1964, p. 1.)

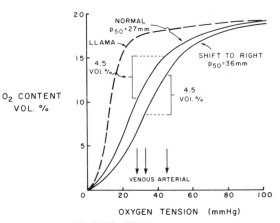

Figure 2–29 At low arterial oxygen tension (i.e., 45 mm.) the delivery of 4.5 volume percent of oxygen from normal hemoglobin with a P_{50} of 27 mm. will reduce venous oxygen tension to 28 mm. A shift to the right, however, will permit the delivery of the same volume of oxygen with less reduction in venous oxygen tension (33 mm.). Nevertheless, the well-adapted llama has a left-shifted dissociation curve.

diffusing area and reduction of the alveolar-capillary gradient. The most important reduction occurs in the arterial-venous gradient, permitting unloading of oxygen throughout the length of the capillary at a relatively high pressure. Since the tissue demands for oxygen are not reduced, the maintenance of a shallow gradient demands an increased flow of oxygen-carrying red blood cells through the tissues. Although an increase in cardiac output would accomplish just this, the added workload on a vital organ is unacceptable for chronic adjustments. Of more importance for the maintenance of an increased oxygen flow to the tissue is an increase in the red blood cell count.

Tissue hypoxia will lead to the release of erythropoietin, which in turn will increase the rate of red cell production and enhance the oxygen-carrying capacity of blood. Furthermore, the increased rate of red cell production will cause an increase in blood volume, with dilatation and opening of vessels and an increase in tissue perfusion. This dual effect on oxygen flow probably outweighs the disadvantages derived from the higher viscosity of circulating blood.

A shift in the oxygen dissociation curve to the right would also reduce the arteriovenous gradient and enhance the unloading of oxygen in the tissue capillaries (Fig. 2–29). However, such a shift may significantly reduce the loading of hemoglobin with oxygen in the lungs, an important consideration, as emphasized by Finch and Lenfant, when the ambient oxygen pressure is about one half of normal. Actually, the curve is shifted to the left during initial adaptation to high altitudes because of acute hyperventilation alkalosis. After a few days, the alkalosis has initiated increased intracellular 2,3-DPG formation, and the curve shifts back to normal, where it remains during prolonged acclimatization. If is of interest that animals indigenous to high altitudes, such as llamas and vicuñas, have hemoglobins with high affinity for oxygen (Fig. 2–29), suggesting that loading with oxygen in the lungs is more important than unloading in the tissues for survival at high altitudes. This suggestion has been supported by Hebbel and associates, who studied two children with the high oxygen-affinity hemoglobin, Andrew-Minneapolis. These youngsters were transported to Leadville, Colorado, at 3100 m. and, when tested immediately after arrival, were found to be preadapted and able to perform strenuous physical activities with little mobilization of cardiovascular reserve. How these "human llamas" and their Andean counterparts can release enough oxygen in the tissues from their high-affinity hemoglobins is still a question. Maybe they have an unusually high density of capillaries and myoglobin in their tissues, or, more likely, their intracellular electron chains may be set for a low oxygen pressure, as has been proposed by Robin to explain prolonged anoxic survival by whales and turtles.

The clinical manifestation of chronic high altitude acclimatization is dominated by ruddy cyanosis and physiologic emphysema. The vascular enlargement can be observed readily in the conjunctiva, mucous membrane, and skin and may contribute to the remarkable capacity of Sherpas to walk barefoot and sleep on ice and snow.

The blood studies reveal a normochromic and normocytic erythrocytosis, with increased red cell mass but no significant increase in granulocyte or platelet counts. <u>The plasma iron concentration is normal in contradistinction to polycythemia vera, in which it is usually low</u>. This difference may be due merely to blood loss and to therapeutic phlebotomies in polycythemia vera, but it has been suggested that tissue hypoxia as experienced at high altitudes enhances intestinal iron absorption. Erythropoietin titers in plasma and urine are increased, also in contradistinction to polycythemia vera, in which they are extremely low.

It is difficult to evaluate the biologic cost of chronic acclimatization to high altitudes, since very few reliable data on the longevity and morbidity of high altitude dwellers exist. However, the compensatory reserves are undoubtedly decreased, and the effect of cardiopulmonary disorders must be more serious than at sea level. Chronic mountain sickness (Monge's disease) is caused by an acquired refractoriness of the respiratory center leading to relative alveolar hypoventilation and excessive tissue hypoxia. Since this in turn will cause an increase in an already expanded red cell mass and higher blood viscosity, cardiovascular decompensation occurs. Therapeutic venesection provides symptomatic relief, but the individuals suffering from Monge's disease usually need to be brought down to sea level for permanent improvement.

2) **Pulmonary Disease.** Chronic pulmonary disease associated with cyanosis, clubbing, and arterial oxygen unsaturation is not always accompanied by an increase in hemoglobin concentration (Fig. 2–30). In some cases a concomitant increase in plasma volume may conceal the effect of an increased red cell mass, but <u>in most cases true secondary erythrocytosis does not occur.</u> The release of erythropoietin appears to be commensurate to the degree of tissue hypoxia, but for unknown reasons there is an unresponsiveness of the stem cells to this hormone or an impairment in the subsequent proliferation of nucleated red cells.

3) **Cardiovascular Disease.** Right-to-left shunt in congenital heart disease is characteristically associated with cyanosis, clubbing, and often extreme secondary appropriate erythrocytosis. Despite high hematocrit, hyperviscosity symptoms are rarely present, probably owing to the simultaneous increase in total blood volume.

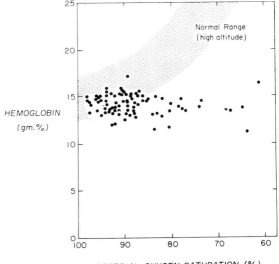

Figure 2–30 Hemoglobin concentrations of patients with various degrees of arterial oxygen desaturation due to chronic pulmonary disease. (Redrawn from Gallo, R. C., et al.: Arch. Intern. Med., *113*:559, 1964. Copyright 1964, American Medical Association.)

Whether or not to perform phlebotomy on "blue babies" prior to surgery is still an unanswered question, but most surgeons feel more comfortable if the hematocrit is brought down below 60 percent by judicious phlebotomies. It certainly will provide a little more reserve if fluid intake becomes inadequate.

In acquired heart disease with chronic decompensation, erythrokinetic studies by Chodos and coworkers have shown that a mild increase in red cell production and red cell mass is usually present. However, the increased plasma volume prevents an accurate assessment of the size of the red cell mass from hematocrit determinations alone.

4) **Alveolar Hypoventilation.** Alveolar hypoventilation, whether related to central or peripheral impairment, causes arterial hypoxemia, cyanosis, and secondary erythrocytosis. Its two most colorful variants are Monge's chronic mountain sickness (see earlier) and the Pickwickian syndrome. In the latter syndrome, catchingly named by Ratto and coworkers, obesity, peripheral hypoventilation, hypercapnia, somnolence, and central hypoventilation are involved in a vicious circle leading to the proverbial somnolent cyanosis of Mrs. Wardle's boy, Joe.

5) **Defective Oxygen Transport.** Secondary erythrocytosis is occasionally observed in patients with cyanosis due to acquired or congenital <u>methemoglobinemia.</u> However, the eryth-

ropoietic response in these patients is less than would be anticipated in cyanotic patients. Cyanosis may actually be present with as little as 1.5 gm. of methemoglobin per 100 ml. in the circulation, an amount that in itself should not result in significant tissue hypoxia. An increase in oxygen affinity is also present in hemoglobin partially combined with carbon monoxide and is probably responsible for the erythrocytosis observed in heavy smokers.

Familial erythrocytosis has been described in a number of individuals with abnormal hemoglobins. In most of these cases, the amino acid substitution occurs in the contact area between the alpha and beta chains. Such substitutions interfere with the release of oxygen to the tissues, decrease the P_{50}, and result in a compensatory erythrocytosis despite fully oxygenated arterial blood.

Drug-Induced Tissue Hypoxia. Although a number of drugs and chemicals can induce histiotoxic anoxia, only cobalt has convincingly been associated with the development of a secondary appropriate erythrocytosis. Several studies have shown that cobalt administration causes the release of erythropoietin and that this release presumably is related to its inhibitory effect on intracellular oxidative metabolism in the kidneys. Since histiotoxic anoxia is generalized (Fig. 2–11), the use of cobalt in the treatment of refractory anemias is of little benefit to patients. Their oxygen-carrying capacity may increase, but merely enough to counteract the effect of the additional tissue hypoxia induced by cobalt.

Inappropriate Secondary Erythrocytosis (Table 2–10)

Renal Disorders. A partial obstruction of the renal artery or its tributaries may cause localized renal hypoxia, the stimulus for erythropoietin production. However, an impaired blood supply to the kidneys usually reduces oxygen consumption and it is only the rare patient who develops enough renal hypoxia to respond with an increased release of erythropoietin and a secondary polycythemia. It is of potential importance that intrarenal vascular obstruction as observed in transplanted kidneys undergoing rejection may cause the release of erythropoietin. Unfortunately, the current assays are too laborious to permit the erythropoietin titers to be used to detect threatening rejection. However, the appearance of an increased number of nucleated red cells or reticulocytes in the circulating blood, presumably caused by the release of

Table 2–10 INAPPROPRIATE SECONDARY POLYCYTHEMIA

Location	Pathologic Condition	Number of Case Reports Until 1972
Kidney		
	Hypernephroma	118
	Other tumors	13
	Hydronephrosis	14
	Cystic disease	35
	Renal artery stenosis	2
	Transplantation rejection	7
	Bartter's syndrome	1
Liver		
	Hepatoma	64
Uterus		
	Leiomyoma	24
Cerebellum		
	Hemangioblastoma	50
Adrenal Gland		
	Pheochromocytoma	5

(Data from Thorling, E. B.: Scand. J. Haematol., Suppl. 17, 1972.)

erythropoietin, has been claimed to be a useful warning signal.

A more common cause of secondary erythrocytosis is the presence of space-occupying renal lesions. These lesions can be cysts, either solitary or part of polycystic renal disease, hydronephrosis, or a variety of renal neoplasms. Erythropoietin assays of cyst fluid have disclosed the presence of erythropoietin, and it has been proposed that the tubular lining of cysts is capable of secreting erythropoietin. With regard to the neoplasms, assays of tumor extracts—especially extracts of hypernephromas—for erythropoietin have occasionally been positive. However, the fact that so many histologically different lesions can lead to an excessive production of erythropoietin has raised the suspicion that it is not only the tumor cells that are engaged in inappropriate erythropoietin production but also the adjoining normal parenchyma that secretes this hormone in response to pressure-induced hypoxia.

Successful removal of renal tumors in patients with polycythemia usually results in normalization of the red blood cell count. Subsequent metastases in the opposite kidney or elsewhere have occasionally been associated with a recurrence of the polycythemia. A mild to moderate erythrocytosis occurs in about 10 percent of patients after renal transplantation. It is not seen in patients previously nephrectomized and it appears to be caused by sustained and inappropriate erythropoietin production by the remnant, otherwise inactive kidneys (Dagher et al., 1979).

In a number of cases erythrocytosis and elevated erythropoietin titers have been observed in young individuals with no evidence of tissue hypoxia or lesions potentially capable of inappropriate erythropoietin production. It has been proposed that the erythropoietin is derived from kidneys with congenital vascular abnormalities, but in view of its unsettled pathogenesis this condition has been called essential erythrocytosis (see Fig. 2–25).

2) **Extrarenal Disorders.** Cerebellar hemangioblastomas are an infrequent cause of secondary inappropriate erythrocytosis. Cyst fluid from the tumor has, in a few cases, been shown to contain erythropoietin stimulatory material indistinguishable from erythropoietin. However, the proximity of the tumor to the respiratory center and to the hypothalamus has also suggested that central hypoventilation plays a role or that a hypothetical hypothalamic-renal connection is involved. In areas such as Hong Kong with a high incidence of hepatocarcinoma 10 percent of afflicted patients develop erythrocytosis. The most favored explanation is that the tumor is responsible for inappropriate secretion of erythropoietin, an explanation supported by the finding that the liver normally produces small amounts of extrarenal erythropoietin. The rare erythrocytosis observed in patients with large uterine myomas may be caused by mechanical interference with renal blood supply. An inappropriate neoplastic production of erythropoietin by these fibrous, differentiated tumors seems unlikely in view of their histologic character.

The occasional association with certain endocrine lesions such as Cushing's syndrome and pheochromocytomas is intriguing but has not been too informative. Although androgen-producing lesions have not been associated with erythrocytosis, androgens have empirically been found to be potent stimulators of erythropoiesis. This was first pointed out by Kennedy and coworkers, who in the late 1950s observed the development of plethora and high hematocrits in women treated with androgens for breast cancer. The effect appears to be mediated via a release of renal erythropoietin as well as via a direct action of androgens on the bone marrow stem cell pool.

Anemia of Renal Disease

Anemia is a hallmark of chronic renal disease and is roughly proportional to the degree of renal failure as measured by urea or creatinine retention. Since the pathogenesis of the anemia and the uremia is related to the failure of many independent functions, it is actually surprising that the proportionality is as good as depicted in Figure 2–31. The two major failing functions are the renal excretory function and the renal endocrine function.

Failure of Renal Excretory Function

Hemolysis. The red cell of patients with uremia frequently shows multiple tiny spicules (Fig. 2–32). The presence of this so-called "burring" has been related to the accumulation of toxic end products in the circulation and has been thought to be responsible for an impaired sodium-potassium pump activity and a shortened red cell life span. However, the correlation between azotemia and red cell life span is poor (Fig. 2–33), and when hemolysis occurs, it is often related more closely to

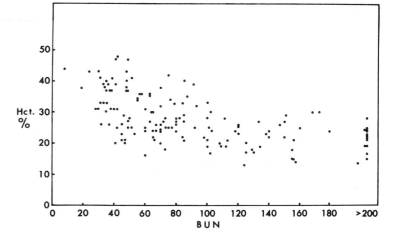

Figure 2–31 Relationship between hematocrit and BUN in 152 patients with various degrees of renal failure and uremia. (From Erslev, A. J.: Arch. Intern. Med., *126*:774, 1970. Reprinted from Wesson, L. G. [Ed.]: Physiology of the Human Kidney, 1969, by permission of Grune & Stratton, Inc., New York.)

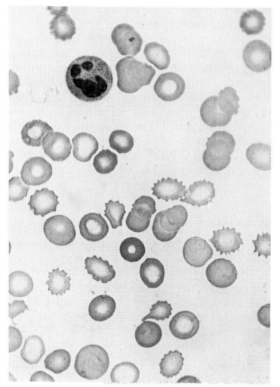

Figure 2–32 Burr cells in smear of blood from a patient with severe uremia.

changes in the microvasculature than to the degree of uremia. Indeed, extensive red cell fragmentation and hemolysis can be observed in patients with malignant vascular hypertension or with inflammatory vascular changes (hemolytic uremic syndrome) and with only

mildly elevated BUN or creatinine concentrations. At present, it seems most reasonable to relate the premature destruction of red cells in chronic renal disease to mechanical disruption of metabolically fragile red cells.

Bleeding Tendency. As a manifestation of chronic renal disease, purpura is almost as characteristic as pallor. In addition to subcutaneous bleedings, gastrointestinal and uterine hemorrhage may cause a considerable loss of blood and increase the demands for an accelerated rate of red cell production. Iatrogenic blood loss should also not be forgotten. Patients with chronic renal disease are usually monitored by multiple laboratory tests and, if also hemodialyzed, may lose some blood in the dialysis coil. All in all, iron deficiency is one of the most common—but fortunately very treatable—problems in patients with chronic renal disease. The pathogenesis of the bleeding tendency is poorly understood, since thrombocytopenia and coagulation factor deficiency, when present, are rarely severe enough to be responsible for overt blood loss. Studies by Horowitz and coworkers, however, suggest that certain retention products may affect normal platelet function and cause an abnormal bleeding time, clot retraction, platelet adhesion, and platelet aggregation. The responsible toxic factor is believed to be a guanidino compound, and intensive dialysis has been found to reduce the bleeding tendency.

Responsiveness to Erythropoietin. In chronic renal failure there is both inadequate production of erythropoietin (see later) and decreased bone marrow response to erythro-

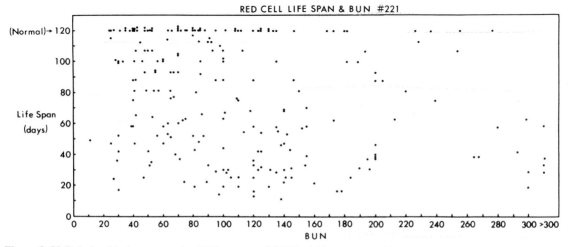

Figure 2–33 Relationship between red cell life span and BUN of 221 patients with various degrees of renal failure and uremia. (From Erslev, A. J.: Arch. Intern. Med., *126*:774, 1970. Copyright 1970, American Medical Association.)

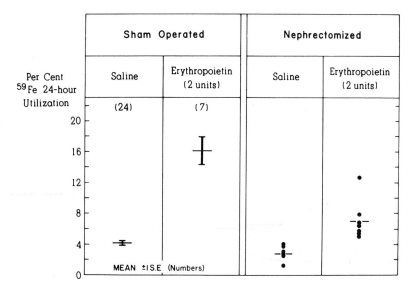

	Sham Operated		Nephrectomized	
Per Cent 59Fe 24-hour Utilization	Saline	Erythropoietin (2 units)	Saline	Erythropoietin (2 units)

Figure 2–34 Erythropoietic response of normal and nephrectomized rats to the same amount of erythropoietin. On day 0, the animals were transfused with 20 ml. per kg. of rat red cells. On day 3, they were either nephrectomized or sham operated and then given 2 units erythropoietin subcutaneously. On day 4, ^{59}Fe was injected intravenously and its utilization determined 24 hours later.

poietin (Fig. 2–34). The reason is not known, but the degree of responsiveness appears to be related to the severity of uremia and is mediated by a still elusive uremic toxin. It seems probable that the improvement in erythropoietic function found after intensive dialysis, especially after peritoneal dialysis, is caused by an increased response to available erythropoietin rather than to an increased production of erythropoietin. Because of this refractory condition, it is anticipated that much more erythropoietin will be needed to abolish the anemia of chronic renal disease than is required for normal erythropoietic maintenance.

Failure of Renal Endocrine Function

The various effects of uremia on the rate of red cell destruction and production result in an increased demand for erythropoietin. This demand could easily be met by a normal kidney but apparently not by an abnormal one. Impaired renal tissue is not capable of producing normal quantities of erythropoietin unless stimulated by intensive anemic hypoxia, and a balance between the rates of red cell destruction and red cell production is not achieved except at anemic levels. Under conditions of progressive kidney failure, the hypoxic stimulus needed to produce adequate amounts of renal erythropoietin becomes greater and the anemia more severe. However, even anephric individuals continue to manufacture red blood cells (Fig. 2–35). This residual erythropoietic activity appears to be generated by the release of extrarenal erythropoietin, but the hemoglobin concentration that can be maintained in anephric patients is usually too low to be compatible with life and has to be augmented by transfusions.

Anemia of Chronic Disease

Although one of the most common anemias, the anemia of chronic disorders is of relatively little clinical significance, since it is rarely severe enough to cause symptoms or demand active transfusion therapy. However, it probably has been treated by more unneeded and ineffective hematinics than any other anemia, and the pathogenesis of this refractory anemia is still a fascinating enigma. (See the 1983 review by Lee and the 1983 monograph by Reizenstein.)

During the early part of this century, anemia was an invariable complication of many chronic debilitating infections, such as tuberculosis, osteomyelitis, and brucellosis, and it was known as *anemia of chronic infection*. With the change in the ecology of disease, it was realized that a similar anemia also occurred in patients with chronic, noninfectious diseases, such as rheumatoid arthritis, lymphomas, and disseminated carcinomas, and the anemia was given the noncommittal name of *anemia of chronic disorders*. It is characterized by a moderate reduction in hemoglobin concentration, a reduction in the level of both serum iron and iron-binding capacity, an increased amount of storage iron in the macrophages of the bone marrow, and a normal or elevated serum ferritin concentration.

The presence of decreased amounts of cir-

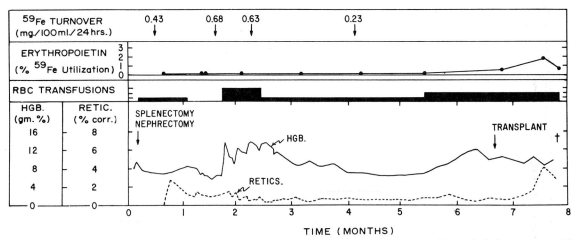

Figure 2–35 Erythropoietic status of a patient who underwent nephrectomy and splenectomy 7 months before a successful kidney transplantation. Although erythropoietin levels were unmeasurable, reticulocytes were produced throughout the anephric period.

culating iron, despite abundant iron stores, is probably caused by a defective iron release mechanism by the macrophages. This defect may in turn be caused by interleukin-1 released from activated monocytes or macrophages. It has been proposed by Konijn and Hershko that apoferritin behaves as an acute-phase protein and that its synthesis is augmented by interleukin-1, effectively trapping macrophage iron in inflammatory conditions. The erythroid cells in the bone marrow apparently can handle available iron, and the utilization of radioactive iron is normal. However, the reutilization of iron is decreased (Fig. 2–36), indicating that hemoglobin iron, which normally is reutilized after being processed by the macrophages, is trapped in these cells and removed from the

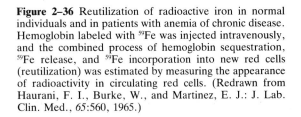

Figure 2–36 Reutilization of radioactive iron in normal individuals and in patients with anemia of chronic disease. Hemoglobin labeled with ^{59}Fe was injected intravenously, and the combined process of hemoglobin sequestration, ^{59}Fe release, and ^{59}Fe incorporation into new red cells (reutilization) was estimated by measuring the appearance of radioactivity in circulating red cells. (Redrawn from Haurani, F. I., Burke, W., and Martinez, E. J.: J. Lab. Clin. Med., 65:560, 1965.)

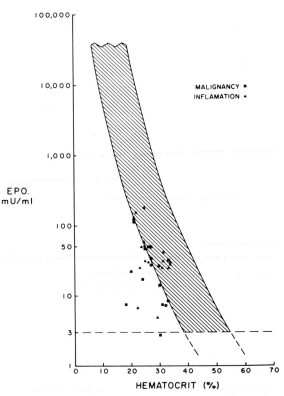

Figure 2–37 Erythropoietin titers of patients with anemias (hematocrit less than 35) due to malignancy or inflammation, in the absence of renal disease. The cross-hatched area represents erythropoietin concentrations in normals and in patients with uncomplicated anemias.

dynamic iron economy of the body. This relative iron deficiency is aggravated by a moderate shortening of the red blood cell life span, resulting in a mild anemia. However, it has always been a puzzle why the anemia of chronic disorders does not display the morphologic characteristics of an iron deficiency anemia but is usually normocytic and normochromic, as if the basic defect resides in the stem cells. Various studies have shown that in some patients there is an element of stem cell failure secondary to a reduced production of erythropoietin (Fig. 2–37). No renal injury or abnormality can be held responsible for this deficiency, and studies of red cells have shown that their oxygen affinity is normal. However, acute and chronic illnesses may be associated with a defect in the peripheral transformation of the thyroid hormone T_4 to the metabolically active T_3. Such defects may cause a relative hypothyroidism, and it seems possible that the low erythropoietin production in some patients with chronic illnesses is caused by decreased metabolic demands rather than by renal dysfunction. It also seems clear, however, that the anemia of chronic disease is not a homogenous entity and that its pathogenesis may be as divergent as its etiology.

Anemia of Endocrine Disorders

Pituitary and Thyroid Dysfunction

Pituitary and thyroid dysfunction or ablation are characteristically associated with a moderate normochromic, normocytic anemia. Although many attempts have been made to assign a specific erythropoietic effect to the thyroid, pituitary, or hypothalamic secretions, most current studies indicate that the anemia is an appropriate response to a decreased cellular demand for oxygen. The administration of thyroid hormones will increase this demand, and the rate of red cell production will respond appropriately. It is questionable whether the administration of growth hormone, ACTH, or gonadal hormones is of additional benefit. In many cases of myxedema or other hypothyroid conditions, the anemia is somewhat atypical because of associated nutritional deficiencies. Malabsorption of B_{12} or folic acid may lead to a megaloblastic, macrocytic blood picture, and the frequent uterine bleedings in hypothyroid females may lead to an iron-deficient, microcytic, hypochromic anemia. Even in hypothyroid men, the common achlorhydria may result in malabsorption of iron and an iron-deficiency anemia.

Despite the erythropoietic effect of increased oxygen consumption induced by thyroid hormones, patients with hyperthyroidism or thyrotoxicosis are rarely erythrocytotic. This may be explained by the fact that thyroid hormones also increase cardiac output and tissue perfusion, making an increase in red cell mass less needed. Nevertheless, direct measurements by Muldowney and coworkers of red cell mass and plasma volume suggest that the absence of a high hematocrit in these conditions is caused by a concomitant increase in plasma volume, and that hyperthyroidism may cause true secondary polycythemia as defined by an increased red cell mass.

Gonadal Dysfunction

In normal mature men the hemoglobin concentration is about 1 to 2 gm. higher than in normal females, whereas the male hemoglobin concentration in childhood, in advanced age, and in gonadal deficiency states is similar to that of females. This phenomenon has led to the assumption that physiologic excretions of androgens have an erythropoietic effect on the bone marrow. Conversely, it has been postulated that physiologic doses of estrogens cause a slight suppression of red cell production. Many experimental data on castrated animals have been marshaled to support these contentions, but unfortunately many studies were

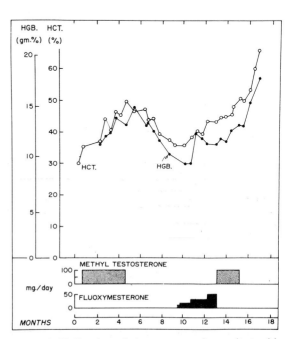

Figure 2–38 Erythropoietic response of a patient with myelofibrosis to various androgen preparations. (Redrawn from Gardner, F. H., and Pringle, J. C.: N. Engl. J. Med., *264*:103, 1961.)

designed to prove rather than to test, and the erythropoietic effects of physiologic doses of gonadal hormones are still not quite clear. More impressive are the data indicating that androgens in pharmacologic doses can stimulate red cell production and even cause full-blown secondary polycythemia (Fig. 2–38). This effect may be mediated by a release of renal erythropoietin or by an enhanced effect of erythropoietin on the bone marrow or by both mechanisms, as suggested by Shahidi and Diamond.

Pregnancy

Anemia of pregnancy is most often caused by an iron deficiency, and the routine use of iron in prenatal care is definitely in order. However, even under conditions of adequate iron intake, a mild anemia is present during the third trimester in almost all pregnant women. This anemia is normochromic and normocytic and unresponsive to any kind of treatment. Measurements of the red cell mass have shown it not to be caused by a lack of red cells but rather by an increase in plasma resulting in a dilution anemia. The red cell mass actually increases about 20 percent during pregnancy, but the plasma volume increases even more. The physiologic effect of such an increase in blood volume is very advantageous for oxygen transport (Fig. 2–21), and despite the moderate decrease in hemoglobin concentration, the pregnant woman and her fetus are undoubtedly well provided with oxygen for their metabolic demands.

Pure Red Cell Aplasia

Pure red cell aplasia is an unusual but dramatic disease characterized by severe anemia due to the isolated depletion of the erythroid tissue and is believed to be related to an immunologic dysfunction. The production and turnover of erythropoietin appear to be normal, but the bone marrow response to this hormone is inadequate, as evidenced by the absence of proerythroblasts and other nucleated red blood cells despite high plasma titers of erythropoietin (See 1983 review by Sieff).

An acute, self-limited form of pure red cell aplasia has been reported following "virus" infections in patients with hereditary spherocytosis or other congenital hemolytic disorders. The predominance of reports dealing with such

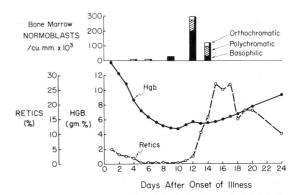

Figure 2–39 Acute aplastic crisis following a brief febrile illness in a patient with hereditary spherocytosis. (Redrawn from Owren, P. A.: Blood, *3*:231, 1948, by permission of Grune & Stratton, Inc., New York.)

patients may be due to the fact that a brief period of erythroid aplasia in a patient with a short red cell life span will have a much more noticeable effect on the hemoglobin concentration than the same period of aplasia would have if the red cell life span were normal (Fig. 2–39). Consequently, it is assumed that brief periods of asymptomatic erythroid aplasia may actually be quite common and if properly looked for will be found in many normals suffering from upper respiratory infections or viral gastroenteritis. The exact pathogenetic mechanism is unknown, but it has been proposed that the erythroid cells or their immediate erythropoietin-sensitive progenitors are affected by a virus-related antibody.

Chronic pure red cell aplasia is a far more unusual disorder, but its relationship to thymic tumors has caused a flurry of interest regarding its pathogenesis.

Thymomas are present in about 30 to 50 percent of cases, and although thymectomy is rarely of dramatic benefit, "spontaneous" recoveries have been described in patients who have undergone thymectomy. Since so-called "autoimmune disorders" are frequently associated with thymus abnormalities, it is of additional pathogenetic importance that prednisone may occasionally cause a striking reticulocyte response (Fig. 2–40) and that remissions may be induced by the therapeutic use of immunosuppressive drugs. Studies by Krantz and Kuo have demonstrated antibodies directed against erythroid bone marrow cells in the serum of some patients. These antibodies presumably coat and possibly reject the erythroid cells or the erythropoietin-responsive progenitor cells, and their presence could ex-

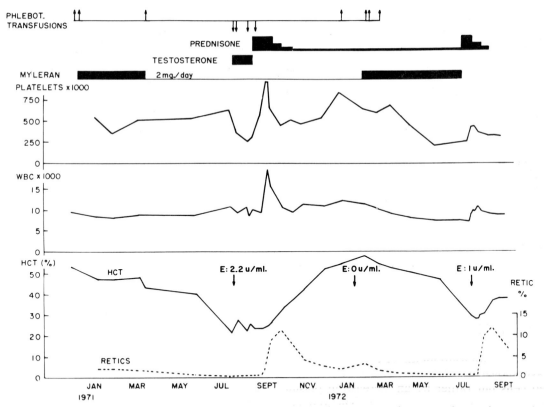

Figure 2–40 A patient with polycythemia vera, disseminated lupus erythematosus, and recurrent bouts of pure red cell aplasia. In each instance, prednisone medication caused a striking increase in reticulocytes, followed by a return of the hematocrit to normal or even polycythemic values. E = erythropoetin.

plain the development of a pure red cell aplasia. The existence of antibodies directed against erythropoietin has also been reported, but since the erythropoietin titer is usually very high, these reports are difficult to accept. The cause-effect relationship of the autoantibodies to the thymic tumor is not clear, but it has been suggested that the tumor destroys normal thymic function and permits the survival of lymphocytic clones programmed to produce autoantibodies. Further studies of this fascinating disease may well lead to concepts of importance for the management not only of patients with pure red cell aplasia but also of patients with other autoimmune diseases.

References

Adamson, J. W., Fialkow, P. J., Murphy, S., Prechal, J. F., and Steinman, L.: Polycythemia vera: stem cell and probable clonal origin of the disease. N. Engl. J. Med., *295*:913, 1976.

Alter, B. P., Potter, N. U., and Li, F. P.: Classification and aetiology of the aplastic anemias. Clin. Haematol, *7*:431, 1978.

Alter, B. P.: Fetal erythropoiesis in stress hematopoiesis. Exp. Hematol., *7*:200, 1979.

Appelbaum, F. R., and Fefer, A.: The pathogenesis of aplastic anemia. Semin. Hematol., *18*:241, 1981.

Berk, P., et al.: Increased incidence of acute leukemia in polycythemia vera associated with chlorambucil therapy. N. Engl. J. Med., *304*:441, 1981.

Camitta, B. H., Storb, R., and Thomas, E. D.: Aplastic anemia. N. Engl. J. Med., *306*:645, 712, 1982.

Champlin, R. et al.: Antithymocyte globulin treatment in patients with aplastic anemia. N. Engl. J. Med., *309*:113, 1983.

Chodos, R. B., Wells, R., Jr., and Chaffee, W. R.: A study of ferrokinetics and red cell survival in congestive heart failure. Am. J. Med., *36*:553, 1964.

Cronkite, E. P.,, and Bond, V. P.: Radiation Injury in Man. Springfield, Ill., Charles C Thomas, 1960.

Dagher, F. J., et al.: Are the native kidneys responsible for erythropoiesis in renal allorecipients? Transplantation, *28*:496, 1979.

Eaves, C. J., and Eaves, A. C.: Erythropoietin (EP) dose-response curves for three classes of erythroid progenitors in normal human marrow and in patients with polycythemia vera. Blood, *52*:1196, 1978.

Erslev, A. J.: Erythroid adaptation to altitude. Blood Cells, *7*:495, 1981.

Erslev, A. J., et al.: Plasma erythropoietin in polycythemia. Am. J. Med., *66*:243, 1979.

Fialkow, P. J.: Polycythemia vera: the in vitro response of normal and abnormal stem cell lines to erythropoietin. J. Clin. Invest., *61*:1044, 1978.

Finch, C. A., and Lenfant, C.: Oxygen transport in man. N. Engl. J. Med., *286*:407, 1972.

Gardner, F. H., Nathan, D. G., Piomelli, S., and Cummins, F. J.: The erythrocythaemic effects of androgen. Br. J. Haematol., *14*:611, 1968.

Hebbel, R. P., et al.: Human llamas. Adaptation to altitude in subjects with high hemoglobin oxygen affinity. J. Clin. Invest., *62*:593, 1978.

Hellman, S., and Mauch, P.: Implications of a proliferative limitation on hematopoietic stem cells. *In* Young, N. S., et al. [eds.]: Aplastic Anemia. New York, Liss Inc., 1984, p. 51.

Horowitz, H. J., Stein, J. M., Cohen, B. D., and White, J. M.: Further studies on the platelet-inhibitory effect of guanidinosuccinic acid and its role in uremic bleeding. Am. J. Med., *49*:336, 1970.

Kennedy, B. J., and Gilbertson, A. J.: Increased erythropoiesis induced by androgenic-hormone therapy. N. Engl. J. Med., *256*:719, 1957.

Kirschbaum, J. D., Matsno, T., Sato, K., et al.: A study of aplastic anemia in an autopsy series with special reference to atomic bomb survivors in Hiroshima and Nagasaki. Blood, *38*:17, 1971.

Knospe, W. H., Blom, J., and Crosby, W. H.: Regeneration of locally irradiated bone marrow. II. Induction of regeneration in permanently aplastic medullary cavities. Blood, *31*:400, 1968.

Koeffler, H., and Goldwasser, E.: Erythropoietin radioimmunoassay in evaluating patients with polycythemia. Ann. Intern. Med., *94*:44, 1981.

Konijn, A. M., and Hershko, C.: Ferritin synthesis in inflammation. I. Pathogenesis of impaired iron release. Br. J. Haematol., *37*:7, 1977.

Krantz, S. B., and Kuo, V.: Studies on red cell aplasia. II. Report of a second patient with an antibody to erythroblast nuclei and a remission after immunosuppressive therapy. Blood, *34*:1, 1969.

Lee, G. R.: The anemia of chronic disease. Semin. Hematol., *20*:61, 1983.

Lewis, S. M., and Dacie, J. V.: The aplastic anemia: paroxysmal nocturnal hemoglobinuria syndrome. Br. J. Haematol., *13*:236, 1967.

Martland, H. S.: The occurrence of malignancy in radioactive persons. Am. J. Cancer, *15*:2435, 1931.

Miller, M. E.: Thymic dysplasia ("Swiss agammaglobulinemia"). I. Graft vs. host reaction following bone marrow transfusion. J. Pediatr., *70*:730, 1967.

Moore, L. G., and Brewer, G. J.: Beneficial effect of rightward hemoglobin-oxygen dissociation curve shift for short-term high-altitude adaptation. J. Lab. Clin. Med., *98*:145, 1981.

Muldowney, F. P., Crooks, J., and Wayne, E. J.: The total red cell mass in thyrotoxicosis and myxoedema. Clin. Sci., *18*:309, 1957.

Ratto, O., Brescoe, W. A., Morton, J. W., and Comroe, J. H., Jr.: Anoxemia secondary to polycythemia and polycythemia secondary to anoxemia. Am. J. Med., *19*:958, 1955.

Reizenstein, P.: The Hematologic Stress Syndrome. New York, Praeger, 1983.

Robin, E. D.: Of men and mitochondria. Coping with hypoxic dysoxia. Am. Rev. Respir. Dis., *122*:517, 1980.

Schafer, A. J.: Bleeding and thrombosis in myeloproliferative disorders. Blood *64*:1, 1984.

Shahidi, N. T., and Diamond, L. K.: Testosterone-induced remission in aplastic anemia of both acquired and congenital types. N. Engl. J. Med., *264*:953, 1961.

Sieff, S.: Pure red cell aplasia. Br. J. Haematol., *54*:331, 1983.

Spaet, T. H., Bauer, S., and Melamed, S.: Hemorrhagic thrombocythemia. A blood coagulation disorder. Arch. Intern. Med., *98*:377, 1956.

Storb, R., et al.: Marrow transplantation for aplastic anemia. Sem. Hematol., *21*:27, 1984.

Toyama, K., et al.: Erythropoietin levels in the course of a patient with erythropoietin-producing renal cell carcinoma and transplantation of this tumor in nude mice. Blood, *54*:245, 1979.

Vincent, P. C., and de Gruchy, G. C.: Complications and treatment of acquired aplastic anemia. Br. J. Haematol., *13*:977, 1967.

Wilson, F. D., et al.: Cytogenetic studies on bone marrow fibroblasts from a male-female hematopoietic chimera: evidence that stromal elements in human transplantation recipients are of host type. Transplantation, *25*:87, 1978.

Young, N. S., Humphries, K., and Levine, A. S.: Aplastic Anemia. Stem Cell Biology and Advances in Treatment. New York, Liss Inc., 1984.

Yunis, A. A., Smith, U. S., and Restrepo, A.: Reversible bone marrow suppression from chloramphenicol. A consequence of mitochondrial injury. Arch. Intern. Med., *125*:272, 1970.

DNA Disorders

ROLE OF VITAMIN B₁₂ AND FOLIC ACID

The identification of vitamin B_{12} and folates as important anti-anemia principles ranks among modern medicine's greatest triumphs. The exemplary clinical investigations of Minot and Murphy and of Castle in the 1920s and 1930s were the first of a steady stream of basic and applied research accomplishments, the most recent of which has been the synthesis of vitamin B_{12} in the laboratory. Castle (1980) has recounted the history of this fascinating chain of discoveries extending for more than a century after Addison's clinical description of pernicious anemia in 1849.

B_{12} and folates participate as factors in a wide variety of biochemical reactions in the body. In some respects, their biochemical reactions are interrelated. Their essential role in DNA synthesis explains why deficiencies of either or both lead to "megaloblastic anemia" (see 1982 review by Carmel) and to disturbances in cell division not only in the marrow but also in other proliferating cell populations, such as the gastrointestinal epithelium. Nervous tissue, which is not in a state of cellular proliferation, also has an important requirement for vitamin B_{12}.

Vitamin B_{12} (molecular weight 1355) is built asymmetrically around cobalt much like heme

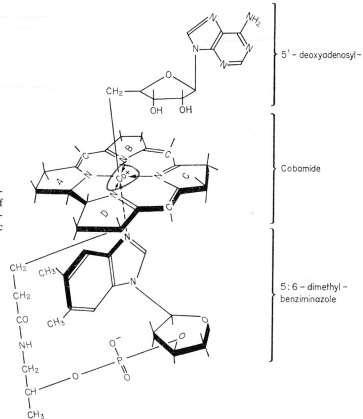

Figure 2–41 Structure of deoxyadenosyl cobalamin, a physiologically active form of vitamin B_{12}. (From Chanarin, I.: The Megaloblastic Anemias. Blackwell Scientific Publications, Oxford, 1979, p. 8.)

5' - deoxyadenosyl-

Cobamide

5:6 - dimethyl - benziminazole

is built around iron. Cobalt, like iron, has six coordinate positions, four of which are bound to nitrogen atoms in a planar tetrapyrrole corrin ring (Fig. 2–41). Below and almost perpendicular to the plane of the corrin ring, a benzimidazole nucleotide occupies the fifth coordinate position, also in a nitrogen linkage. The sixth position is ionic, and in "cyanocobalamin," the parent compound of the family of vitamin B_{12} relatives, it is occupied by cyanide. The presence of the cyanide ligand in this position, however, is an artifact of isolation. The physiologically active coenzyme forms of the vitamin contain either a methyl or a deoxyadenosyl group in this position. Cyanocobalamin, as well as its relative hydroxycobalamin, is readily converted to these active forms within the body.

The absorption of vitamin B_{12} is dependent on a unique mechanism unshared by any other essential nutrient (Seetharam and Alpers, 1982). The parietal cells of the stomach produce, along with hydrochloric acid, a glycoprotein known as *intrinsic factor (IF)*, which tightly and specifically binds B_{12}, the *extrinsic factor*, after it has been ingested and is released from complexes in foodstuffs (Fig. 2–42). IF has a molecular weight of about 44,000 and binds B_{12} on a mole-for-mole basis. The binding occurs with the benzimidazole nucleotide moiety of B_{12} and is independent of the specific chemical form of the vitamin. Dimers are formed when the vitamin is bound. It then travels down the length of the intestinal tract,

protected in the IF complex from the degradative activities of digestive enzymes. Specific receptors on the surface of the microvilli of the terminal ileum take up the IF-B_{12} complex in a process dependent upon a pH above 6.5 as well as upon divalent cations (Fig. 2–43). It is still uncertain whether the entire complex enters the cell or whether IF is released back into the lumen after the vitamin is removed.

After a dose of 1 μg. of B_{12}, about 60 to 80 percent is absorbed. However, the proportion absorbed decreases as the amount of ingested B_{12} increases. About 1 to 5 μg. is absorbed from a dietary intake of 5 to 30 μg. per day. A tiny amount of B_{12}, less than 1 percent, is absorbed in an IF-independent manner, but this is too small to be of physiologic significance. There is a substantial excretion of B_{12} from the biliary tract into the intestinal lumen, but this is efficiently reabsorbed in an IF-dependent enterohepatic circuit and thus is not lost to the body economy.

In addition to IF, other specific vitamin B_{12}–binding proteins are important to the body economy. The members of a family of "R-binders" (R for rapid electrophoretic mobility), found in plasma, saliva, milk, and other body fluids, share a common protein structure but differ in their carbohydrate content. Transcobalamin (TC) I and III are R-binders found in plasma. Most of the B_{12} present in plasma is attached to TC I and has a relatively slow rate of turnover. TC III contains only a minor fraction of the plasma vitamin B_{12} and appears to arise from granulocytes largely as a result of in vitro cell lysis. A third plasma binder, TC II, lacks carbohydrate and, like IF, differs in its protein make-up from the R-binders. TC II accounts for most of the unsaturated plasma vitamin B_{12}–binding capacity and is responsible for binding newly absorbed vitamin B_{12} and rapidly transporting it to the tissues, so its turnover rate is many times more rapid than that of TC I.

Much remains to be learned about the biologic roles of the vitamin B_{12}–binding proteins. TC I seems to be dispensable, since its congenital absence causes no clinically important abnormality. In contrast, congenital lack of TC II leads to megaloblastic anemia (Seligman et al., 1980; Hall, 1981). Striking elevations of the plasma R-binders and vitamin B_{12} levels are observed in patients with chronic myelogenous leukemia, in individuals with other myeloproliferative syndromes, and occasionally in patients with cancer.

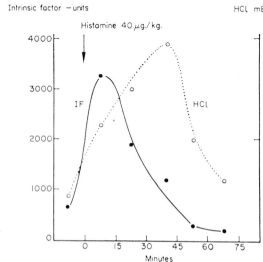

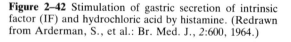

Figure 2–42 Stimulation of gastric secretion of intrinsic factor (IF) and hydrochloric acid by histamine. (Redrawn from Arderman, S., et al.: Br. Med. J., *2*:600, 1964.)

Figure 2–43 Hypothetical model of vitamin B_{12} uptake by receptors in the ileal mucosa. The intrinsic factor (IF) B_{12} complex travels down the gut lumen as a dimer. A specific receptor at the mucosal surface consists of two types of subunits. The α subunits are hydrophilic, face the lumen, and bind the IF-B_{12} complex. The β subunits are transmembrane anchors. The binding is calcium-dependent and induces a conformational change in the receptor that opens a channel for B_{12} transport into the mucosal cell. IF free of its B_{12} is released because of its lower equilibrium constant. (Adapted from Gräsbeck, R., and Kouvonen, I.: Trends Biochem. Sci., 8:203, 1983.)

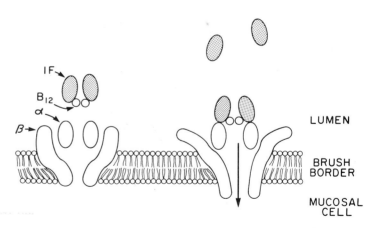

Folic acid (pteroylmonoglutamic acid) consists of pteroic acid in combination with only one molecule of L-glutamic acid (Fig. 2–44). However, the term *folates* refers to a large family of related compounds containing as many as six or seven L-glutamic acid residues locked in gamma glutamyl polypeptide linkage. Most food folate is in the polyglutamate

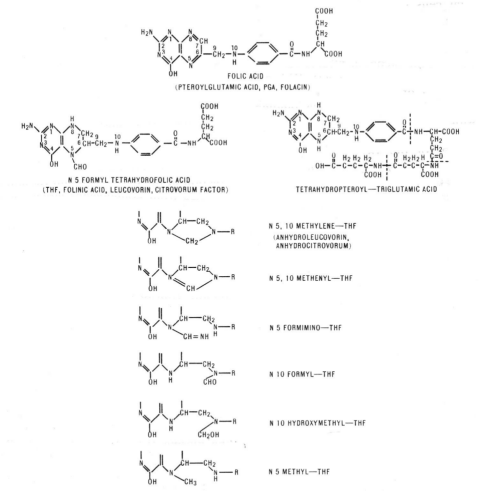

Figure 2–44 Structure of folic acid and its derivatives. Tetrahydrofolate is abbreviated here as THF and in the text as FH_4. (From Harris, J. W., and Kellermeyer, R. W.: The Red Cell. Cambridge, Harvard University Press, 1970, p. 395.)

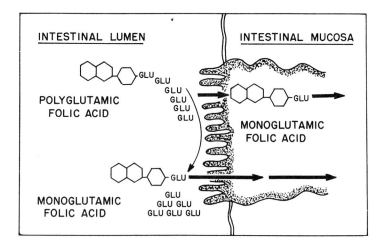

Figure 2–45 Intestinal absorption of the folate derivatives in food, present largely in polyglutamate form. The site of action of the enzyme conjugase, which degrades the polyglutamate to the monoglutamate, is not known but may actually be within the mucosal cell rather than in the intestinal lumen. Folate appears in the plasma as the reduced monoglutamate N_5 methyl tetrahydrofolate. (From Streiff, R. R.: J.A.M.A., *214*:105, 1970. Copyright 1970 by the American Medical Association.)

form and must be broken down in the intestine to the monoglutamate to permit efficient absorption. This is accomplished by the intestinal enzyme *conjugase,* more appropriately designated as gamma glutamyl carboxypeptidase (Fig. 2–45).

Following its absorption, folic acid is reduced by the enzyme *dihydrofolate reductase.* The reduction is accomplished in two steps, each involving the addition of two hydrogen atoms to yield biologically active tetrahydrofolate (FH_4). Dihydrofolate reductase is inhibited by minute concentrations of the antifolate compound *methotrexate,* an effective chemotherapeutic agent used in the treatment of neoplastic diseases (Jolivet et al., 1983).

Reduced folates, acting out their roles as agents of single carbon unit transfer, are methylated in a variety of ways. The active carbon may exist in one of several different chemical states (methyl, formyl, hydroxymethyl, methylene, methenyl, formimino), and it may be attached at several alternative sites on the parent FH_4 molecule (Fig. 2–44).

In addition to folic acid itself, the only other pharmacologically available folate is the N^5 formyl derivative known as *folinic acid* (also called *citrovorum factor,* or *leucovorin*). This agent is of use as an antidote for methotrexate toxicity, against which folic acid, the biologically inactive precursor of FH_4, is ineffective.

Plasma folate occurs almost entirely as the monoglutamate form of methyl FH_4, but following its uptake into cells the molecular size is once again increased by the enzymatic addition of multiple glutamic acid residues. This conversion (or reconversion) to the polyglutamate form markedly enhances coenzymatic activity (Hoffbrand, 1975). Thus the intra-

cellular pool of reduced and methylated polyglutamates is the principal source of folate biologic activity. Folate-binding proteins are present in extacellular fluids as well as on cell membranes and inside cells. Their physiologic roles are still not clearly understood (Wagner, 1982).

Although B_{12} and folates participate as cofactors in a number of biochemical reactions involving transfer of carbon or hydrogen atoms, their roles in DNA synthesis are of par-

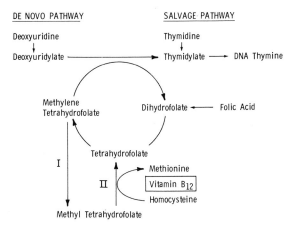

Figure 2–46 The methyl tetrahydrofolate "trap" hypothesis. Elevated plasma N_5 methyl tetrahydrofolate levels are observed in patients with vitamin B_{12} deficiency due to an inability to convert this, the major extracellular form, to tetrahydrofolate and other active coenzymic intracellular forms. Because of this lack of active intracellular folates (and specifically of $N_{5, 10}$ methylene tetrahydrofolate), there is a deficient conversion of deoxyuridylate to thymidylate and consequently also of DNA synthesis. The unutilized folate is "trapped" as N_5 methyl tetrahydrofolate. (Redrawn from Waxman, S., et al.: J. Clin. Invest., *48*:284, 1969.)

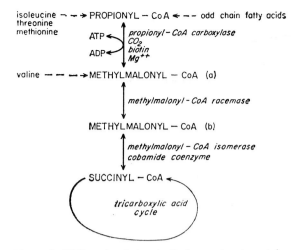

isoleucine ¬ → → PROPIONYL – CoA ← – – odd chain fatty acids
threonine
methionine

ATP ⤵
ADP ⤴ *propionyl-CoA carboxylase*
CO₂
biotin
Mg⁺⁺

valine – – – → METHYLMALONYL – CoA (a)

methylmalonyl-CoA racemase

METHYLMALONYL – CoA (b)

methylmalonyl – CoA isomerase
cobamide coenzyme

SUCCINYL – CoA ←

tricarboxylic acid cycle

Figure 2–47 The role of vitamin B_{12} in propionate metabolism. The cobamide coenzyme is deoxyadenosyl cobalamin. (From Rosenberg, L. E., et al.: Science, *162*:805, 1968. Copyright 1968 by the American Association for the Advancement of Science.)

ticular interest with respect to the pathogenesis of megaloblastic anemia. Patients with B_{12} deficiency show hematologic response to treatment with large doses of folic acid (although their neurologic symptoms may worsen). This clinical observation has for a long time aroused interest in the hypothesis that B_{12} and folates are interrelated in their roles as coenzymes in DNA synthesis. Several findings have shed some light on this interrelationship. Plasma levels of methyl FH_4 tend to be elevated in patients with B_{12} deficiency, whereas intracellular polyglutamate folates are decreased. This has suggested that B_{12} may play a role in cellular uptake of methyl FH_4 monoglutamate or in the conversion of monoglutamate to polyglutamate folate derivatives. However, the reciprocal changes in plasma and intracellular folate levels may also be explained by the methyl FH_4 "trap" hypothesis, as explained in Figure 2–46.

The biochemical action of B_{12} in the nervous tissue is still controversial, but circumstantial evidence has pointed to its role in propionate metabolism (Fig. 2–47). Deoxyadenosyl cobalamin acts as cofactor in the rearrangement of active methylmalonate, formed as a result of carboxylation of propionate, to succinate. Indeed, increased urinary excretion of methylmalonate is a reliable indicator of B_{12} deficiency. An increase in the serum concentration as well as the urinary excretion is also seen in methylmalonic acidemia, a rare inherited de-

fect of B_{12} conversion to its active deoxyadenosyl coenzyme form (Matsui et al., 1983).

Although folate lack is not notable for the presence of neurologic sequelae, except inasmuch as other vitamin deficiencies may coexist, rare congenital deficiencies of the intermediary steps of folate metabolism may cause mental retardation and other neurologic problems early in infancy. This observation has stimulated interest in the possibility that folates are of importance in the normal development of the nervous tissue (Erbe, 1975).

GENERAL EFFECTS OF MEGALOBLASTIC ANEMIA

The signs and symptoms of megaloblastic anemia are primarily related to the hemopoietic and gastrointestinal systems, although the neurologic system is also affected in B_{12} deficiency. The degree of anemia may be quite profound, but its onset is very slow and as a result it is amazingly well tolerated, unless congestive heart failure or angina pectoris supervenes. The sclerae are often slightly icteric, *jaundiced* the tongue is usually atrophic and smooth, and splenomegaly may be present. There may be vague gastrointestinal complaints. The neurologic signs of B_{12} deficiencies include a spastic and incoordinae gait, paresthesias, and sometimes mental changes. Increased reflexes, Babinski signs, and loss of position and vibration sense are indicative of posterior and lateral column demyelination (Fig. 2–48). Decreased reflexes and hypesthesia are signs of peripheral

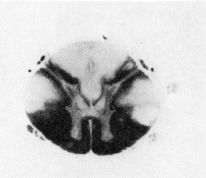

Figure 2–48 Degeneration of the posterior and lateral columns of the spinal cord in vitamin B_{12} deficiency. (From Chanarin, I.: The Megaloblastic Anemias. Oxford, Blackwell Scientific Publications, 1979, p. 371.)

neuropathy, and altered behavior and impaired mentation may indicate cerebral involvement.

The deficiency affects all the proliferating hemopoietic elements, and therefore pancytopenia is commonly observed, but granulocytopenia and thrombocytopenia are usually not so severe that infectious susceptibility or hem-

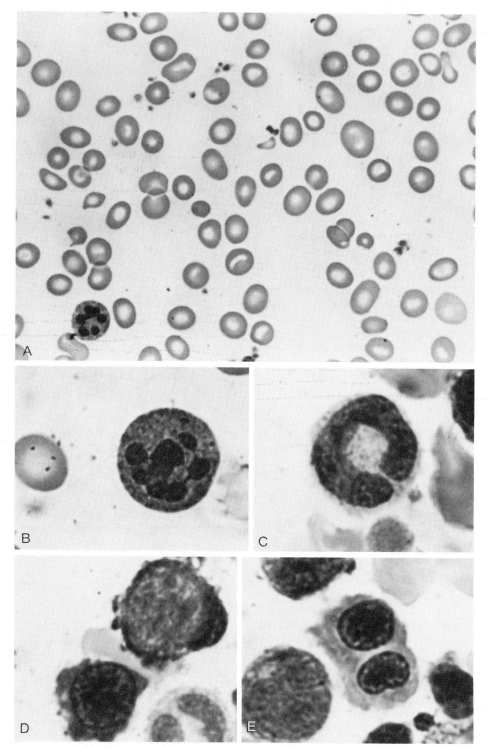

Figure 2–49 Morphologic signs of megaloblastic anemia. *A,* Blood film shows ovalmacrocytosis and anisocytosis. At greater magnification: *B,* hypersegmented blood neutrophil; *C,* large C-shaped marrow band; *D* and *E,* characteristic changes in marrow nucleated erythroid cells at various maturation stages.

orrhage results. The anemia is macrocytic, but wide variations of erythrocyte size on either side of the mean are characteristic, and indeed some erythrocytes are microcytic. The presence of "macro-ovalocytes" is a particularly valuable morphologic sign. Mature segmented neutrophils have a greater than normal mean number of lobes per nucleus; a few may contain as many as 7 or 8 (Fig. 2–49).

Not all macrocytic conditions are megaloblastic. An increase in mean corpuscular volume may be seen with reticulocytosis or if there is acquisition of excessive membrane surface area owing to plasma lipid abnormalities (Table 2–11).

When the anemia is severe, megaloblastic erythroid precursors are found in the circulation, and a small proportion of mature erythrocytes contains nuclear remnants (Howell-Jolly bodies, Cabot's rings). The reticulocytes are not increased, and polychromasia is not prominent. Distinctive morphologic changes are also seen in the gastrointestinal epithelial cells, but the diagnosis rests on the finding of "megaloblastic" changes in the marrow. This term was originally applied to erythroid precursors only, but today it is used to refer to changes in all three cell lines—granulocytic and megakaryocytic as well as erythroid. The entire erythroid line of maturation is altered to form a "megaloblastic series." There is the appearance of a "maturation arrest" because

Table 2–11 SOME CAUSES OF MACROCYTIC ERYTHROCYTES

Impairment of DNA synthesis
 Vitamin B_{12} deficiency
 Folate deficiency
 Chemotherapy
  Antimetabolites (e.g., 6-mercaptopurine, methotrexate)
  Alkylating agents (e.g., cyclophosphamide)
 Primary refractory anemias
  Aplastic anemia
  Sideroblastic anemia
  Erythroleukemia and other myelogenous leukemia variants
  Refractory megaloblastic anemias (acquired)
 Rare hereditary blocks in DNA synthesis (e.g., orotic aciduria)
Reticulocytosis
 Hemolytic anemia
 Response to acute blood loss
Surface membrane excess
 Liver disease
 Chronic alcoholism
 Obstructive jaundice
 Postsplenectomy
 Hereditary lecithin: cholesterol acyl transferase (LCAT) deficiency

of the marked shift to the left, with large numbers of early erythroid precursors having intensely basophilic cytoplasm. The arrest in nuclear development is reflected in an abnormally finely divided and open pattern of the nuclear chromatin. Hemoglobin formation proceeds in the cytoplasm, however, and "nuclear-cytoplasmic dissociation" is observed. The entire series of cells is larger than normal, and mature cells emerge as macrocytic erythrocytes. The marrow granulocytic precursors also show distinctive changes, in particular large horseshoe- and C-shaped nuclear forms at the band stage of maturation. The marrow shows a marked overall increase in cellularity (Fig. 2–49).

The deficient marrow, driven by the stimulus of "poietins," reacts with a hypercellular proliferative response. However, the defect in nuclear development leads to intramedullary destruction of the blood cell precursors. Heme catabolism from the breakdown of erythroid precursors in the marrow is the major factor contributing to the signs of hemolysis—the elevated serum indirect bilirubin, the absence of plasma haptoglobin, and the elevation of serum lactic dehydrogenase to levels rarely seen even in the hemolytic anemias. Megaloblastic anemia is a classic example of the pathophysiology of ineffective erythropoiesis. The number of reticulocytes in the peripheral blood is not elevated despite intense erythroid hyperplasia in the marrow. The serum iron concentration is raised, and its rate of clearance from the circulation to the erythroid marrow is increased, with only small amounts appearing over subsequent days in the newly formed erythrocytes (Fig. 2–26). The amount of radioactive label appearing in the "early bilirubin" peak after administration of a tagged heme precursor is markedly increased (see Fig. 2–85).

Serum concentrations of vitamin B_{12} are less than 120 pg. per ml. in deficient states. The absorptive defect is characterized by the Schilling test, in which urinary excretion of radioactive B_{12} is measured following oral ingestion of a small labeled test dose, given without (Stage I) or with (Stage II) intrinsic factor. Two hours after the test dose, a large nonradioactive "flushing" dose is injected parenterally. Urinary excretion less than 7 percent of the administered test dose is found when there is an absorptive defect. A twofold enhancement by intrinsic factor indicates that the defect is intrinsic factor–dependent. The accuracy of the test depends on adequate renal function.

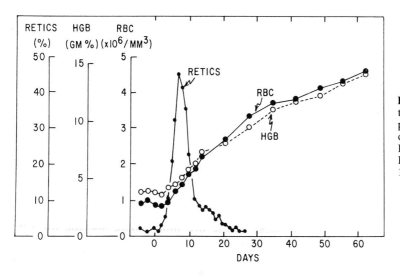

Figure 2–50 Hematologic response to treatment of vitamin B_{12} deficiency in a patient with pernicious anemia. (Redrawn from Castle, W. B. *In* Cecil and Loeb [Eds.]: A Textbook of Medicine. Philadelphia, W. B. Saunders Co., 1959, p. 1131.)

In folate deficiency, the serum concentration of the vitamin is below 2.0 ng. per ml. Red cell folate concentration more accurately reflects tissue stores and is less than 135 ng. per ml. packed cells in deficient states.

With treatment, the signs promptly revert to normal within several days. The serum iron concentration decreases and its utilization for the production of circulating erythrocytes becomes effective, the jaundice disappears, the elevated serum lactic dehydrogenase falls, and megaloblastic cells are no longer seen in the marrow. The reticulocyte count becomes elevated within 3 to 4 days, reaches a peak at 7 to 10 days, and then falls (Fig. 2–50). The reticulocyte response is the most reliable early sign of response, and in the more anemic individuals it may peak at 25 to 50 percent. The neurologic symptoms of B_{12} lack are reversed, unless they have progressed to an advanced degree of severity. Pharmacologic doses of folic acid will produce a hematologic response in the B_{12}-deficient patient while worsening the neurologic complications. Presumably, the folate causes a fall in serum B_{12} level, with a diversion of available B_{12} away from neural to hemopoietic tissue. Large doses of B_{12} will also give a hematologic response in the folate-deficient patient. Response to therapy is specific if the administered dose is limited to the range of the minimal daily requirement, about 1 μg. per day of B_{12} or 50 μg. per day of folate.

VITAMIN B_{12} DEFICIENCY

Dietary Lack. Inadequate intake is an exceptionally rare cause of B_{12} deficiency, since this vitamin is present in a wide variety of products of animal origin—meat, fish, eggs, butter, milk, and cheese—and the minimal daily requirement of 1 to 5 μg. is readily met unless a strict vegetarian diet is followed. Even then, the total body stores of 2000 to 5000 μg. are well conserved, with a loss of only 0.1 percent per day of the total body pool, and the earliest signs of B_{12} deficiency are not seen until after 10 to 20 years on such a diet.

Intrinsic Factor Lack. The term *pernicious anemia (PA)* no longer seems appropriate, considering the fact that the condition can now be effectively cured. However, its historical roots are deep and it is probably acceptable to continue to use this term but only for megaloblastic anemia caused by a lack of intrinsic factor.

Congenital PA is a rare autosomal recessive condition that is apparently clinically manifest only in the homozygous state. There is an isolated lack of IF without insufficiency of gastric acid or pepsin. Passively acquired B_{12} stores present at birth are exhausted in 2 or 3 years, and anemia then develops.

Adult PA is a disorder of mature and older adults. Genetic factors still not well defined play some role, since there is a significant intrafamilial occurrence as well as an ethnic predilection for individuals of northern and western European background. The absence of IF in the gastric juice is always found in association with atrophic gastritis, and there is accordingly a lack of gastric acidity and pepsin, even after stimulation with histamine. Atrophic gastritis is not uncommon in the general population, and its incidence increases with age. Why certain affected persons develop pernicious anemia is still uncertain, but the

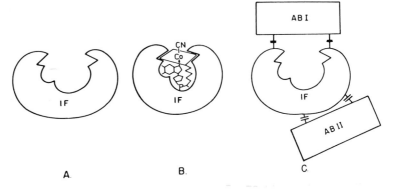

Figure 2–51 Anti-intrinsic factor antibodies of the blocking (AB I) and binding (AB II) types. (From Gräsbeck, R.: Progr. Hematol., *6*:233, 1969. By permission of Grune & Stratton, Inc., New York.)

following evidence supports an autoimmune theory of pathogenesis:

1. The histologic appearance of lymphocytic infiltration of the gastric mucosa suggests a local immunologic process.

2. Antibodies that react against the cytoplasm of the gastric parietal cell are present in the serum of 90 percent of patients with adult PA (DeAizpurua et al., 1983). A significant incidence of such antibodies is present, however, in patients who do not have PA. These include 60 percent of all individuals with atrophic gastritis, 30 percent of blood relatives of PA patients, and slightly less than 10 percent of a control population. PA patients frequently have serum antibodies directed against parenchymal endocrine glands, most notably the acinar cells of the thyroid. Conversely, patients with primary myxedema and Hashimoto's thyroiditis have a 30 percent incidence of antiparietal cell serum antibodies and a 12 percent incidence of coexisting PA.

3. About 75 percent of PA patients have anti-IF antibodies in serum, saliva, and gastric juice. These are much more specific for PA and are rarely found in its absence. These antibodies are polyclonal and may be either IgG or IgA. They apparently react at two different sites on the IF molecule (Fig. 2–51). "Blocking" antibodies prevent the binding of B_{12} to IF, presumably by obstructing the site of attachment. "Binding" antibodies do not interfere with the attachment of B_{12} to IF, but they do impede absorption in the ileum.

Whether these various autoimmune phenomena associated with PA are cause or effect remains uncertain, but the properties of the anti-IF antibodies present in gastric secretions clearly suggest a role in its pathogenesis.

Pernicious anemia patients who stop their treatment do not relapse for an average of over 5 years, a sign of how avidly the body's stores of B_{12} are guarded (Savage and Lindenbaum, 1983). Similarly, total gastrectomy will predictably produce megaloblastic anemia after 5 or 6 years, but partial gastrectomy in most instances does not deplete IF sufficiently to lead to frank megaloblastosis. With the

Figure 2–52 Serum vitamin B_{12} levels at various intervals after subtotal gastrectomy. Patients with B_{12} deficiency megaloblastic anemia have values in the range of 0 to 100 pg. per ml. (Redrawn from Hines, J. D., et al.: Am. J. Med., *43*:555, 1967.)

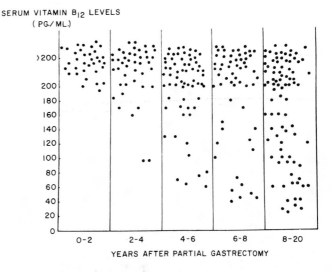

passage of years, however, an increasing proportion of partial gastrectomy patients develop low serum B_{12} levels, some of whom have mild megaloblastic changes in the marrow (Fig. 2–52). Iron deficiency is the commonest cause of postgastrectomy anemia, and its presence may mask concomitant megaloblastosis, the signs of which are brought out following iron repletion. Coexistence of thalassemia trait may exert a similar confounding effect on the expression of megaloblastic erythropoiesis on the red cell indices.

Decreased Ileal Absorption. Ablation of the specific site of B_{12} absorption in the terminal ileum by surgical resection or by such diseases as regional ileitis, lymphoma, and tuberculosis leads to B_{12} deficiency without an associated lack of IF or of gastric acid. Certain drugs (neomycin, colchicine, para-amino salicylate) reportedly interfere with B_{12} absorption by mechanisms that remain obscure. The gastrointestinal epithelial changes of tropical sprue are extensive and commonly cause B_{12} deficiency, especially in chronic cases. The megaloblastic alterations of B_{12} or folate deficiency themselves cause sufficient epithelial change to interfere with ileal absorption. Indeed, patients with folate deficiency tend to have lower than normal serum concentrations of B_{12}, with spontaneous correction after folate repletion (Fig. 2–53). Poor absorption may also occur consequent to pancreatic insufficiency, primarily because pancreatic enzymes are required to cleave R-binder B_{12} complexes and make the vitamin available for attachment to IF. *Imerslund's syndrome* is a rare congenital deficiency of the receptor site in the terminal ileum causing megaloblastic anemia in children. IF secretion is normal. Renal structural abnormalities and proteinuria are also commonly present.

Decreased Availability. Decreased serum B_{12} levels and megaloblastic anemia are found in association with anatomic abnormalities of the gastrointestinal tract that lead to stasis and pooling of the luminal contents. Such "blind loop syndromes"—strictures, surgically created bypasses, fistulas, and large diverticula—have in common the presence of bacterial overgrowth along with steatorrhea. The anemia does not respond to orally administered B_{12}, but parenteral replacement is effective. Intrinsic factor is present in normal amounts, indicating that the IF-B_{12} complex is unavailable for absorption in the terminal ileum. The finding that therapy with broad-spectrum antibiotics causes disappearance of the stigmata of B_{12} lack provides strong evidence that bacterial utilization is responsible for the deficiency. A similar mechanism explains the megaloblastic anemia associated with the fish tapeworm *(Diphyllobothrium latum)*. Infestation occurs as a result of ingestion of improperly cooked fresh-water fish. The worms grow to great lengths in the intestinal tract and effectively compete with the host for available IF-B_{12} complex. The disorder is especially common in Finland.

FOLATE DEFICIENCY

Dietary Lack. Poor nutrition—an unusual cause of B_{12} deficiency—frequently gives rise to folate depletion. The elderly recluse, the "tea and toast" faddist, and the alcoholic are prototypes of deficiency in the United States. In other countries, excessive cooking of food, often limited in amount and diversity, destroys labile folates and causes leeching out of the soluble folates in the cooking water. Newborns procure sufficient amounts even from deficient mothers but develop megaloblastic anemia when they reach the 2-year stage of rapid growth if they are raised on low-folate diets, such as goat's milk or boiled milk. Folates are present in many different foodstuffs—leafy green vegetables, fruits, meats, eggs—and food intake must be severely limited in diversity in order to fall short of the minimal daily requirement of 50 μg. Lack of ascorbate, thiamine, and other essential nutrients often coexists. In alcoholics, poor diet is not the only factor, since ethanol seems to interfere with

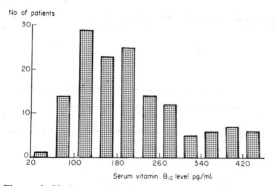

Figure 2–53 Serum vitamin B_{12} levels in patients with megaloblastic anemia due to folate deficiency. The normal range of values is 200 to 800 pg. per ml. (Redrawn from Mollin, D. L., Waters, A. H., and Harriss, E. *In* Heinrich, H. C. [Ed.]: 2 Europaisches Symposium. Hamburg, 1961, Stuttgart, Enke. Reprinted in Chanarin, I.: The Megaloblastic Anemias. Philadelphia, F. A. Davis Co., 1969.)

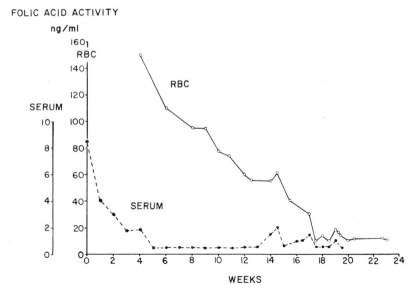

FOLIC ACID ACTIVITY

Figure 2–54 The fall in serum folate and red cell folate in a subject placed on a folate-deficient diet. (Redrawn from Herbert, V.: Trans. Am. Assoc. Phys., 75:307, 1962.)

folate absorption, its intermediary metabolism, and its hepatic storage (Hillman and Steinberg, 1982; Lindenbaum, 1980). It also exerts a direct toxic suppression on the bone marrow elements (Larkin and Watson-Williams, 1984).

The sequence of events after limitation of folate intake has been studied experimentally by Herbert (1962) (Fig. 2–54). The serum folate concentration is the most sensitive indicator of deficiency, falling within a month of deficient intake. Red cell folate concentration is more stubbornly defended, but it also falls as megaloblastic anemia appears after 3 to 4 months of deficiency. Folate stores are neither as ample (relative to daily requirement) nor as avidly guarded as B_{12} stores.

The minimal daily requirement of folate increases during pregnancy to about 400 μg. Serum folate levels tend to fall as pregnancy proceeds to term. A diet that maintains body folate in a marginal state of balance will prove inadequate in the face of such an increase in demands, and thus folate deficiency is the commonest cause of megaloblastic anemia in pregnancy. Conditions of increased cellular proliferation, such as hemolytic anemia and exfoliative skin disease, as well as thyrotoxicosis also raise the minimal requirement for folate.

Malabsorption. "Blind loop syndromes," which bring on B_{12} deficiency because of bacterial utilization, are not associated with folate lack. Possibly, bacterial synthesis in the stagnant loop may actually add to the body's supply. However, gastrointestinal disorders affecting extensive areas of absorptive surface, with attendant malabsorption, frequently lead to folate deficiency (Halsted, 1980). Gluten-sensitive enteropathy (non-tropical sprue) most severely affects the upper reaches of the bowel—the duodenum and jejunum—where folate absorption normally is maximal, sparing the terminal ileum along with B_{12} absorption in many instances. In tropical sprue, the involvement extends throughout the gut, affecting B_{12} as well as folate absorption. Folic acid therapy often improves the malabsorption along with the megaloblastic anemia in tropical sprue, but in nontropical sprue improvement in gastrointestinal function is achieved by elimination of gluten from the diet. Oral therapy with folic acid—the monoglutamate form—is effective, suggesting that the polyglutamates of food are not absorbed as well.

Other gastrointestinal disorders associated with malabsorption are lymphoma, scleroderma, amyloidosis, and Whipple's disease. Malabsorption may also follow extensive surgical resection. In addition to deficiencies of folate or B_{12} or both, iron lack is commonly present in malabsorption syndromes, giving the picture of a combined deficiency anemia.

Drugs. Patients on phenytoin therapy have a significant incidence of low serum folate levels and of megaloblastic anemia that responds readily to oral folic acid therapy. The notion that this agent interferes with the absorption of food folates by inhibiting intestinal conjugase activity has not yet withstood the test of scientific confirmation. Some evidence suggests that it may interfere with folate intermediary metabolism. The mechanism of megaloblastic anemia produced by the antimalarial pyrimethamine is more closely akin to that of methotrexate as a competitive inhibitor of folate metabolism. Trimethoprim is an antifolate antibiotic that can be safely used in humans because of its selectivity for bacterial dihydrofolate reductase.

MISCELLANEOUS MEGALOBLASTIC ANEMIAS

Therapy of neoplastic disease often leads to megaloblastic bone marrow and macrocytic red cells. Some of the cytotoxic agents in use that predictably inhibit nucleotide synthesis with secondary megaloblastic change are the antifolates (methotrexate), purine inhibitors (6-mercaptopurine, thioguanine, azathioprine), pyrimidine inhibitors (5-fluorouracil), and other inhibitors of DNA synthesis (cytosine arabinoside, hydroxyurea). *Primary refractory megaloblastic anemia* may represent a nuclear maturation defect of a myelodysplastic syndrome. When such a defect affects both the erythroid and granulocytic precursors with an increase in marrow myeloblasts, it is known as *erythroleukemia (Di Guglielmo's syndrome,* or, more commonly today, *refractory anemia with excess blasts)*. Ringed sideroblasts are frequently seen. Conversion to acute myelogenous leukemia is not uncommon. In some proliferative disorders of the bone marrow, local shortages are brought on by the increased requirements of the abnormal proliferation, causing morphologic signs of deficiency in neighboring cells. *Hereditary orotic aciduria* is a rare megaloblastic anemia of childhood caused by an inherited block in pyrimidine synthesis.

References

Carmel, R.: Megaloblastic anemia: vitamin B_{12} and folate. Curr. Hematol., 2:243, 1982.

Castle, W. B.: The conquest of pernicious anemia. *In* Wintrobe, M. M. (Ed.): Blood, Pure and Eloquent. New York, McGraw-Hill Book Co., 1980, p. 283.

DeAizpurua, H. J., Cosgrove, L. J., Ungar, B., and Toh, B. H.: Autoantibodies cytoxic to gastric parietal cells in serum of patients with pernicious anemia. N. Engl. J. Med., 309:625, 1983.

Erbe, R. W.: Inborn errors of folate metabolism. N. Engl. J. Med., 293:753, 1975.

Hall, C. A.: Congenital disorders of vitamin B_{12} transport and their contributions to concepts. Yale J. Biol. Med., 54:485, 1981.

Halsted, C. H.: Intestinal absorption and malabsorption of folates. Ann. Rev. Med., 31:79, 1980.

Herbert, V.: Experimental nutritional folate deficiency in man. Trans. Am. Assoc. Physicians, 75:307, 1962.

Hillman, R. S., and Steinberg, S. E.: The effects of alcohol on folate metabolism. Ann. Rev. Med., 33:345, 1982.

Hoffbrand, A. V.: Synthesis and breakdown of natural folates (folate polyglutamates). Progr. Hematol., 9:85, 1975.

Jolivet, J., Cowan, K. H., Curt, G. A., et al.: The pharmacology and clinical use of methotrexate. New Engl. J. Med., 309:1094, 1983.

Larkin, E. C., and Watson-Williams, E. J.: Alcohol and the blood. Med. Clin. N.A., 68:105, 1984.

Lindenbaum, J.: Folate and vitamin B_{12} deficiencies in alcoholism. Semin. Hematol., 17:119, 1980.

Matsui, S. M., Mahoney, M. J., and Rosenberg, L. E.: The natural history of the inherited methylmalonic acidemias. N. Engl. J. Med., 308:857, 1983.

Savage, D., and Lindenbaum, J.: Relapses after interruption of cyanocobalamin therapy in patients with pernicious anemia. Am. J. Med., 74:765, 1983.

Seetharam, B., and Alpers, D. H.: Absorption and transport of cobalamin (vitamin B_{12}). Ann. Rev. Nutr., 2:343, 1982.

Seligman, P. A., Steiner, L. L., and Allen, R. H.: Studies of a patient with megaloblastic anemia and an abnormal transcobalamin II. N. Engl. J. Med., 303:1209, 1980.

Wagner, C.: Cellular folate binding proteins: function and significance. Ann. Rev. Nutr., 2:229, 1982.

Heme and Globin Disorders

HEMOGLOBIN SYNTHESIS

The circulating erythrocyte is the most specialized of the body's cells—95 percent of its cytoplasm consists of the respiratory pigment hemoglobin packed into the cell interior at a concentration almost five times that of the proteins of the exterior plasma. The formation of hemoglobin begins at the earliest precursor stage of the developing erythroid cell and is completed when the anucleate reticulocyte matures to an erythrocyte. No additional hemoglobin is produced during the 120-day period of the erythrocyte's life span in the circulation. The biosynthesis of hemoglobin is a complex series of distinct but delicately coordinated biochemical events, so well balanced that component parts are brought together in an assembly-line fashion, without significant shortages or surpluses, to form the completed molecule. Heme is formed in a sequential series of enzymatically controlled reactions. Dissimilar polypeptide globin subunits under separate genetic control are assembled on polyribosomes. The finished molecule has two pairs of such subunits, each linked with its own prosthetic heme group into a tetrameric macromolecule.

General Effects of Disorders of Hemoglobin Synthesis

Deficiency in the quantity of hemoglobin leads to microcytic, hypochromic anemia. The hemoglobin lack comes either from a lack of heme, as an iron deficiency, or from insufficient globin, to which the designation *thalassemia* is given. Qualitative abnormalities of the hemoglobin may alter the internal consistency of the erythrocyte cytoplasm and cause increased cell rigidity, which leads to premature destruction and hemolysis. Abnormal hemoglobin oxygen affinity or oxidation state gives rise to cyanosis or erythrocytosis. Many abnormal hemoglobins produce no pathophysiologic abnormality because they function quite normally.

PORPHYRIN

Of all the tissues in the body, the erythroid marrow and the liver are the pre-eminent porphyrin producers. The synthesis begins on the mitochondria and requires energy. The intermediate steps take place in the cytosol, and the process is completed once again on the mitochondria with the insertion of iron into the completed porphyrin molecule to form heme. The brightly colored finished product contains four pyrrole rings connected into a larger cyclic tetrapyrrole structure by methene bridges. Side chains are attached to the ring structure: 4 methyl, 2 vinyl, and 2 propionyl. The structure of heme is shown in Figure 2–55.

The biochemical steps in heme synthesis are outlined in Figure 2–56. Active succinate is

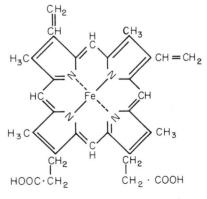

HEME (FERROPROTOPORHYRIN 9)

Figure 2–55 The structure of heme. (From Harris, J. W., and Kellermeyer, R. W.: The Red Cell. Cambridge, Harvard University Press, 1970, p. 3.)

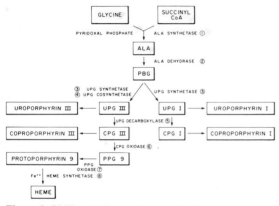

Figure 2–56 The synthesis of heme. Eight enzymatic steps are indicated. The initial step (1) is energy-requiring, takes place on mitochondria, and uses pyridoxal phosphate as a cofactor. The final steps (6, 7, and 8) are also mitochondrial. The intermediate enzymes (2 through 5) are in the cytosol. CPG oxidase (6) performs an oxidative decarboxylation.

Enzymatic deficiencies in hereditary porphyria are as follows: acute intermittent porphyria (3); erythropoietic porphyria (4); porphyria cutanea tarda (5); hereditary coproporphyria (6); hereditary protoporphyria (8); variegate porphyria (7 or 8). In lead poisoning, decreased activity of (2) and (8) are most pronounced, although (1) and (6) are also inhibited. As another example of "toxic" porphyria, the chemical compound hexachlorobenzene inhibits (5) and produces a clinical picture resembling porphyria cutanea tarda. The enzymatic lack in the various porphyria states is associated with induction of increased ALA synthetase activity due to the lack of feedback control and consequent overproduction of porphyrin precursors synthesized proximal to the site of the enzymatic block.

Abbreviations are as follows: ALA = δ amino levulinic acid; PBG = porphobilinogen; UPG = uroporphyrinogen; CPG = coproporphyrinogen; PPG = protoporphyrinogen.

joined to glycine to form delta-aminolevulinic acid (ALA). This enzymatic step, controlled by ALA synthetase, is both rate-limiting and regulatory. It is subject to negative feedback inhibition, and, as will be subsequently explained, in a variety of deficiencies of enzymes in the porphyrin synthetic pathway, the lack of end product causes deficient inhibition along with marked overproduction of precursors synthesized at sites above the block. Pyridoxal phosphate, the active form of the vitamin pyridoxine, is also required for this initial synthetic step.

Monopyrrole porphobilinogen rings are then formed by head-to-tail linkages of two ALA molecules. Four porphobilinogens in turn condense into the cyclic tetrapyrrole structure, which then undergoes progressive decarboxylation from uroporphyrinogen (containing eight carboxyl side chains) to coproporphyrinogen (containing four carboxyl side chains) to protoporphyrinogen (containing two carboxyl side chains). Progressive decarboxylation is associated with an increased degree of insolubility that determines fecal as opposed to urinary excretion, with the less soluble being predominantly fecal and the more soluble urinary (Table 2–12). Oxidation converts these colorless heme precursors into the brightly colored uroporphyrins, coproporphyrins, and protoporphyrins.

The porphyrins may exist in a variety of isomeric states, depending on the position of the side chains, but only a limited number of isomers are of biologic significance. The uro- and copro- derivatives are found biologically only as the I and III isomers. In the formation of uroporphyrinogen from porphobilinogen, a cosynthetase operating in conjunction with a synthetase directs the bulk of synthesis to the III isomer, which serves exclusively as heme precursor. In the absence of cosynthetase, uroporphyrinogen I is preferentially formed, and this does not fulfill the requirements of heme synthesis. Following consecutive conversions from uroporphyrinogen III to coproporphyrinogen III to protoporphyrinogen 9 to protoporphyrin 9, four of the six coordinate positions of ferrous iron are chelated to the completed tetrapyrrole to form heme, ready for combination with globin or other apoproteins.

Table 2–12 PORPHYRIN AND PORPHYRIN PRECURSORS IN HUMANS*

	Urine μg./24 hrs.	Stool μg./gm. dry wt.	Erythrocytes μg./100 ml. cells
ALA	4000	—	—
PBG	1500	—	—
Uroporphyrin	50	5	Trace
Coproporphyrin	300	50	3
Protoporphyrin	—	120	80

*Values are upper limits of normal. Abbreviations as in Figure 2–56. (Data from Meyer, U. A., and Schmid, R. The porphyrias. *In* Stanbury, J. B., Wyngaarden, J. B., and Frederickson, D. S. [Eds.]: The Metabolic Basis of Inherited Disease. 4th ed. New York, McGraw-Hill Book Co., 1978, p. 1176.)

General Effects of Disorders of Porphyrin Synthesis

The porphyrias are caused by inherited or acquired blocks in the enzymatic steps governing heme synthesis, but the most pronounced consequence of the block is overproduction of the heme precursors above the site of the block (Goldberg and Moore, 1980). The liver is most commonly the major site of the defect with sparing of the erythroid cells ("hepatic porphyrias"), although in some conditions the erythroid tissue is affected. It is surprising that in those states affecting the erythroid cells heme synthesis is sufficient to meet almost completely the needs of hemoglobin synthesis, and hypochromia of the erythrocytes is either absent or minimal. Specific diagnosis is usually accomplished by quantification and characterization of the various heme precursors in the urine, feces, erythrocytes, and liver. Direct enzyme analysis of a variety of tissues, including red cells, hepatocytes, and cultured fibroblasts, may reveal latent as well as symptomatic cases. The characteristics of the porphyrias are summarized in Table 2–13.

Pink or red urine may be observed if there is sufficient concentration of a colored derivative—uroporphyrin or coproporphyrin or both. The freshly passed urine is colorless, however, if the increase affects primarily colorless reduced precursors. In the case of protoporphyr-

ia the urine is normal; excretion is via the fecal route because of the insolubility of this derivative. One detects deposition of the colored derivatives in tissue slices by observing the emission of red fluorescence upon exposure to ultraviolet light. Indeed, cutaneous absorption of light in the 400 nm. wavelength range produces photosensitive skin reactions with symptoms that range from mild itching and burning to erythema, edema, blistering, and eventually even scarring and disfigurement involving exposed areas, such as the face and the backs of the hands. Damage to other tissues may also occur, as will be subsequently discussed.

Inherited Disorders of Porphyrin Synthesis

Acute Intermittent Porphyria. This is an autosomal dominant hepatic disorder of the synthesis of uroporphyrinogen synthetase. The resulting block leads to overproduction of proximal, potentially neurotoxic monopyrroles and underproduction of distal light-sensitive porphyrins. The overproduction of ALA and porphobilinogen in the liver is associated with acute attacks of abdominal pain, polyneuropathy, and neuropsychiatric disturbances, sometimes with a fatal outcome, but with relative freedom from symptoms between episodes. In some instances the attacks are pro-

Table 2–13 CLASSIFICATION OF PORPHYRIAS*

Condition	Photosensitivity	Tissue Primarily Involved Erythroid	Hepatic	Biochemical Abnormalities Useful in Diagnosis
Hereditary				
Acute intermittent porphyria	−	−	+	Increased urinary ALA and PBG.
Erythropoietic porphyria	+	+	−	Increased urinary and erythrocyte uroporphyrin I and coproporphyrin I.
Porphyria cutanea tarda	+	−	+	Increased urinary uroporphyrin I>III and coproporphyrin I and III. (Porphyrins also increased in liver, along with excess iron.)
Coproporphyria	+	−	+	Increased fecal and urinary coproporphyrin III. Increased urinary ALA and PBG during acute attacks.
Variegate porphyria	+	−	+	Increased fecal protoporphyrin 9 and coproporphyrin III. Increased urinary coproporphyrin III and, during acute attacks, ALA and PBG.
Protoporphyria	+	+	+	Increased erythrocyte and fecal protoporphyrin 9.
Acquired				
Lead poisoning	−	+	?	Increased urinary ALA and coproporphyrin III. Increased erythrocyte protoporphyrin 9.
Hexachlorobenzene toxicity	+	−	+	Increased urinary uroporphyrin I and III and coproporphyrin I and III.

*Abbreviations as in Figure 2–56. Enzyme defects are listed in the legend to Figure 2–56. All inherited conditions are autosomal dominant, except erythropoietic porphyria, which is autosomal recessive.

voked by any of a variety of medications, such as barbiturates, estrogens, or sulfa drugs, which further increase ALA synthetase activity. Fasting also provokes attacks, whereas a high-carbohydrate diet appears to be of value in their prevention. There have been reports that intravenously administered heme derivatives successfully terminate attacks by means of end product inhibition of ALA synthetase activity. It has still not been conclusively established that the neuropathic symptoms are caused by the increased monopyrroles, but they remain the prime suspects. Freshly passed urine is colorless but may darken after several hours' standing owing to spontaneous oxidation of porphobilinogen to porphobilin. In addition to the classic acute intermittent porphyria, there are two variants, also autosomal dominant with late onset, *variegate porphyria* and *hereditary coproporphyria*. These variants are distinguished by light-sensitive skin, with more marked lesions in the variegate variety, and by the increased excretion of porphyrin precursors further along the pathway of synthesis in addition to ALA and urobilinogen (Table 2–13). The acute attacks resemble those of acute intermittent porphyria.

Congenital Erythropoietic Porphyria. This disorder is a rare but dramatic autosomal recessive condition in which a block in the production of normal III isomer porphyrins leads to an increase in light-sensitive uroporphyrin and coproporphyrin I isomers. It affects primarily the erythroid cells, but red staining of all the tissues and of the urine is prominent. The onset is usually in childhood. Photosensitivity is especially severe, and there are signs of hemolysis along with splenomegaly.

Porphyria Cutanea Tarda. This condition, also a hepatic porphyria, presumably originates from a combination of inherited enzyme deficiency in addition to other factors essential to the expression of the clinical signs and symptoms, which typically do not begin until middle age. Among the acquired factors, alcoholism and liver disease and exposure to certain medications, especially estrogen, are commonly observed, but increased liver iron is always present, often along with elevation of the plasma iron concentration and increased saturation of the plasma iron binding protein. The excess liver iron is of pathogenetic importance, since its removal by a series of phlebotomies ameliorates both the clinical and biochemical manifestations of the disorder (Fig. 2–57). Although the primary deficiency involves uroporphyrinogen decarboxylase, co-

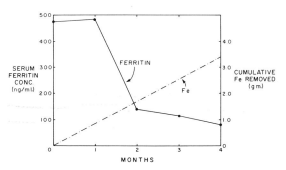

Figure 2–57 Decrease in serum ferritin concentration as iron stores were reduced by weekly phlebotomy in a patient with porphyria cutanea tarda. Initial liver biopsy documented markedly increased hepatocellular iron. The reduction in iron stores resulted in a marked decrease in the urinary porphyrin excretion (normal serum ferritin concentration 12 to 200 ng./ml.).

synthetase also appears to be in some manner affected, since urinary uroporphyrin I excretion exceeds that of uroporphyrin III. Urine urobilinogen excretion may be normal or, if elevated, commensurate with the degree of liver dysfunction. In addition to the symptoms of liver disease, photosensitivity and red urine are usually present.

Hereditary Protoporphyria. This disorder is associated with high tissue concentrations of protoporphyrin 9 in both erythrocytes and liver due to a decrease in heme synthetase. Symptoms may be entirely absent, but mild photosensitivity is often present from childhood. Cholelithiasis commonly occurs as a result of the high concentration of this relatively insoluble porphyrin in the bile. In some cases of long duration, chronic liver disease has developed. The excess porphyrin is excreted exclusively via the fecal route; the urine is normal. Mild anemia may be present, but there are no clinical signs of hemolysis, despite the fact that photohemolysis is demonstrable in vitro.

Acquired Disorders of Porphyrin Synthesis

Lead Intoxication. In lead intoxication several of the enzymes controlling heme synthesis are inhibited (see Fig. 2–56). Depression of ALA dehydrase activity is one of the earliest changes. Heme synthetase is also readily depressed. Increases in urinary ALA and in erythrocyte protoporphyrin levels are accordingly observed early in the course of the disease. Urinary coproporphyrin III is also frequently increased, whereas urinary porphobilinogen is normal or only slightly increased. Photosensitivity is not a feature of lead toxicity because the increased intraerythrocytic protoporphyrin occurs as a zinc complex tightly bound to hemoglobin, in contrast to hereditary protoporphyria, in which the protoporphyrin is loosely bound and passes out of the erythrocytes into the skin and other tissues, causing light sensitivity. Increased amounts of ferritin and hemosiderin accumulate in the erythroid precursors because of the blocks in heme synthesis. The erythrocytes are slightly hypochromic, and a significant proportion of them show punctate basophilic stippling due to the presence of aggregated incompletely degraded ribosomes. The defect in ribosomal ribonucleic acid degradation is apparently due to reduced levels of pyrimidine-5'-nucleotidase. Hereditary lack of this enzyme is also associated with basophilic stippling. The anemia of lead toxicity is mild, and the erythrocyte life span only slightly or moderately shortened. The neurologic symptoms are the most significant aspects of the disease—encephalopathy in the child and peripheral motor neuropathy in the adult. Abdominal pain as well as renal disease may also occur. The people of the world's industrialized regions have higher blood levels than those living in the more remote areas. This has increased fears about the possible public health hazards of lead (Chisholm, 1973; Mahaffey et al., 1982).

Hexachlorobenzene Intoxication. Toxic exposure to hexachlorobenzene mimics porphyria cutanea tarda. Affected individuals are photosensitive and have red urine. The resemblance is explained by the observation that the same enzyme, uroporphyrinogen decarboxylase, is depressed in both conditions. The original clinical observations, made following an outbreak in Turkey, have served to stimulate interest in experimental porphyria induced by this and other chemical agents.

IRON

Normal Iron Metabolism

Iron is by far the most abundant heavy metal in the body. It is needed chiefly for hemoglobin synthesis. About 1 mg. is required for each ml. of red cells produced, adding up to a daily need of 20 to 25 mg. for erythropoiesis. Almost all of this iron is obtained through recycling, and only about 5 percent, or 1 mg. per day, is newly absorbed to balance losses incurred via fecal and urinary excretion and in sweat and desquamated skin (Finch and Huebers, 1982). The average menstruating female loses about twice this amount and so must absorb more to maintain balance. Menstrual loss of blood, however, is difficult to estimate and varies a great deal from woman to woman.

Absorption by the gastrointestinal epithelial cell is finely tuned to admit just enough iron to cover losses, without permitting either excess or deficiency of body iron to develop (Charlton and Bothwell, 1983). Absorption normally admits about 5 to 10 percent of a total dietary intake of 10 to 20 mg. per day. The physiologic signal between the size of the body iron supply and the gastrointestinal mucosal cell is still only vaguely understood. The mucosal cell itself appears to act as a "ferrostat" by reflecting within its own cytoplasm the state of the body store of iron. A high concentration of cytoplasmic iron, present presumably almost entirely as ferritin, discourages further uptake, whereas an iron-poor intracellular environment encourages uptake by the mucosal cell for passage onward to the plasma for binding to transferrin. Indeed, evidence suggests that a transferrin pool within the intestinal lumen binds iron and modulates transport across the brush border into the cell. A reciprocal relationship between intestinal transferrin concentration and the cell store of iron would then regulate the iron absorption, with higher transferrin levels promoting absorption when there is iron lack and lower levels decreasing iron absorption when iron is plentiful in the mucosal cell (Fig. 2–58). However, the absorption of iron is also increased in response to increased erythropoietic activity, even without iron deficiency. Since the intestinal mucosal cells are in a constant state of renewal—proliferating from the crypts out toward the tips of the villi, where they are shed into the lumen—they contribute to iron loss in the feces.

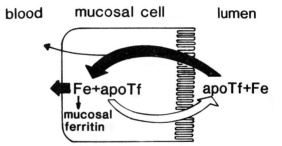

Figure 2–58 Model for the regulation of iron absorption. (From Huebers, H. A., et al.: Blood, *61*:289, 1983.)

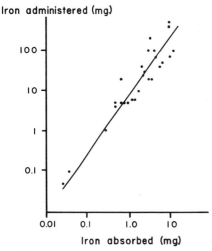

Figure 2–59 Augmentation of absolute amount of iron absorbed with increasing doses administered. (Redrawn from Bothwell, T. H., and Finch, C. A.: Iron Metabolism. Boston, Little, Brown & Co., 1962, p. 98.)

The amount of iron absorbed increases with the dose administered up to doses of about 100 mg. (Fig. 2–59). At higher doses, the mucosal cell acts as a barrier to avert excessive iron absorption, and the proportion of iron absorbed decreases. However, the barrier is not absolute, and increasing amounts of iron ingested are met by increasing increments absorbed, even though the proportion absorbed falls off. The mucosal barrier is temporarily raised following recently ingested iron, and thus more iron will be absorbed from appropriately spaced doses than from an equivalent amount given as a single dose (Fig. 2–60).

Iron absorption occurs primarily in the duodenum and upper jejunum. At neutral and alkaline pH, ferric iron forms insoluble compounds inaccessible to absorption. Acid gastric juice is therefore important for the solubilization of ingested iron (Fig. 2–61). Ferrous iron is more efficiently absorbed than ferric iron, and substances that reduce iron such as ascorbic acid thus promote its absorption. Chelation with low molecular weight substances, such as fructose, amino acids, and even ascorbic acid, may promote iron solubility and therefore its absorption. Other chelators present in foodstuffs, however, hinder iron absorption. These include phytates, phosphates, and tannates in foods such as grains, milk, and tea.

The organic forms of food iron are generally less well absorbed than inorganic medicinal ferrous sulfate. However, meat is an excellent source of iron. Most meat iron is complexed into the heme prosthetic group of myoglobin. Heme iron is efficiently absorbed by a mechanism independent of chelators and reducers. However, much of the world's population subsists on foods of plant origin that provide iron with a much lower level of bioavailability than that associated with meat iron.

Effete red cells that have lived out their 120-day life span are taken up by the phagocytic

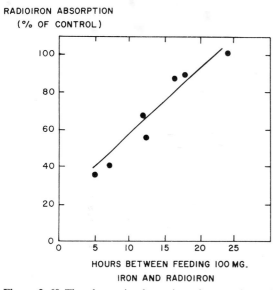

Figure 2–60 The change in absorption of a test dose of radioactive iron at intervals after an initial loading dose of nonradioactive iron. (Redrawn from Stewart, W. B., et al.: J. Exper. Med., 92:375, 1950.)

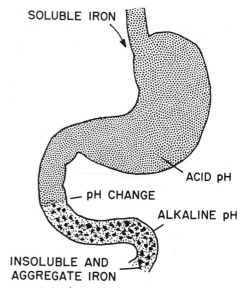

Figure 2–61 Relation of pH to the maximal site of iron absorption in the upper duodenum. (Finch, C. A.: Iron Metabolism. *In* Nutrition Today. Summer 1969, p. 4. Copyright by Nutrition Today, Inc. Reprinted with permission.)

Figure 2–62 Structure of ferritin. A series of identical subunits is assembled to form a protein shell (apoferritin). An iron micelle, containing up to 4000 atoms of iron, is formed inside. Iron can be removed, leaving behind an intact apoferritin shell.

There is a group of isoferritins that differ depending on the tissue of origin. Thus, for example, ferritin extracted from macrophages differs from that found in erythroid cells or heart. Ferritin found in plasma also differs from that found in tissues, especially in its low iron content. It appears to originate predominantly from macrophages rather than from parenchymal cells.

(Reprinted from Pape, L., et al.: Biochemistry, 7:606, 1968. Copyright 1968, American Chemical Society. Reprinted by permission of the copyright owner.)

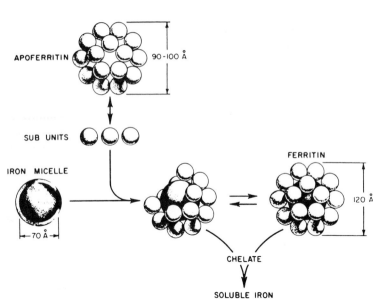

macrophages, chiefly in the spleen, liver, and bone marrow. Inside these phagocytic cells, the hemoglobin is broken down into its essential constituents. The iron taken from the degraded heme is saved and packed in extremely high concentration inside apoferritin protein shells to form molecules of ferritin, each of which may contain as many as 4000 atoms of iron (Fig. 2–62). Ferritin molecules in turn are compressed within lysosomes into still larger amorphous aggregates of insoluble material called hemosiderin. These form granules visible by light microscopy. Thus it is as ferritin and hemosiderin, chiefly in macrophages, that the bulk of the reserve iron is stored. It is from these depots that iron recycles, fulfilling the continuing need for iron in the production of red cells (Fig. 2–63).

The storage iron most recently obtained from degraded heme is the first to be reutilized for hemoglobin synthesis; the chronologically more archaic iron depots may remain untouched for very long periods of time. In a normal adult with 2500-ml. red cell mass, 2500 mg. of iron circulates as hemoglobin while another 500 to 1500 mg. is present as storage iron. Although the vast bulk of the storage iron is found in macrophages, ferritin is detectable in many of the tissues of the body, including erythroblasts and the intestinal epithelial cells. Other significant pools of body iron are in myoglobin (130 mg.) and a variety

Figure 2–63 Metabolic pathways of iron. The bulk of body iron turnover goes to erythropoiesis in the marrow and is reutilized from hemoglobin degraded in macrophages located primarily in the liver, spleen, and marrow. Only a small proportion of the iron is newly absorbed from dietary sources to make up for excretory losses. Cell-to-cell interaction between erythroid precursors and macrophages takes place in the marrow with possible exchange of ferritin iron. The direction of this exchange is still uncertain, but most evidence suggests that marrow (and splenic) macrophages remove excess ferritin and hemosiderin iron from erythroid cells. Transferrin mediates iron transport from macrophages and the intestinal mucosa to immature erythroid cells. It also delivers iron to hepatic and other parenchymal cells, but at a much lower rate.

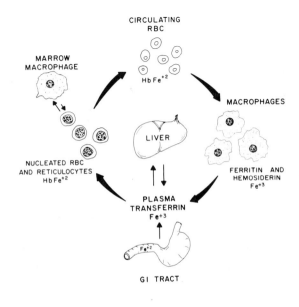

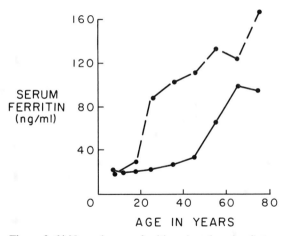

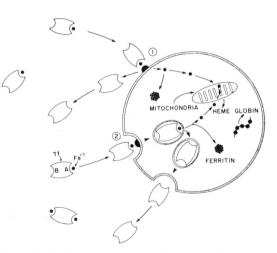

Figure 2–64 Normal serum ferritin values for men (interrupted line) and women (solid line) at different ages, showing lower iron stores in the young of both sexes and in women of childbearing age. (Adapted from Cook, J. D., et al.: Blood, *48*:451, 1976.)

Figure 2–65 Schematic representation of the delivery of iron to erythroid precursors. *A* and *B* indicate the two iron-binding sites on the transferrin molecule. Transferrin preferentially delivers its iron to receptors present on the surface of nucleated erythroid cells and on reticulocytes but absent from mature erythrocytes. The presence of an anion, physiologically probably bicarbonate, is necessary to establish the extraordinarily high affinity between transferrin and Fe^{+3}; in its absence, virtually no binding takes place. The cell frees iron from transferrin by removing the anion. Two mechanisms for delivery have been postulated. Pathway (1) depicts the transferrin iron complex binding with a specific cell surface receptor, followed by release of apotransferrin and cellular uptake of iron. Pathway (2) depicts pinocytosis of the transferrin-iron complex, release of iron, and then ejection of the iron-free transferrin back to the plasma. Iron is transported within the cell to mitochondria for heme synthesis and is stored as ferritin and hemosiderin.

of enzymes, including the cytochromes, catalase, and peroxidase (8 mg.).

The size of the body's pool of storage iron is conveniently assessed by measurement of the concentration of serum ferritin. In normal individuals, each 1 ng./ml. of serum ferritin represents about 10 mg. of storage iron (Fig. 2–64). Ferritin found in plasma differs from that in the cells of the tissues; it has a low iron content and exists partly in a glycosylated form. Storage iron may also be evaluated directly on tissue samples such as bone marrow and liver. In some pathologic states, measurement of serum ferritin may be unreliable, and tissue analysis is required for accurate assessment of iron stores. Investigators have applied the magnetic properties of iron to obtain accurate measurements of the amount of iron present in the liver by a noninvasive procedure.

Iron is taken from storage depots and transported back to erythroid precursors by a highly specialized plasma protein, transferrin. Stored in ferritin in the trivalent state, the iron is first reduced to the ferrous form for removal from the apoferritin shell and then it is carried in plasma in the ferric state, up to two atoms per molecule of transferrin. The normal concentration of iron in plasma is about 100 μg. per 100 ml., one third the total binding capacity of available transferrin. The total amount of iron in the transferrin pool is about 4 to 5 mg., approximately half intravascular and half extravascular. Although this transferrin-bound iron is only 1 percent of that in the body, its metabolic rate of turnover is extremely rapid—

50 percent of it is cleared from the intravascular space every 60 to 120 minutes. Transferrin molecules deliver their iron at the surface of the erythroid precursors and return empty to the macrophages to pick up another load (Fig. 2–65).

It has been proposed that the two iron-binding sites on the transferrin molecule, site A and site B, are unequal in their affinity for ferric iron and subserve different physiologic functions. However, most of the available evidence indicates that both sites function equally under physiologic conditions. The more heavily iron-laden the transferrin pool becomes, the more iron is delivered to parenchymal cells (Huebers and Finch, 1984).

The rate of disappearance of radioactive iron from the plasma as well as its reappearance in the circulating red cells as newly produced labeled hemoglobin is a convenient method for measuring the functional state of erythropoiesis (see Fig. 2–26). In hypoplastic conditions the utilization of iron is depressed, causing a rise in its plasma concentration along with a decrease in the rate at which it is cleared from the plasma. In iron deficiency the clearance rate is more rapid than normal, as it is in conditions associated with increased proliferation of red cell precursors in the marrow, such as hemolytic anemia. The reappearance of the tracer in the blood erythrocytes is a measure of red cell production. When erythropoiesis is efficient, about 80 percent of the radioiron is incorporated into circulating erythrocytes over a 10 day period. When erythrocyte production is impaired owing to a hypoplastic or to a hyperplastic but inefficient marrow, this figure is considerably reduced. Examples of inefficient marrows are those associated with megaloblastic anemia and with thalassemia major. In these conditions the clearance rate of radioiron from the plasma is rapid, but its incorporation into circulating erythrocytes is poor. A labile pool of storage iron contributes a minor slow component to the plasma radioiron disappearance curve. The anatomic location and biochemical nature of this labile pool are still not known, but this may be the iron that inflicts toxic damage upon the body cells in states of iron overload. Although the labile storage pool constitutes only a minor fraction of the total stores of iron, it appears to be the physiologic form of iron accessible to chelation therapy.

Iron Lack

General Effects. The first change in the development of iron deficiency is the loss of storage iron from the macrophages of the spleen, liver, and bone marrow. A decrease in plasma ferritin concentration parallels this loss. After the stores of iron are used up, the plasma iron concentration falls, at the same time stimulating an increase in the synthesis of transferrin. The saturation of transferrin with iron thus falls from 30 percent to values often below 10 percent (Fig. 2–66). Erythrocyte protoporphyrin levels are increased secondary to the intracellular deficit of sufficient iron for heme synthesis. Anemia is the last change to be observed. At first, the erythrocytes may be normocytic and normochromic and show only a few shape changes, but microcytic, hypochromic, and misshapen erythrocytes emerge as significant anemia develops (Fig. 2–67). Even with only a moderate degree of anemia, the deficit in body iron is thus already advanced.

Iron-deficiency anemia must be distinguished from other causes of microcytosis (Cook, 1982). A low serum ferritin level establishes the presence of iron deficiency, but when there is coexistence of liver disease, malignancy or other chronic disease, the level may

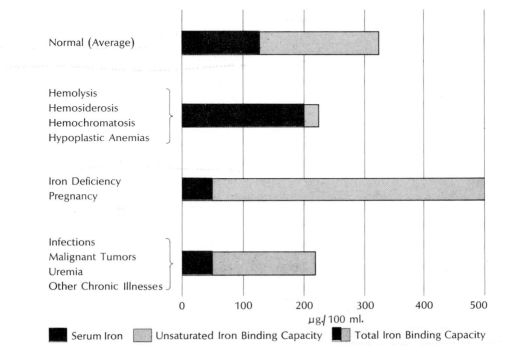

Figure 2–66 The changes in serum iron and iron-binding capacity in various disorders. The total transferrin concentration is expressed as total iron-binding capacity in μg. iron bound per 100 ml. plasma. (From McIntyre, P.: Hosp. Pract., 7(3):101, 1972.)

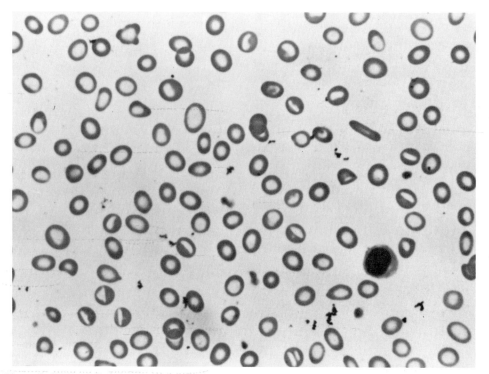

Figure 2–67 Blood film showing abnormal red cell morphology in patient with iron-deficiency anemia.

be within the normal range despite iron-deficient erythropoiesis. Low serum iron concentration is a hallmark of both iron lack and anemia of chronic disease; however, serum transferrin concentration, expressed as iron-binding capacity, rises in iron deficiency but falls in chronic disease anemia (Lee, 1983). Examination of bone marrow for stainable iron is a convenient means of rapidly distinguishing these two conditions; if iron stores are preserved, iron deficiency can be excluded as the cause of the anemia. Thalassemia trait is characterized by its familial character, normal iron studies, and sometimes by abnormal hemoglobin analysis, depending on the type of thalassemia (Table 2–14). Sideroblastic anemias result in the production of microcytic erythrocytes, but they are usually a minor

population, and the mean corpuscular red cell volume in most cases is normal or increased. Lead poisoning may cause slight microcytosis. In small children, lead poisoning is commonly associated with iron deficiency.

Whether iron deficiency without anemia causes significant symptoms remains a controversial issue. The activities of certain iron-containing enzymes decrease, but this change may not be of pathophysiologic significance. When anemia develops it is often well tolerated, except when there is acute blood loss or cardiovascular limitation. Changes in epithelial tissues complicate more protracted deficiency. There is inversion of the normal curvature of the fingernails ("spooning"), which also become more brittle; hair splits and breaks off; and a smooth red tongue reflects glossitis.

Table 2–14 MICROCYTIC ANEMIA

	Iron Deficiency	Chronic Disease	Thalassemia Trait
RBC morphology	Abnormal	Normal	Abnormal
Bone marrow iron	Absent	Present	Present
Serum iron	Low	Low	Normal
Total iron-binding capacity	High	Low	Normal
Saturation (%)	Very low	Low	Normal
Serum ferritin	<12 ng./ml.	Normal or high	Normal
Sedimentation rate	Normal	Increased	Normal
Hemoglobin A_2	Low or normal	Normal	Increased in β Normal in α

Dysphagia with web formation in the upper esophagus rarely complicates iron lack of many years' duration. Atrophic gastritis with anacidity is frequently associated with iron deficiency, but whether gastritis is primarily the result of iron deficiency (through secondary epithelial changes) or the cause of it (through impaired absorption of food iron) or both is not clear.

Infants with iron-deficiency anemia frequently have detectable occult blood in the feces without demonstrable gastrointestinal disease, presumably because of mucosal friability secondary to the deficient state. Mucosal changes secondary to iron deficiency in infants reportedly may be of sufficient magnitude to cause malabsorption. Significant weight gain occurs after treatment of small children with iron-deficiency anemia. Whether or not iron deficiency in this age group affects intelligence or behavior is still uncertain. A moderately elevated platelet count is often seen in infants with iron-deficiency anemia. Thrombocytosis in iron-deficient adults seems to be less prominent and more often explainable on the basis of reactive changes to hemorrhage, tumor, or other underlying disorders.

Unusual appetites or cravings (pica) are an especially intriguing effect of iron deficiency (Danford, 1982). Common examples are ice-chewing and starch- or clay-eating, depending on demographic and cultural circumstances. Iron-deficient children with pica may develop lead poisoning because of ingestion of lead-based paint. These unusual eating patterns usually respond to treatment of the iron deficiency.

Pathogenesis. Iron deficiency always arises because of the inability of diet and absorption to keep pace with the increased requirements imposed either by the expansion of the red cell mass or by blood loss. The requirement for iron is so great and the amount available so limited that iron deficiency affects a large proportion of the world's population. In some underdeveloped regions, over 50 percent of the women and children are iron-deficient. Even in developed regions, there is a 10 to 20 percent incidence among women of childbearing age and children. In the economically less developed parts of the world, the diet consists largely of cereals, relatively poor sources of dietary iron. The hookworm, estimated to infest almost a half billion of the world's people, further burdens body iron balance because of the gastrointestinal blood loss caused by this parasite. Some countries have initiated programs of iron fortification of food in an effort to reduce the prevalence of iron deficiency, but such programs are still the subject of some controversy because of the possibility of promoting hemochromatosis in population groups in which there is a significant prevalence of the gene for this disorder.

The growth spurt of the 2-year-old and of the adolescent are common times for iron deficiency to appear. The well-nourished infant fed on cow's milk is particularly susceptible because such a diet, although adequate in calories, is a poor source of iron. Iron deficiency is very rare at the time of birth, even if the mother is iron-deficient. However, the rapid growth that follows premature birth requires iron supplementation during the first weeks of life to prevent the development of anemia. Pregnancy creates a fourfold increase in the daily iron requirement (Fig. 2–68). The maternal red cell mass expands by about 20 percent, or by 400 mg. of iron, and the fetus requires an additional 300 mg. In calculating net iron loss in the mother, one must add the

Figure 2–68 The change in iron requirement during pregnancy. (Redrawn from Bothwell, T. H., and Finch, C. A.: Iron Metabolism. Boston, Little, Brown & Co., 1962, p. 309.)

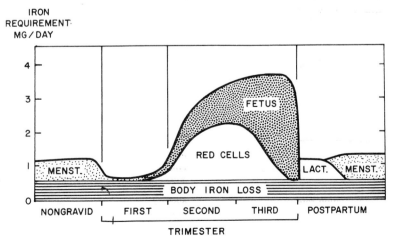

amount of iron lost as a result of bleeding during delivery to the iron in the fetus and placenta. Iron needed for lactation is about equal to what would have been lost during menstruation.

Iron-deficiency anemia is especially common after gastrectomy for a number of reasons, including lack of gastric acidity needed for absorption of food (but not medicinal) iron, rapid gastrointestinal transit time, and gastrointestinal blood loss related to peptic ulcer disease. Surgical bypass of the duodenum, a major site of iron absorption along with the upper jejunum, may be still another factor, as in the Billroth type II operation.

Intestinal malabsorption syndromes from a variety of underlying causes may limit procurement of iron as well as other nutrients from the diet; but if the duodenal surface is well preserved, sufficient iron may be absorbed to meet requirements.

Blood loss is the most important factor in the development of iron deficiency. Identification of its origin may bring to light the presence of unsuspected but significant underlying disease, such as carcinoma of the colon. Hiatal hernia, hemorrhagic gastritis, peptic ulcer disease, and esophageal varices are particularly frequent causes of upper gastrointestinal bleeding. Chronic aspirin users develop iron-deficiency anemia because of increased gastrointestinal blood loss with or without demonstrable underlying disease. Menorrhagia, often associated with uterine fibroids, is the most frequent cause in premenopausal females. Sources of urinary blood loss include renal tumors as well as the hemoglobinuria and hemosiderinuria associated with chronic intravascular hemolysis. Vasculitis of the pulmonary vessels with chronic hemorrhage into the lungs will cause pulmonary macrophages to become iron-laden in *Goodpasture's syndrome*. However, iron is not efficiently reutilized from these cells, and an iron-deficient bone marrow with microcytic, hypochromic anemia ensues.

Iron Excess

General Effects. The accumulation of excessive quantities of iron in the body ultimately originates from increased absorption or from parenteral administration as transfusions or as pharmacologic iron complexes. The capacity of the macrophages to gather the extra iron within their protective confines is immense, but ultimately transferrin saturation rises, its

synthesis is inhibited, and the plasma iron concentration approaches 200 µg. per 100 ml. with near 100 percent saturation of the iron-binding capacity (Fig. 2–66). As the transferrin saturation rises above 50 percent, parenchymal cells are no longer protected from pathologic iron uptake and damage occurs over the years to various organs, especially the liver, heart, pancreas, pituitary, and synovial tissues. Signs of chronic liver disease appear, along with those of heart failure, diabetes mellitus, and endocrine insufficiency. A characteristic form of arthropathy may develop. The term *hemochromatosis* is used to describe the disease that arises from such chronic iron overexposure. Grayish pigmentation of the skin is caused by deposition of melanin in the deeper layers of the epidermis. Deposits of iron are seen in the glandular structures of the skin.

Acute iron poisoning occurs chiefly in children who accidentally swallow an overdose of iron pills. Nausea, vomiting, and intestinal bleeding are soon followed by vascular collapse and shock, with a high likelihood of a fatal outcome.

The detection of iron overload would be best accomplished by the direct measurement of total body iron stores, but no satisfactory technique is available for this. A rise in the plasma iron concentration and an increase in transferrin saturation are associated with increased iron stores, but similar changes are seen secondary to altered bone marrow function, such as hypoplastic and megaloblastic anemia. Furthermore, the hypoferremic response to inflammation may depress an elevated plasma iron level and mask a state of iron overload.

A time-honored but cumbersome method of measuring iron stores uses quantitative phlebotomy carried out over many months to the point of early iron-deficiency anemia, a sign that the iron stores initially present have been depleted. The total amount of hemoglobin iron removed (assuming 1 mg. Fe per ml. erythrocytes) is roughly equivalent to the iron stores initially present.

One may assess a "labile" intracellular pool of iron by measuring the urinary excretion of iron for 24 hours after a single injection of the chelating agent desferrioxamine (DFOM). The normal individual excretes about 0.5 mg., whereas the iron-loaded patient may excrete up to 10 to 20 mg. This labile pool is thought to be physiologically chelated within cells to low molecular weight substances, since the other biologic forms of iron (ferritin, transferrin, heme) are not significantly available for DFOM chelation.

The concentration of ferritin in plasma may be extraordinarily high in iron-overloaded states, but normal values also are observed. Breakdown of normal hepatic or neoplastic parenchymal cells may cause release of ferritin into the plasma. Thus, elevated plasma ferritin levels also occur in patients with acute or chronic liver disease, leukemia, or cancer. Plasma ferritin measurements are useful in the detection of iron deficiency and of iron excess and in following changes on body iron status, but one must use caution to interpret the value correctly.

Perhaps the most sensitive method for the early detection of iron overload is direct measurement on samples obtained by liver biopsy. Estimation is made microscopically after suitable staining or by chemical measurement. Although bone marrow iron content is invaluable in the detection of iron deficiency, it is less helpful in hemochromatosis, as discussed subsequently.

Pathogenesis. An increase in the body content of iron in *primary familial hemochromatosis* occurs because of an inappropriate and as yet unexplained increase in iron absorption by the intestinal mucosal cells (Edwards et al., 1982). An increase in liver iron, predominantly in the hepatocytes, may be the sole manifestation early in the course of the disease, but elevation of the plasma iron and increased saturation of transferrin are also often present initially. Iron-loading in macrophages and elevation of the plasma ferritin occur later. In advanced stages, the body may contain 30 to 40 gm. of iron. The fact that macrophage and intestinal mucosal cell iron content do not appear increased early in the disease has led to the postulate that the primary defect may be a deficient rate of ferritin synthesis in these sites, with breakdown of the mucosal barrier against increased absorption and reduction of the normal protective storage function of the macrophages, with consequent iron-loading of transferrin and of parenchymal cells, especially hepatic. In point of fact, however, the basic biochemical abnormality causing this disorder remains unknown. Erythrocyte morphology is normal, and erythropoiesis is unaffected. Indeed, anemia is noteworthy for its absence. The gene for hemochromatosis is located on the short arm of chromosome 6, closely linked with the HLA locus. Because of this linkage, it has been possible to trace the segregation of the gene in families by using HLA haplotype analysis (Fig. 2–69). In Caucasian populations, 8 to 10 percent of the population are heterozygous, a surprisingly high incidence. However, most heterozygotes show no abnormalities clinically or biochemically, and although there is a modest excess in iron accumulation in the body, it is self-limited and does not progress to cause any pathologic consequences. The frequency of homozygosity is about 2 or 3 per thousand, and these individuals are at high risk of developing biochemical abnormalities of iron excess that, if allowed to proceed untreated, will progress from the latent phase to hemochromatosis.

It is still uncertain whether or not increased

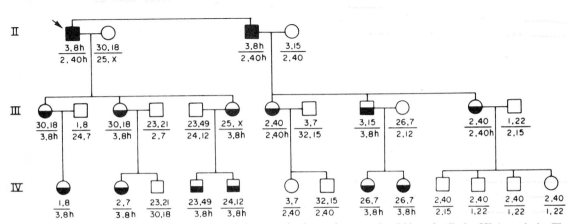

Figure 2–69 Demonstration of the segregation of the gene for hemochromatosis within a family by HLA analysis. The propositus (arrow) is homozygous. By haplotype analysis, family heterozygotes may be identified. The hemochromatosis genes are designated by the letter "h." (Adapted from Edwards, C. Q., et al.: Clin. Haematol., *11*:414, 1982.)

oral intake of iron, dietary or medicinal, can cause hemochromatosis without the interaction of some other factor, such as familial hemochromatosis, thalassemia, or liver cirrhosis. A small proportion of patients with cirrhosis develop increased iron absorption, but the pathogenesis of this increase is obscure. The Kaffir beer prepared in iron vessels and consumed by the Bantus of Southern Africa does appear to be one form of dietary iron that is absorbed in sufficient amounts to cause hemochromatosis.

Iron overload due to chronic transfusion (transfusion hemosiderosis) contrasts with primary hemochromatosis inasmuch as iron-loading occurs first in the macrophages and only later in the parenchymal cells (Schafer et al., 1981). Plasma ferritin is elevated early in the course of the iron overload, and a rise in the plasma iron and an increase in transferrin saturation occur later. The iron overload may be readily detected in bone marrow macrophages or circulating blood monocytes, which are not reliable parameters of iron overload in early primary hemochromatosis.

Iron overload also complicates disorders of erythropoiesis in which iron is not properly utilized for hemoglobin formation. The increased iron absorption is apparently related to the hyperplastic, although ineffective, erythropoiesis characterizing these conditions, the best examples of which are sideroblastic anemia and thalassemia major and intermedia. Red cell morphology is abnormal. The anemia is of any degree from minimal to severe. An excessive number of hemosiderin granules accumulates in the cytoplasm of erythroid precursor cells as well as in mature erythrocytes, where their presence becomes much more obvious after splenectomy. The term *sideroblast* is applied to any nucleated erythroid precursor that contains stainable iron granules. In normal marrow about 25 percent of erythroid precursors are sideroblasts containing two or three small cytoplasmic granules. The number and size of such iron granules as well as the proportion of erythroid cells containing them increase in a number of states of increased erythropoiesis, including hemolytic anemia and megaloblastic anemia. However, in the marrow of certain iron-loading anemias there are seen a large number of *ringed sideroblasts*, erythroid cells in which a necklace of iron granules surrounds the nucleus. To these conditions the term *sideroblastic anemia* is applied. The ringed configuration is presumably related to the fact that the iron accumulation is concentrated on the mitochondria, which cling to

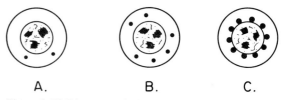

A.   B.   C.

Figure 2–70 Diagrammatic representation of sideroblasts. Iron granules in the cytoplasm are identified by means of an iron stain. *A*, Normal nucleated erythroid cell containing two small cytoplasmic hemosiderin granules. *B*, Nucleated erythroid cell with an increased number of cytoplasmic iron granules, a nonspecific alteration. *C*, Ringed sideroblast.

the nuclear membranes in the fixed and stained preparations (Fig. 2–70).

The *sideroblastic anemias* are classified as primary or secondary and hereditary or acquired (Bottomley, 1982). Hypochromic, small, misshapen erythrocytes are seen in the midst of a population of normocytic or even macrocytic cells. Hereditary sex-linked hypochromic anemia is usually first detected in young adult or adolescent males, whereas primary acquired sideroblastic anemia is seen in patients of either sex over the age of 60 years (Beris et al., 1983). Occasionally, with observation the latter condition will ultimately prove to be a secondary variety associated with a myeloproliferative syndrome culminating in acute myelogenous leukemia. The condition can also occur secondary to certain drugs (isoniazid, cycloserine, chloramphenicol) or to alcoholic excess, but reversibility averts the development of hemochromatosis. Rare ringed sideroblasts are occasionally seen in the marrow of patients with certain chronic diseases, but hyperferremia and iron-loading do not complicate the picture and they should not be designated as sideroblastic anemia.

Some of the sideroblastic anemias are pyridoxine-responsive, as described by Harris (1964). The doses required are pharmacologic, and signs of pyridoxine deficiency are absent. Anemia is improved, and the serum iron decreases. The response is not complete, although it is generally more satisfactory in the hereditary than in the primary acquired cases. The explanation of responsiveness may reside in a defect in conversion of pyridoxine to its active form, pyridoxal phosphate, which is required for the first step in heme synthesis on the mitochondria, upon which iron accumulates. Various studies have provided some evidence for superior therapeutic efficacy of pyridoxal phosphate, but it would appear that the entire group of disorders is at present too heterogeneous to be properly analyzed until a more precise biochemical classification is achieved. Indeed, megaloblastic erythropoiesis and macrocytic erythrocytes are also sometimes observed along with a degree of folic acid responsiveness.

Hemochromatosis is a major cause of morbidity and mortality in thalassemia, a primary deficiency of globin synthesis. Erythroid cells are iron-loaded, but ringed sideroblasts are not prominent. Transfusional hemosiderosis contributes to the iron load in thalassemia major as well as in any anemia of sufficient severity to require chronic transfusion therapy.

Primary hemochromatosis is treated with removal of iron by repeated phlebotomy over a long period of time, until iron stores become depleted and the serum iron falls. This approach has also been used in hemochromatosis secondary to iron-loading erythrocyte disorders in which the anemia is mild. Patients with thalassemia major require chelation therapy with desferrioxamine (DFOM), since they will not tolerate phlebotomy (Propper and Nathan, 1982). When DFOM is administered by prolonged subcutaneous or intravenous infusions given on an almost daily basis, iron overload may be reversed and iron balance restored, but the procedure is expensive and cumbersome. In the meantime, the search for an effective oral iron chelating agent continues. Iron chelators may be lifesaving in the treatment of acute iron poisoning.

GLOBIN

Normal Structure

The primary structure and production rate of globin molecules are under genetic control. Specific amino acid sequences are governed by the triplet code of DNA bases passed down in the chromosomes from generation to generation. The rate at which globin polypeptide chains are synthesized is a function of the rate at which the DNA code is transcribed into mature messenger RNA. The sequence of translational events that follow modifies the production rate of the completed chains. These include the initiation and assembly on, and the release of the polypeptide chains from, the messenger RNA–polyribosome complex upon which the amino acids are joined together in proper sequence.

A variety of genetic loci direct globin synthesis. The α and β chains of normal adult hemoglobin (Hb A) are produced in matched amounts, but under the control of separate genes located far apart from one another on different chromosomes (the α genes on chromosome 16 and the non-α genes on chromosome 11). The δ chain closely resembles the β chain, to which it is genetically linked on chromosome 11, but it is synthesized at only 1/40 the rate of β chains. Thus, the concentration of Hb A_2 ($\alpha_2\delta_2$) in the normal adult is only about 2.5 percent of the total hemoglobin. Alpha chains are synthesized from early embryonic life on but are combined with different chains according to the stage of development (Table 2–15). The ζ and ϵ globin chains are embryonic products produced during the first trimester of intrauterine development. Beyond the first trimester, α and γ chain synthesis predominates in the formation of fetal hemoglobin (Hb F ($\alpha_2\gamma_2$), which makes up 75 to 90 percent of the total hemoglobin at birth. Two genetic loci govern the production of different types of γ chains, one with glycine at the 136 position Gγ, the other with alanine Aγ. Although the synthesis of adult type β chains is begun early in intrauterine development, predominance is not established until its synthetic rate sharply rises in the weeks just preceding birth. Hb A then gradually replaces Hb F in the circulating erythrocytes until the normal adult level of Hb F (<2 percent) is attained, usually at about 6 months of age, although slight elevations may persist for 2 years (Fig. 2–71).

Thanks largely to the work of Perutz, the three-dimensional fine structure of the hemoglobin molecule is well understood. The α and β subunits, similar but not identical in size and shape, possess a complementariness of structure that causes them to associate spontaneously with each other and form a dimer that

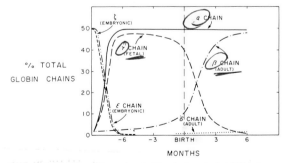

Figure 2–71 The change in globin chains during intrauterine development. (Redrawn from Bunn, H. F., Forget, B. G., and Ranney, H. M.: Human Hemoglobins. Philadelphia, W. B. Saunders Co., 1977, p. 107.)

constitutes the basis of both the function of the molecule as an oxygen transporter and its physicochemical stability. Unpaired, the subunits not only are incapable of oxygen transport but also are extremely unstable. The stability of the dimer $(\alpha_1\beta_1)$ comes from the extensive area of surface contact between the two subunits, involving 34 amino acid residues in the contact site. When two dimers come together to form the complete tetrameric configuration, an "asymmetric" contact point forms between the α chain of one dimer and the β chain of the other. This asymmetric $(\alpha_1\beta_2)$ contact area is somewhat less extensive, involving only 19 amino acid sites, but this region is important in the regulation of the normal sigmoid shape of the hemoglobin oxygen dissociation curve. It is at this point that the allosteric properties of hemoglobin, as it combines with its substrate oxygen, are modulated. The initial attachment of oxygen to the α chain heme causes its iron to "snap back" as if released from a position under tension. This signal then sends a "shock wave" through the molecule that increases the affinity of the β chain heme groups for oxygen atoms, producing the upward inflection of the oxygen association curve and at the same time causing the β chains to move closer by 7 Å. The β chains shift back apart when oxygen is removed (Fig. 2–16). These intramolecular changes have led to the use of the terms *tense (T)* and *relaxed (R)* to describe the allosteric configurational states of deoxy- and oxyhemoglobin, respectively. The salt bridges that stabilize the T form are broken when the molecule combines with oxygen. The binding of low molecular weight phosphates, such as 2,3-diphosphoglycerate, takes place in the cleft between the two β chains when they are in the deoxy-configuration, diminishing the oxygen affinity of the hemoglobin.

The globular subunit, which is divided into eight helical regions designated by the letters *A* through *H*, is physiologically submerged in an aqueous medium with which it blends be-cause it carries all its hydrophilic groupings on its exterior surface. These include hydroxyl groups, such as those of serine and threonine, as well as polar carboxyl and amino groups. The molecular interior is arid and is lined with hydrophobic nonpolar groups. Each subunit has its heme group neatly tucked into a *heme pocket* that dips down from the molecular surface and is also completely lined with hydrophobic groups that exclude water from the region. The heme comes into contact at about 60 atomic sites with the surface of the pocket. The fifth coordinate position of the heme iron is bound to the *proximal histidine* residue (β^{92} and α^{87}). Molecular oxygen is carried between the sixth coordinate position of iron and the *distal histidine* (β^{63} and α^{58}) (see Fig. 2–15).

Globin Genes

Remarkable advances have occurred during the past few years in our knowledge of the fine points of gene structure. Indeed, investigation of a variety of thalassemia syndromes has revealed how different mutant nucleotide base substitutions can drastically reduce the rate of—or even abolish—globin chain synthesis.

The normal layout of the globin genes is shown in Figure 2–72, the alpha genes on chromosome 16 and the non-alpha on chromosome 11. There are two alpha genes on each chromosome, or a total of four in the normal diploid nucleated erythroid cell.

Within each gene there are *intervening sequences* of nucleotides *(introns)* that do not code for any protein structure. The remainder of the gene *(exons)* bears the code. The entire gene is transcribed into mRNA, but the intervening sequences must be removed by processing that occurs in the cell nucleus (Fig. 2–73). The ends of the remaining mRNA are spliced together and the processed product moves out into the cytoplasm, freed of its intervening sequences, to carry out its predestined role in protein synthesis.

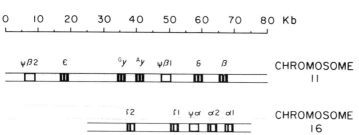

Figure 2–72 Map of the globin genes. The top line is the scale measured in Kilobases (Kb.), or 1000 base pairs. Transcription of mRNA takes place from the 5' to the 3' end, corresponding to amino and carboxyl ends of the coded protein, respectively. The middle line shows the non–alpha globin genes on the short arm of chromosome 11. The lower line shows the alpha genes on chromosome 16. Regions of the gene that code for the primary structure of globin chains are shown in black, and the intervening sequences are demonstrated in white. The all white boxes are pseudogenes (ψ), evolutionary remnants of globin genes that are not expressed. (Adapted from Benz, E. J., Jr., and Forget, B. G.: Ann. Rev. Med., *33*:364, 1982.)

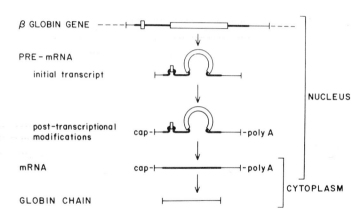

Figure 2–73 Messenger RNA processing. Intervening sequences (white boxes) are spliced out. The mRNA bearing the code for protein synthesis (heavy black line) is ligated together and then moves out into the cytoplasm as mature mRNA. The thin continuous lines are mRNA sequences not translated into protein but important for initiation and termination of transcription. (From Benz, E. J., Jr., and Forget, B. G.: Ann. Rev. Med., *33*:365, 1982.)

The details of mRNA transcription are shown in Figure 2–74. There are two small regions of particular nucleotide sequences ("boxes") upstream from the point at which transcription begins *(CCAAT box and ATA box)*. These regions are important to the rate and accuracy of transcription. At a specific point downstream from these sites the mRNA strand is started. The first nucleotide serves as a signal for adding a 5'-CAP structure. This is followed by a brief stretch of nontranslated sequences until an initiating codon is reached, which is the signal to start polypeptide translation. Specific sequences signal the exact splice sites for the removal of the intervening sequences. Another codon appears at the end of the gene, signaling for termination of polypeptide translation. This is followed by another brief stretch of nontranslated sequences. Finally, a polyadenylate tail is added to the mRNA under the direction of still another specific signal.

From the foregoing discussion, it is evident that a nucleotide base substitution may influence globin chain production even though it is located outside the DNA region that actually codes for the protein primary structure.

Hemoglobinopathy Due to Structural Defects (Table 2–15)

Nomenclature. In the years that followed the first description of sickle hemoglobin (HbS) in 1949 it became evident that the letters in the alphabet would not be sufficient to accommodate names for the large number of mutant hemoglobins being discovered, now including over 300 variants. Family names and then place names were given as trivial expressions, to be followed by a specific designation of the amino acid substitution that characterized the abnormal hemoglobin. For example, *Hb Philly* was first observed in Philadelphia. It has normal α chains, but the β chains are affected by an inherited abnormality of the thirty-fifth amino acid from the N-terminal end of the β chains, at which phenylalanine is found in place of tyrosine (Fig. 2–75). This abnormal hemoglobin is thus designated α_2

Figure 2–74 Structure of an individual globin gene, showing in detail the promotor boxes upstream from the point at which mRNA transcription is started ("CAP" site). Specific nucleotide sequences mark the splice sites for removing intervening sequences during mRNA processing. Other codons signal for initiation and termination of polypeptide synthesis, as well as for addition of the polyadenylate tail. U = uracil; T = thymine; G = guanine; C = cytosine; A = adenine. (From Benz, E. J., Jr., and Forget, B. G.: Ann. Rev. Med., *33*:366, 1982.)

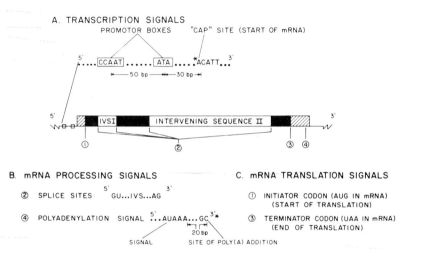

Table 2–15 SELECTED HEMOGLOBINS—THEIR STRUCTURES AND STRUCTURAL MUTATIONS

Normal Amino Acid Sequence	
HbA	$\alpha_2 \beta_2$
Hb A$_2$	$\alpha_2 \delta_2$
Hb F	$\alpha_2 \gamma_2$
Hb H	β_4
Hb Bart's	γ_4
Hb Portland	$\zeta_2 \gamma_2$
Hb Gower-1	$\zeta_2 \epsilon_2$
Hb Gower-2	$\alpha_2 \epsilon_2$
Methemoglobinemia	
Hb M Boston	$\alpha_2^{58\ his\to tyr} \beta_2$
Hb M Iwate	$\alpha_2^{87\ his\to tyr} \beta_2$
Hb M Saskatoon	$\alpha_2 \beta_2^{63\ his\to tyr}$
Hb M Hyde Park	$\alpha_2 \beta_2^{92\ his\to tyr}$
Increased Oxygen Affinity with Erythrocytosis	
Hb Chesapeake	$\alpha_2^{92\ arg\to leu} \beta_2$
Hb Rainier	$\alpha_2 \beta_2^{145\ tyr\to his}$
Hb Hiroshima	$\alpha_2 \beta_2^{143\ his\to asp}$
Decreased Oxygen Affinity with Cyanosis	
Hb Kansas	$\alpha_2 \beta_2^{102\ asn\to thr}$
Unstable Hemoglobin with Hemolytic Anemia	
Hb Torino	$\alpha_2^{43\ phe\to val} \beta_2$
Hb Hammersmith	$\alpha_2 \beta_2^{42\ phe\to ser}$
Hb Zürich	$\alpha_2 \beta_2^{63\ his\to arg}$
Hb Tacoma	$\alpha_2 \beta_2^{30\ arg\to ser}$
Hb Philly	$\alpha_2 \beta_2^{35\ tyr\to phe}$
Hb Freiburg	$\alpha_2 \beta_2^{23\ val\to o}$
Hb Gun Hill	$\alpha_2 \beta_2^{93-97\to o}$
Hb Genova	$\alpha_2 \beta_2^{28\ leu\to pro}$
Hb Seattle	$\alpha_2 \beta_2^{76\ ala\to glu}$
"Exterior" Mutants	
Hb S	$\alpha_2 \beta_2^{6\ glu\to val}$
Hb C	$\alpha_2 \beta_2^{6\ glu\to lys}$
Hb E	$\alpha_2 \beta_2^{26\ glu\to lys}$
Hb C Harlem	$\alpha_2 \beta_2^{6\ glu\to val;\ 73\ asp\to asn}$
Hb Korle-bu	$\alpha_2 \beta_2^{73\ asp\to asn}$
Hb G Accra	$\alpha_2 \beta_2^{79\ asp\to asn}$
Hb D Punjab	$\alpha_2 \beta_2^{121\ glu\to gln}$
Mutants with Low Synthetic Rate	
Hb Lepore	$\alpha_2\ \delta\text{-}\beta_2$ (fusion gene)
Hb Constant Spring	$\alpha_2^{141\to172} \beta_2$

Globin polypeptide subunits, each under the control of separate genes, are designated alpha (α), beta (β), gamma (γ), delta (δ), epsilon (ϵ), or zeta (ζ). The subscript refers to the number of subunits. The superscript indicates the mutation site.

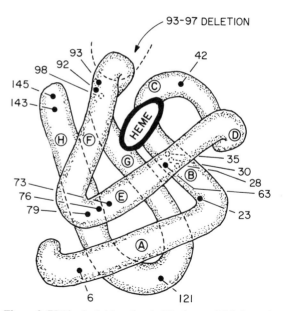

Figure 2–75 The β globin subunit. The letters "A" through "H" indicate the eight helical regions. The numbered positions indicate amino acid sites discussed in the text and in Table 2–15. (Redrawn from Giblett, E. R.: Genetic Markers in Human Blood. Oxford, Blackwell Scientific Publications Ltd., 1969.)

$\beta_2^{35tyr\to phe}$. Mutations of the β chain outnumber those of the α chain. Abnormal δ and γ chains have also been discovered. Many abnormal hemoglobins produce no abnormality in erythrocyte appearance or function and are not pathogenetic. Some are harmful only in the homozygous state, whereas others are lethal in the homozygous state and thus are observed only in heterozygous carriers.

Structural alterations in the primary structure of the globin chains are most commonly the result of single-base substitutions in the DNA nucleotide sequence changing the triplet code from that for one amino acid to that for another. Other mechanisms include deletion of codons, fusion genes (as in Hb Lepore, described further on), and frame shift mutations in which a single-base deletion changes the coding order of the nucleotide triplets that follow.

Methemoglobinemia. A substitution of tyrosine for histidine at either the proximal or distal histidine residues of either the α or the β chains locks the heme iron into a trivalent state resistant to the action of the enzyme methemoglobin reductase, which has the responsibility of maintaining the iron atoms of hemoglobin in the ferrous state. The affected heme groups in half the molecule are incapable of oxygen transport, whereas the unaffected pair of hemes retains the ability to combine reversibly with oxygen. In the α chain methemoglobinemias, the normal β partner has a somewhat decreased affinity for oxygen because of the absence of the "signal" that is normally sent across to the β chain from the α when it first combines with oxygen. In the β chain mutants, the oxygen affinity of the unaffected α subunit is more nearly normal. Inheritance is autosomal dominant and homozygosity is apparently lethal, in contrast to inherited deficiency of methemoglobin reductase, which is an autosomal recessive state. The methemoglobinemia of mutant hemoglobins is resistant to therapy, whereas that oc-

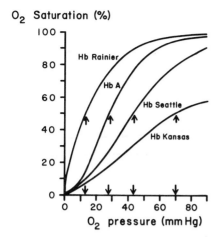

Figure 2–76 Examples of hemoglobins with abnormal oxygen affinity. Arrows indicate P_{50}. (Reproduced with permission from "Abnormal Hemoglobins with High and Low Oxygen Affinity" by G. Stamatoyannopoulos, A. J. Bellingham, C. Lenfant and C. A. Finch, Annual Review of Medicine, Volume 22. Copyright © 1971 by Annual Reviews Inc. All rights reserved.)

curring as a result of deficiency of the enzyme responds to treatment with such reducing agents as methylene blue and ascorbic acid.

High-Affinity Hemoglobin with Erythrocytosis. Mutant hemoglobins that raise the hemoglobin oxygen affinity shift the oxygen dissociation curve to the left, impeding oxygen unloading at the tissues (Fig. 2–76). The erythropoietin response evokes a secondary form of polycythemia that is familial and benign and is unassociated with increases in the platelet or leukocyte count. The mutation sites affect either the area of $\alpha_1\beta_2$ subunit contact or the C-terminal ends of the β chains close to the cove where low molecular weight phosphates are bound. Mutants such as Hb Chesapeake, which are located at the $\alpha_1\beta_2$ contact, have a raised oxygen affinity along with a loss in the normal sigmoid contour of the oxygen dissociation curve, but their Bohr effect is preserved. In Hb Hiroshima and Hb Rainier, which affect the C-terminal region of the β subunits, the Bohr effect is impaired. These substitutions presumably raise oxygen affinity by interfering with low molecular weight phosphate-binding and allosteric movements.

Low-Affinity Hemoglobin with Cyanosis. Hb Kansas is a mutation at the $\alpha_1\beta_2$ contact that causes a lowered oxygen affinity (Fig. 2–76). Cyanosis is reversed if the patient is placed in an atmosphere of sufficiently high partial pressure of oxygen. Oxygen unloading is facilitated in the tissues, with a decreased

stimulus to erythropoietin secretion causing a mild but "physiologic" anemia.

Unstable Hemoglobin with Congenital Heinz Body Hemolytic Anemia. Amino acid replacements that loosen the attachment of heme in its pocket or that interfere with the dimeric association of the subunits at the $\alpha_1\beta_1$ contact region cause the mutant hemoglobin to be inordinately susceptible to oxidation. Water entry into normally hydrophobic regions is followed by conversion to methemoglobin and oxidation of the hemoglobin into insoluble lumps. These impede erythrocyte pliability and cause hemolysis. The intact spleen plucks these precipitates from the erythrocytes. After splenectomy, a large proportion of the circulating erythrocytes contains Heinz bodies (intracellular inclusions of precipitated hemoglobin). The replacement of one hydrophobic amino acid for another inside the heme pocket, as in Hb Torino, causes only mild hemolysis, but when a hydrophilic group is placed into the heme pocket lining, as in the case of serine in Hb Hammersmith, heme loss is marked and hemolysis severe. A gross deletion of a block of five amino acids adjacent to the proximal histidine residue in Hb Gun Hill produces gross molecular distortion with heme-deficient globin subunits and marked hemoglobin instability. Hb Zürich affects the distal histidine residue of the β chain, which is replaced by arginine. The polar group of arginine lies poised just outside the heme pocket and leads to very mild hemolysis unless the patient is given certain "oxidant" drugs, such as sulfonamides, which explosively provoke episodes of severe hemolysis. Hb Philly and Hb Tacoma are unstable because they affect the $\alpha_1\beta_1$ contact area. The globin subunit also cannot bear disruption of its helical regions without suffering molecular instability. The insertion of the hydroxyl group of proline into the B helix of the β chains in Hb Genova breaks up the regular helical structure and causes a gross alteration in molecular configuration with hemolysis.

The oxygen affinity of the unstable hemoglobins may be raised or lowered, with an effect on the level of hemoglobin at which the patient compensates. When the affinity is high, the erythropoietin response is greater, and the degree of anemia is less than in those mutants with a lowered affinity, in which compensation is achieved at a lower concentration of circulating hemoglobin. The severity of the hemolytic process obviously also determines the severity of the anemia.

Exterior Mutants. Mutants placed on the hydrophilic exterior of the molecule do not alter either the oxygen affinity or the oxidative stability of the molecule. Relatively few of the more than 50 variants described in this class of abnormal hemoglobins cause any significant signs. Two major exceptions are the most common structural hemoglobinopathies, Hb S and Hb C. Both these hemoglobins are substituted at the 6 position from the N-terminal end of the β chain, where glutamic acid is replaced by valine in the case of Hb S and by lysine in the case of Hb C. Hb E, prevalent in Southeast Asia, also has a lysine in place of glutamic acid, but the affected site is 26 from the N-terminus of the β chain.

Since the amino acid substitutions of Hb S and Hb C are associated with a progressively less negative charge (from negatively charged glutamic acid to neutral valine to positively charged lysine), these hemoglobins are readily separated by electrophoresis. Other abnormal hemoglobins in which the amino acid substitution does not change the molecular charge may not be separable by this technique. The detection of Hb S is also facilitated by microscopic demonstration of sickling of deoxygenated erythrocytes, reduced solubility of deoxygenated solutions, and mechanical instability with vigorous agitation.

Erythrocytes that contain Hb S undergo jagged distortion of their membranes under reduced partial pressure of oxygen, a phenomenon known as *sickling* (Fig. 2–77). The sickling is visualized by electron microscopy as a

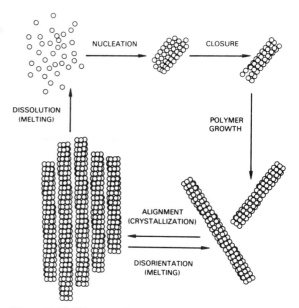

Figure 2–78 Diagram of polymerization of deoxy Hb S. The initial nucleation phase is followed by growth and alignment. The individual fibers appear to contain an inner core of four strands and an outer layer of 10 strands. "Melting" is caused by oxygenation as well as by lowering the temperature. (From Beck, W. S. [Ed.]: Hematology. 3rd ed. Cambridge, MA, The MIT Press, 1981, p. 148.)

linear molecular stacking of hemoglobin molecules, the filaments intertwining into cable-like structures illustrated in Figure 2–78. The process is reversible, and as the oxygen tension is raised, the semisolid gelled hemoglobin liquefies once again, and the cell reassumes its normal biconcave shape. The reversibility of the process is a function of the allosteric shift of the β chains, with the deoxy T configuration causing a "fit" between the β chains of one molecule and the α chains of the next, on to a linear stacking of molecule upon molecule. With reoxygenation, the β chains relax and move closer together, and the complementariness between adjacent molecules is broken. The erythrocyte membrane may undergo irreversible deformation. The cell will then remain irreversibly sickled, even though the interior structure of the oxyhemoglobin S is not in the gelled state. Sickled erythrocytes seen in routine blood films prepared from blood of sickle cell anemia patients are examples of irreversibly sickled cells.

Murayama (1966) proposed that the substitution of valine with its hydrophobic side chain in place of glutamic acid with its exterior polar carboxyl group causes, in a sense, an interiorization of a portion of the molecular exterior. He suggested that a cyclic hydrophobic valine-

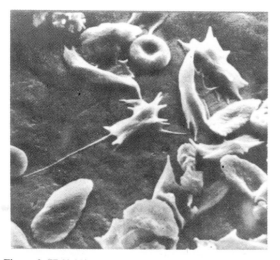

Figure 2–77 Sickled erythrocytes as demonstrated by scanning electron microscopy. (From Jensen, W. N., and Lessin, L. S.: Semin. Hematol., 7:409, 1970. By permission of Grune & Stratton, Inc., New York.)

to-valine bond forms between the 1 and 6 amino acid residues of the β chain of Hb S. This changes the exterior molecular configuration and causes a key and lock arrangement between molecules when the β chains are in the deoxy configuration.

Further considerations of the orientation of tetramers of deoxy Hb S within the multi-stranded sickle fiber lead to the conclusion that there are many contact sites between the entrapped molecules in both horizontal and vertical planes, not just the one area of contact envisioned by Murayama at the site of the amino acid substitution. Wishner and coworkers (1975) have drawn up a model depicting a multiplicity of contact sites with an asymmetric placement of the hemoglobin tetramers within the fibers such that only one of the two substituted valines of deoxy Hb S tetramer is situated at a contact point (Fig. 2–79).

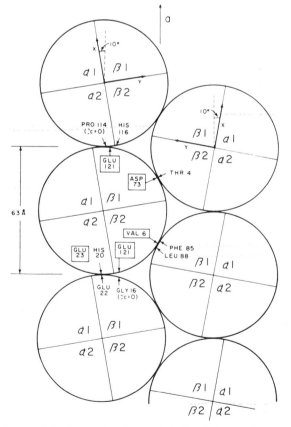

Figure 2–79 Intermolecular contact sites between deoxy Hb S molecules within fibers. The illustration is based on the results of x-ray crystallography of hemoglobin crystals and thus may not necessarily reflect physiologic conditions. (From Wishner, B. C., et al.: J. Mol. Biol., 98:179, 1975. Copyright by Academic Press Inc. [London] Ltd.)

Wishner's model is based on studies of hemoglobin crystals, but it correlates in many respects with clinical observations made in individuals who have inherited another abnormal hemoglobin present in the red cells along with Hb S. For example, Hb C Harlem has two amino acid substitutions in its beta chains, one identical with that of Hb S and the other at the 73 position, where asparagine replaces aspartic acid. Despite the fact that this molecule is more abnormal than Hb S, its presence in patients also heterozygous for Hb S inhibits the sickling process. Another mutant, Hb Korle-bu, has the same property of inhibiting sickle fiber formation. Hb Korle-bu is characterized by the same substitution at position 73 of the beta chain as that found in the Hb C Harlem, but otherwise its structure is normal. From this observation one is led to the conclusion that position 73 of the beta chain is an important site of contact between hemoglobin tetramers in the sickle fiber, as in fact shown in Wishner's model. Analogous observations have been made with a number of other mutant hemoglobins that interact with deoxy Hb S to affect the sickling process.

The presence of fetal hemoglobin together with Hb S also inhibits gelation. Newborn infants do not suffer from sickle cell disease. Symptoms become manifest only as the fetal hemoglobin is replaced by the adult type. Hb F levels are commonly raised in sickle cell anemia to values from 5 to 15 percent, but the fact that it is heterogenously distributed among the erythrocytes explains why its level is not generally related to disease severity. However, those erythrocytes with higher Hb F content do survive longer in the circulation. In the double heterozygous condition of hereditary persistence of fetal hemoglobin and sickle trait, erythrocytes uniformly have 20 to 30 percent Hb F mixed together with Hb S, and the result is a benign condition.

Conversely, Hb C rather strongly interacts with Hb S in the gelation, and its presence in erythrocytes together with Hb S in equal proportions causes significant in vivo sickling in the disorder known as *Hb SC disease* (Ballas et al., 1982). Normal Hb A, which is found in a proportion of about 60:40 relative to that of Hb S in individuals who are carriers of sickle cell trait, also interacts with Hb S in the gelation, but to a much lesser degree.

Heterozygous carriers of the sickle cell trait show no abnormality of erythrocyte morphology, life span, or function, except under certain extenuating circumstances, such as severe hypoxia. At the tips of the papillae in the renal medulla a number of factors combine to produce an optimal environment for erythrocyte sickling. The region is hypoxic and acidotic, with a high salt concentration. Acidosis, by shifting the oxygen dissociation curve to the right, promotes sickling, whereas alkalosis inhibits it. The gelation of deoxy Hb S is also highly dependent on the intracellular hemoglobin concentration, which is raised as water passes out of erythrocytes during their movement through a hyperosmolar environment. As a result, episodes of sickling within the renal medulla may be incurred in individuals with sickle cell trait or other sickle hemoglobinopathies, leading to infarction and hematuria. Low molecular weight phosphates (inorganic phosphate as well as 2,3-DPG) also promote sickling by decreasing the oxygen affinity of the hemoglobin.

Sickle cell anemia is usually a severe disease in which erythrocytic sickling causes chronic hemolytic anemia in a setting of vaso-occlusive phenomena that may affect any organ of the body (Warth and Rucknagel, 1983). Periodic bouts of occlusion of the microvasculature in one or several parts of the body cause "painful crises," which at their worst produce prolonged excruciating pain, sometimes associated with fever. Major arteries and veins may also suffer occlusion. There is a serious susceptibility to infection. Organ damage is cumulative over the years. Death, if not caused by infection, may come unannounced from a major occlusion affecting a vital function, or it may come in more chronic fashion from gradual failure of any one of several organs, such as liver, kidney, or heart. The sickle variants Hb SC disease and Hb S thalassemia also suffer vaso-occlusive phenomena, but symptoms are usually milder. Carriers of sickle cell trait are asymptomatic except for an incidence of hematuria due to renal infarction.

Vascular changes occur in reaction to erythrocytic sickling. These changes are demonstrable in the kidney and are presumably etiologically related to a renal concentrating defect that cannot be reversed in adults despite exchange transfusion of normal for sickle erythrocytes. Vascular changes are also present in the eye, and retinal aneurysms leading to vitreous hemorrhage cause blindness, a complication particularly associated with Hb SC disease.

Therapy over the years has been essentially symptomatic. Acidosis is treated, hydration ensured, and occasionally the sickled erythrocytes replaced by normal transfused cells as a temporary expedient. The search for a pharmacologic agent that would prevent sickling has been elusive. Methemoglobin and such liganded states of hemoglobin as carboxyhemoglobin and cyanmethemoglobin all assume the oxy R configuration and therefore do not sickle, but these altered states of hemoglobin do not function in oxygen transport. Treatment of Hb S erythrocytes with cyanate results in a carbamylation of the hemoglobin molecules that not only inhibits sickling but also results in a marked improvement in the life span of the treated erythrocytes. Cyanate is an example of a class of antisickling agents that inhibit sickling by raising the oxygen affinity of the chemically altered hemoglobin. Carbamylation, alkylation, amidination, and other chemical modifications of hemoglobin may also introduce new configurations at critical contact sites on the molecular surface, causing steric hindrance to fiber formation, much in the same manner that the mutant hemoglobins Hb C Harlem and Hb Korle-bu inhibit sickling. Among the growing list of chemicals that are being found to have significant in vitro antisickling effects, none has yet reached the stage of clinical usefulness in the prevention or reversal of sickling in patients.

Individuals homozygous for Hb C have a mild chronic hemolytic anemia associated with splenomegaly (Fabry et al., 1981). The pathogenesis of the hemolysis apparently lies in the fact that this abnormal hemoglobin spontaneously crystallizes at a slightly lower concentration than Hb A. As red cells age in the circulation they undergo water loss, with concomitant increase in the intracorpuscular concentration of hemoglobin to values approaching 36 gm. per 100 ml. Hb A does not begin to crystallize into an insoluble state until its concentration is over 40 gm. per 100 ml., but Hb C begins to develop this change in physical state at the values physiologically approached during red cell aging in the circulation. At this point, the cell becomes rigid and is subject to entrapment and destruction. The presence of this abnormal hemoglobin within erythrocytes causes a prominent tendency for the central deposition of a mass of hemoglobin into a "target cell" configuration. Intracellular crystals are readily demonstrable in vitro by suspension of the erythrocytes in hypertonic saline, which raises intracorpuscular hemoglobin concentration, or in vivo after removal of the spleen. Heterozygotes have fewer target cells and do not show signs of significant hemolysis.

The pathogenesis of Hb E disease presumably resembles that of Hb C.

Nongenetic Structural Alterations. As red cells age in the circulation, glucose becomes attached to the N-terminal valines of one or both beta chains of hemoglobin in an irreversible ketoamine linkage. Older erythrocytes contain a higher level of glycosylated hemoglobin than young. The average value in normal individuals is about 7 percent of the total hemoglobin. Several different glycosylated components are present, about one third hemoglobins A_{1a} and A_{1b}, and the remainder Hb A_{1c}. The oxygen affinity of the modified hemoglobin is increased because of impaired binding of 2,3-DPG at the blocked N terminus. The level of glycosylated hemoglobin is approximately doubled in patients with diabetes mellitus. Following its level in diabetics may provide a more valid index of the adequacy of treatment than serial blood sugar measurements (Koenig and Cerami, 1980).

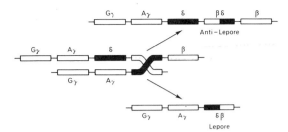

Figure 2–80 Hemoglobin Lepore, an example of a product of a fusion gene. Allelic chromosomes become misaligned. Crossover produces a fusion gene. Lepore hemoglobins resemble δ chain at their amino terminals and β chain at their C terminals. Anti-Lepore hemoglobins have the reciprocal structure, with β structure at their amino terminals. Several different Lepore hemoglobins have been described that differ from one another at the exact point of crossover. Also shown are the positions on the chromosome of the fetal globin genes Gγ and Aγ. (From Wood, W. G., et al.: Progr. Hematol., *10*:43, 1977.)

Hemoglobinopathy Due to Quantitative Defects

The thalassemias are a heterogeneous group of disorders, usually inherited, characterized primarily by a deficiency in the rate of synthesis of specific globin chains (Benz and Forget, 1982). The deficit of one subunit may bring about an imbalance with surplus of another.

The structure-rate hypothesis as conceived by Itano (1957) postulated that the structure of an abnormal globin chain was an important factor that determined its synthetic rate. The fact that Hb S was synthesized at a slightly less efficient rate than Hb A provided support for this theory. Two types of rare structural alterations cause a marked slowing of their synthetic rate. One affects β chain production, and the other α. The first of these, Hb Lepore, is a globin chain that is a hybrid polypeptide consisting of a portion of the δ chain connected to a portion of the β chain to make a completed globin subunit of normal chain length that pairs with α chains in the completed tetrameric hemoglobin molecule. This hybrid globin subunit is the product of a fusion gene that presumably first originated in prior generations by a crossover occurring between homologous chromosomes slightly displaced during synapsis. Several different types of Lepore hemoglobins have been described, differing from one another in the proportion of the molecule that resembles the δ chain (Fig. 2–80). Protein synthesis is normally initiated at the N-terminal end of the molecule, which in the Lepore hemoglobins is always that of the δ portion of the chain, and thus its synthesis takes on the slow character of normal δ chain production. The deficit results in a β-thalassemia syndrome.

Hb Constant Spring, described by Milner and coworkers (1971), is found in trace quantities in association with α-thalassemia states. In contrast to the normal α chain, which has 141 amino acids, this abnormal hemoglobin carries a defect in chain length that causes it to grow to an abnormal length of 172 amino acids—31 too long. The pathogenetic basis of the defect appears to lie in the fact that at position 142 of the messenger RNA, where the triplet codon normally signals "terminate," a mutation signals instead for the insertion of a specific amino acid. Additional amino acids are then added until the next terminating codon is read from the messenger RNA strand at position 173. The defect in chain termination markedly slows its synthetic rate and causes an α-thalassemia syndrome.

Most thalassemia syndromes are not associated with abnormalities in the primary structure of the globin chains. Deletion is the most frequent cause of α-thalassemia, often arising from unequal crossing over by a mechanism similar to that already described for Hb Lepore. A number of different single-base substitutions lead to decreased or absent globin chain production. Examples are (1) conversion of a codon from one that codes for insertion of a specific amino acid in the polypeptide

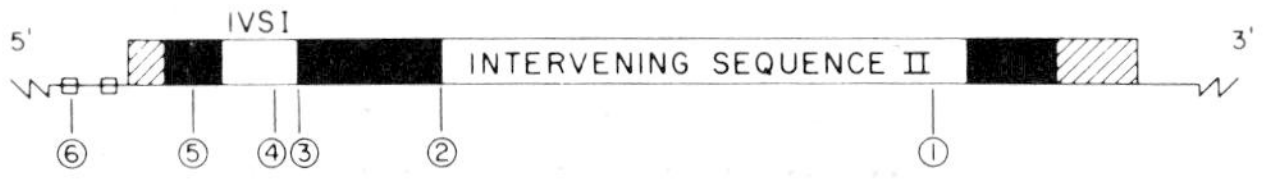

LESION	CONSEQUENCE	SYNDROME	β mRNA
1. Deletion 3'-end into IVS II	No "spliceable" mRNA precursor	β°-thal	Absent
2. Mutation "GT" splice site	β mRNA precursor not processed	β°-thal	Absent
3. Premature terminator codon codon 39	Translation stops prematurely (? mRNA unstable)	β°-thal (Sardinia)	Reduced
4. Base substitution in IVS I	Alternative splice site created; causes abnormally processed mRNA product retaining some IVS I : not translatable.	β⁺-thal	Reduced Abn'l mRNA detectable
5. Like (3), codon 17	Same as (3)	β°-thal (Asia)	Reduced
6. Alteration CCAAT box (CCAAC)	? Inefficient transcription	Normal δ gene ?Hb Lepore	Greatly reduced

Figure 2–81 Examples of gene lesions in β-thalassemia. Each encircled number represents a nucleotide base substitution that markedly reduces the rate of β chain production. (From Benz, E. J., Jr., and Forget, B. G.: Ann. Rev. Med., 33:368, 1982.)

chain to one that instead signals for premature termination; (2) substitution at the splice site of an intervening sequence that prevents normal mRNA processing; and (3) introduction of a false splice site in the middle of an intervening sequence, again causing abnormal mRNA processing. Detailed substitutions are illustrated in Figure 2–81.

Any one or combination of the genes directing globin chain synthesis may hypothetically be affected by a thalassemic lesion causing depressed production rates, but only those affecting the α or the β loci are important. The degree of depression of globin chain formation may be minimal, moderate, or virtually complete, but it is relatively consistent within the affected members of the same family.

In thalassemia trait, the inheritance of normal globin gene loci along with the mutant strain ameliorates the phenotypic expression, and the clinical condition is asymptomatic. Anemia is minimal or mild, the erythrocytes are microcytic and are often present in greater than normal numbers, and the erythrocyte morphology is abnormal. Some thalassemic carrier states are so minimal that they are

completely silent and exhibit no abnormalities whatsoever. The depressed β chain production in the carrier state of β-thalassemia is reflected in an increased proportion of Hb A$_2$ to approximately twice the normal value, with the shortage of β chains altering the ratio of β to δ chain production. A few also have slight elevations of Hb F to about 2 to 6 percent of the total hemoglobin.

Hb F is more elevated and Hb A$_2$ is normal in δβ-thalassemia, in which there is extensive deletion of both the δ and β genes. When the deletion extends still further upstream from the δ locus, the result is a non-thalassemia syndrome called *hereditary persistence of fetal hemoglobin,* in which Hb F production is even greater. These clinical syndromes suggest that somewhere on the DNA between the γ and δ genes there lies a region concerned with the normal suppression of the γ gene, deletion of which results in continued production of fetal hemoglobin. In carriers of α-thalassemia trait, the proportions of Hb A$_2$ and Hb F are not altered, since these hemoglobins, in common with Hb A, are all affected by the shortage of α chains (Weatherall and Clegg, 1981). Table

Table 2–16 HEMOGLOBIN ABNORMALITIES IN THALASSEMIA TRAIT

Type	Hemoglobin A$_2$	Hemoglobin F	Abnormal Hemoglobin
Beta	Increased	Normal or slightly increased	Absent
Delta-beta	Normal	Increased	Absent
Lepore	Normal or decreased	Slightly increased	6%–15% Lepore
Alpha	Normal	Normal	Absent in adults; 1%–6% Bart's in cord blood
Constant Spring	Normal	Normal	1%–2% Constant Spring

Thalassemia is subclassified according to the degree of the genetic deficit of β or α chains. β° is used to designate a more severe defect with absent β chain production. β⁺ is milder. In analogous fashion, α–1 is more severe, and α–2 is milder. (See text.)

2–16 summarizes the hemoglobin abnormalities in various types of thalassemia trait.

Homozygosity for β-thalassemia (Cooley's anemia) is associated with little or no capacity to produce β chains (and thus Hb A) because both alleles responsible for β chain synthesis are affected. Hb F becomes the major hemoglobin type produced, usually exceeding 50 percent and often approaching 95 percent of the total. The Hb A and the Hb F are contained in variable mixtures in the erythrocyte population. The better-filled cells containing more Hb F have a more prolonged survival time than the more empty Hb F–poor cells. The pathogenesis of the severe hemolysis is explained by imbalanced production of α as compared with β chains. The surplus unpaired α chains are extremely unstable and precipitate readily within nucleated erythroid precursor cells, causing marked intramedullary destruction (i.e., ineffective erythropoiesis). Those cell lines that retain a greater capacity of γ chain production not only are better filled with hemoglobin but also have fewer surplus unpaired α chains and thus are less rapidly hemolyzed. The patients are severely anemic, are transfusion-dependent beginning in early childhood, develop massive enlargement of the spleen and of the liver, show prominent signs of extramedullary hemopoiesis, and suffer physical disfigurement because of the bone deformity brought on by the extreme erythroid hyperplasia in the marrow. Iron overload ultimately causes failure of the heart or liver, along with diabetes mellitus. Some apparently homozygous patients have a much milder anemia because one or both of their inherited thalassemic genes are mild or minimal. Patients in such a state, designated *thalassemia intermedia,* are not transfusion-dependent but over the years are apt to develop hemochromatosis.

There are four gradations of severity of α-thalassemia, depending on the number of α gene loci deleted. When all four loci are absent $(--/--)$ the result is a lethal condition of Oriental newborns presenting with hydrops and erythroblastosis fetalis. Because of the lack of α chains, there is no fetal or adult hemoglobin but instead nearly 100 percent Hb Bart's (γ_4), a hemoglobin that lacks α chains and therefore has an oxygen affinity too great to function in oxygen delivery. When three α loci are deleted $(--/-\alpha)$, the newborn has about 20 percent Hb Bart's and grows up to develop Hb H disease. Hb H (β_4) also cannot function in oxygen transport. Hb H is unstable and precipitates in circulating red cells, causing a hemolytic anemia associated with microcytic erythrocytes. Individuals who lack two α loci may have the deletions either on the same chromosome $(--/\alpha\alpha)$ or on the opposite one $(-\alpha/-\alpha)$. In either case, the result is a mild microcytic anemia typical of thalassemia trait. The presence of both deletions on the same chromosome is especially characteristic of Oriental populations and is a prerequisite for the occurrence of the more severe α-thalassemia syndromes described previously. The single gene deletion $(\alpha\alpha/-\alpha)$ causes little or no red cell abnormality, and most of those who inherit it are "silent carriers." The two-gene deletion is called α-thalassemia-1 trait. It is associated with about 5 percent Hb Bart's at birth. The single gene deletion causes about 2 percent Hb Bart's in the cord blood at birth. It is designated α-thalassemia-2 trait.

From the large number of different types of thalassemia affecting the α and β genes, it is evident that a large variety of genetic combinations can be inherited. A few examples of such gene combinations are given in Table 2–17.

Prenatal Diagnosis

One of the practical spinoffs of the advanced genetic technology previously described has been the development of accurate methods for diagnosing hemoglobinopathy during early intrauterine life. The earlier methods used minute samples of fetal blood obtained by amniocentesis or by direct fetoscopy. The pattern

Table 2–17 SOME EXAMPLES OF COMBINATIONS OF THALASSEMIA GENES

Type	Hemoglobin A₂	Hemoglobin F	Abnormal Hemoglobin
Homozygous beta	Normal, decreased, or increased	10%–90% (usually above 35%)	Free alpha chain
Homozygous alpha-1*	Absent	Absent	80%–90% Bart's; remainder H and Portland
Alpha-1 alpha-2	Decreased	Normal	3%–30% H; 0%–5% Bart's
Homozygous delta-beta	Absent	100%	None reported

*These values relate to the newborn. All other values are beyond the newborn period.

of globin chain synthesis was then characterized from the pattern of incorporation of radioactive amino acids. More recently, advances in recombinant DNA technology have permitted accurate diagnosis on nonerythroid fetal cells, such as amniotic fluid fibroblasts and chorionic villi (Boehm et al., 1983). A variety of restriction endonucleases are available to carry out gene analysis, permitting accurate diagnosis of sickle cell anemia or of homozygous thalassemia syndromes early during intrauterine life (Pirastu et al., 1983). Direct identification of deletions or base substitutions including the sickle mutation, have been accomplished. In addition, phenotypically silent DNA polymorphisms that are closely linked to abnormal globin loci have also been used to identify the globin genotype in the fetus. These advances in clinical diagnosis have in turn permitted informed decisions to be made about therapeutic abortion.

Hemoglobinopathy: Population Genetics

Inherited abnormalities of globin chain structure or production rate sporadically affect individuals from all population groups, but by far the most frequently affected are people from tropical or subtropical regions. Incidence figures are highest in Africa, the Mediterranean Basin, the Near and Middle East, and Southeast Asia. Hb S trait reaches its highest frequency in Africa, where it affects 20 to 30 percent or more of the population in regions of West, Central, and East Africa. There is also a significant incidence in the Mediterranean countries and in localized regions of Arabia and India. Hb C trait has a peak prevalence of 10 to 20 percent among West Africans in the region of Ghana. Hb E attains a comparable frequency in areas of Southeast Asia. The α- and β-thalassemia genes are relatively frequent throughout the entire "hemoglobinopathy belt." In the Mediterranean countries, β-thalassemia is more prevalent, with an incidence of about 5 to 15 percent in regions of Italy and Greece. In southeast Asia, α-thalassemia is the more common type, affecting 25 percent of the people of Thailand. African and American blacks also have a high incidence of both types of thalassemia trait. In the United States, about 28 percent of blacks have α-thalassemia trait, most of them silent carriers.

References

Ballas, S., Lewis, C. N., Noone, A. M., et al.: Clinical, hematological, and biochemical features of Hb SC disease. Am. J. Haematol., *13*:37, 1982.

Benz, E. J., Jr., and Forget, B. G.: The thalassemia syndromes: models for the molecular analysis of human disease. Ann. Rev. Med., *33*:363, 1982.

Beris, P., Graf, J., and Miescher, P. A.: Primary acquired sideroblastic and primary acquired refractory anemia. Semin. Hematol., *20*:101, 1983.

Boehm, C. D., Antonarakis, S. E., Phillips, J. A., III, et al.: Prenatal diagnosis using DNA polymorphisms. N. Engl. J. Med., *308*:1054, 1983.

Bottomley, S. S.: Sideroblastic anemia. Clin. Haematol., *11*:389, 1982.

Charlton, R. W., and Bothwell, T. H.: Iron absorption. Ann. Rev. Med., *34*:55, 1983.

Chisholm, J. J., Jr.: The continued hazard of lead poisoning. Hosp. Pract., *8*(11):127, 1973.

Cook, J. D.: Clinical evaluation of iron deficiency. Semin. Hematol., *19*:6, 1982.

Danford, D. E.: Pica and nutrition. Ann. Rev. Nutr., *2*:303, 1982.

Edwards, C. Q., Dadone, M. M., Skolnick, M. H., and Kushner, J. P.: Hereditary hemochromatosis. Clin. Haematol., *11*:411, 1982.

Fabry, M. E., Kaul, D. K., Raventos, C., et al.: Some aspects of the pathophysiology of homozgous Hb CC erythrocytes. J. Clin. Invest., *67*:1284, 1981.

Finch, C. A., and Huebers, H.: Perspectives in iron metabolism. N. Engl. J. Med., *306*:1520, 1982.

Goldberg, A., and Moore, M. R.: The porphyrias. Clin. Haematol., *9*:225, 1980.

Harris, J. W.: Notes and comments on pyridoxine responsive anemia and the role of erythrocyte mitochondria in iron metabolism. Medicine, *43*:803, 1964.

Huebers, H. A., and Finch, C. A.: Transferrin: Physiologic behavior and clinical implications. Blood, *64*:763, 1984.

Itano, H. A.: The human hemoglobins; Their properties and genetic control. Adv. Prot. Chem., *12*:216, 1957.

Koenig, R. J., and Cerami, A.: Hemoglobin A$_{1C}$ and diabetes mellitus. Ann. Rev. Med., *31*:29, 1980.

Lee, G. R.: The anemia of chronic disease. Semin. Hematol., *20*:61, 1983.

Mahaffey, K. R., Annest, J. L., Roberts, J., and Murphy, R. S.: National estimates of blood lead levels—United States 1976–1980. N. Engl. J. Med., *307*:573, 1982.

Milner, P. F., Clegg, J. B., and Weatherall, D. J.: Hemoglobin H disease due to a unique hemoglobin variant with an elongated alpha-chain. Lancet, *1*:729, 1971.

Murayama, M.: Molecular mechanism of red cell "sickling." Science, *153*:145, 1966.

Pirastu, M., Kan, Y. W., Cao, A., et al.: Prenatal diagnosis of β-thalassemia. N. Engl. J. Med., *309*:284, 1983.

Propper, R., and Nathan, D.: Clinical removal of iron. Ann. Rev. Med., *33*:509, 1982.

Schafer, A. I., Cheron, R. G., Dluhy, R., et al.: Clinical consequences of acquired transfusional iron overload in adults. N. Engl. J. Med., *304*:319, 1981.

Warth, J. A., and Rucknagel, D. L.: The increasing complexity of sickle cell anemia. Progr. Hemat., *13*:25, 1983.

Weatherall, D. J., and Clegg, J. B.: The Thalassaemia Syndromes. Oxford, Blackwell Scientific Publ., 1981.

Wishner, B. C., Ward, K. B., Lattman, K. E., and Love, W. E.: Crystal structure of sickle cell deoxyhemoglobin at 5 Å resolution. J. Mol. Biol., *98*:179, 1975.

Survival Disorders

GENERAL SIGNS OF HEMOLYSIS

After a 4-month trip through the streams and bogs of the circulation, the normal erythrocyte ends its life span and is ingested by macrophages. Its death is heralded by cellular changes of aging: loss of surface membrane, decrease of cell water, and decline in activity of several enzyme systems. Premature disappearance of erythrocytes either by hemorrhagic loss from the circulatory compartment or by hemolysis may lead to anemia. Hemolysis occurs when the cell itself is intrinsically defective or when the milieu in which it is bathed contains noxious factors.

When the life span of the erythrocyte is only slightly shortened, the consequence may not be of significance. However, in severe hemolytic states a red cell life span of only $\frac{1}{10}$ to $\frac{1}{20}$ the normal period of 120 days severely strains the capacity of the bone marrow to sustain erythroid cell production at a rate sufficient to maintain a circulating hemoglobin concentration compatible with health. The production of erythroid cells in the marrow is increased to meet the demands of increased erythrocyte turnover. This is reflected in hyperplasia of the erythroid precursor cells. Marrow normally occupied by fat is converted to hypercellular tissue. The proportion of erythroid to granulocytic precursors is increased. Young reticulocytes and sometimes nucleated erythroid cells are released into the circulation. The bone marrow is able to increase red cell production to a limited degree—about six to eight times the normal rate. Therefore, it is possible to compensate for shortened erythrocyte life spans that are $\frac{1}{6}$ to $\frac{1}{8}$ normal.

The hemolytic state is thus not necessarily associated with severe anemia. Indeed, the term *compensated hemolysis* is used to describe hemolytic states that are not associated with anemia at all. However, it is still not clear how the bone marrow, in the absence of the stimulus of anemic hypoxia, maintains a rate of red cell production high enough to compensate fully for the reduced erythrocyte life span.

Acute hemolysis causes a rapid reduction in red cell mass because the bone marrow is caught off guard; there is a 4- to 5-day delay before production is geared up in response to the anemia.

When chronic hemolysis is associated with anemia, the reduced red cell mass turning over at a faster rate represents the balance between production and destruction in a steady-state condition. Limitations upon production may cause anemia even when the degree of erythrocyte hemolysis is moderate. Such limitation occurs secondary to other diseases, such as neoplastic or inflammatory states, or to deficiency of essential nutrients, especially iron and folate. The acute *aplastic crisis* is the most critical imbalance between production and destruction—erythroid precursors suddenly vanish from the marrow, the reticulocyte count drops, and soon after there is a rapid increase in the degree of anemia as the remaining short-lived erythrocytes, no longer being replenished from the marrow, disappear from the circulation. Fortunately, the period of aplasia of red cell formation, probably triggered by a minor infection, is usually short-lived, and recovery is the rule. Similar infections may very likely arrest erythropoiesis in normal individuals, but during the period of marrow arrest the fall in blood count is imperceptible because of the longevity of normal erythrocytes.

In the Wright-stained peripheral blood film, reticulocytes are recognized as polychromatophilic macrocytes. Microspherocytes are small, round, densely stained erythrocytes seen in a variety of hemolytic states. Regular and irregular distortions of the erythrocyte membrane into spurs and burrs and the fracturing of erythrocytes into bits and pieces suggest metabolic or mechanical damage.

The biochemical signs of hemolysis are those of the release and breakdown of the pigment of the red cells. Erythrocyte destruction within the confines of the circulatory system (intra-vascular hemolysis) causes leakage of hemoglobin directly into the plasma. Phagocytosis of intact erythrocytes or of erythrocyte fragments releases hemoglobin inside the phagocytic macrophages, where the heme is degraded to bilirubin (extravascular hemolysis). Hemolytic states are not exclusively intra- or extravascular, but when extensive cell damage causes the erythrocytes to "fall apart" in the circulation, the signs of hemoglobin release into the plasma and urine are marked. Hemoglobin released from erythrocytes into the circulation is first bound to haptoglobin, a plasma protein with α_2 electrophoretic mobility (Fig. 2–82). The complex of hemoglobin with haptoglobin is then rapidly cleared from the plasma into the hepatocytes, promptly reducing the plasma concentration of haptoglobin to near absent levels. Thus, a reduction of the plasma haptoglobin concentration (and of the α_2 fraction of the serum proteins) is often observed in hemolytic states, regardless of pathogenesis. Haptoglobin concentration, however, is subject to rather pronounced increases secondary to many inflammatory and neoplastic states, and its final level represents a balance between those factors promoting its synthesis and those producing its degradation, such as hemolysis. Haptoglobin normally is capable of binding hemoglobin to the extent of about 100 mg. per 100 ml. plasma. When the haptoglobin-binding capacity is exceeded, hemoglobin is lost in the urine. Haptoglobin serves the purpose of conserving iron by preventing its loss in the urine as heme. Oxidized heme, split apart from its

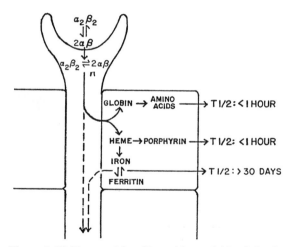

Figure 2–83 The renal handling of hemoglobin. Subunit dissociation into lower molecular weight components permits glomerular filtration. Some of the filtered hemoglobin is taken up into the epithelial cells of the tubules and degraded. The released iron is incorporated into ferritin and hemosiderin. Shedding of renal tubule cells causes persistence of hemosiderinuria for some time after hemoglobinuria has stopped. (From Bunn, H. F., and Jandl, J. H.: J. Exper. Med., *129*:925, 1969.)

globin bond, may also be detected bound to hemopexin, a β-globulin of the plasma, as well as to albumin (as methemalbumin), giving the plasma a dirty brown color. Heme bound to hemopexin is also taken up into the hepatic parenchymal cells. Release of the red cell isozymes of lactic dehydrogenase, LDH-1 and LDH-2, is frequently sufficient to elevate the serum levels of these enzymes.

The detection of free hemoglobin in the plasma and urine indicates that the haptoglobin-binding capacity has been exceeded and that the degree of intravascular hemolysis has been extensive. The free plasma hemoglobin, unattached to high molecular weight haptoglobin, is readily filtered through the glomerulus. Some passes through directly to produce urine positive for the presence of heme pigment. However, hemoglobin is also resorbed into the epithelial cells of the tubules, where its iron is removed and deposited within the cell as ferritin and hemosiderin. These iron-rich proteins are then sloughed with the normal loss of tubule epithelial cells into the urine, where they can be detected in the sediment by the Prussian blue reaction for iron (Fig. 2–83). Hemosiderinuria is a valuable sign that the patient either is suffering from intravascular hemolysis or has recently done so. After the patient's recovery from an acute intravascular hemolytic episode, the urine stain for hemosid-

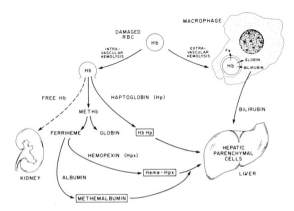

Figure 2–82 Extra- and intravascular disposal of erythrocytes. Intact erythrocytes and cell fragments are removed by extravascular uptake into phagocytic macrophages. Hemoglobin products leaked directly into the circulation are bound to several plasma proteins and redirected into hepatocytes. "Surplus" free hemoglobin is excreted in the urine.

erin will remain positive for some days after hemoglobinuria has stopped.

Myoglobinuria can be distinguished from hemoglobinuria by the solubility of myoglobin at 80 percent ammonium sulfate and by its inability to bind haptoglobin.

Jaundice is a common sign of hemolysis. Often the degree is subclinical and cannot be detected except by chemical measurement of the serum bilirubin concentration. The degree of jaundice is never intense; total serum bilirubin concentrations in excess of 6 mg. per 100 ml. suggest malfunction of the liver or of its biliary drainage system, since the capacity of the normal liver to process bilirubin is immense. Hemolytic jaundice involves primarily elevation of the unconjugated bilirubin (or indirect-reacting fraction). It circulates bound to plasma albumin and therefore is not lost in the urine. After its transport to the liver, bilirubin is processed by the hepatic cells and converted to the water-soluble diglucuronide derivative (direct-reacting, or conjugated), which is the major form excreted in the bile. A portion of this conjugated bilirubin is absorbed and undergoes enterohepatic circulation. Most of it is reduced by colonic bacteria to urobilinogen, which also has an enterohepatic circulation. In hemolysis the output of bile pigments into the intestinal tract is increased in direct proportion to the degree of heme degradation and thus to the extent of the hemolytic process. Measurement of the fecal urobilinogen excretion may be used to quantitate the extent of hemolysis as a function of heme degradation rate, but the procedure is too cumbersome for general use. Urine urobilinogen is likewise increased as a reflection of the increased enterohepatic circulation, but only a small proportion of the total is excreted by this route.

Bilirubin is produced in phagocytic cells throughout the body from degraded heme pigments of a variety of types, chief among which by far is hemoglobin. Phagocytes possess an efficient enzymatic mechanism that rapidly and voraciously strips away the iron for metabolic recycling, digests the globin into its constituent amino acids for re-entry into the body pool, and oxidizes the tetrapyrrole ringed structure of heme into biliverdin (Gemsa et al., 1973). This conversion, mediated by heme oxidase, fractures open one of the four bridges (the α-methene) that hold together the four pyrrole groups into a ringed tetrapyrrole structure. Carbon monoxide is produced in this reaction and is delivered to the lungs for respiratory

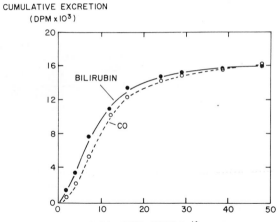

CUMULATIVE EXCRETION (DPM x 10³)

Figure 2–84 Parallel appearance of radioactivity into bilirubin and carbon monoxide after administration of radioactive hematin. (Redrawn from Landaw, S. A., et al.: J. Clin. Invest., *49*:914, 1970.)

excretion, one mole for each mole of heme degraded. Since there is almost no other source of endogenous carbon monoxide, measurement of its production rate accurately quantitates the catabolism of heme compounds and thus also the rate of hemolysis (Fig. 2–84). Biliverdin, a green pigment, is reduced to bilirubin, which is then transferred from the phagocytic cells to the hepatic parenchymal cells for conjugation.

The load of heme pigments normally presented for degradation comes chiefly from dying senescent erythrocytes, but about 15 percent is from other sources, some from the liver and some from the bone marrow (Fig.

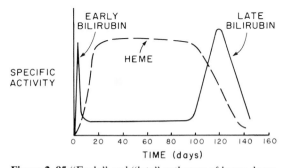

Figure 2–85 "Early" and "late" pathways of heme degradation into bilirubin. The graph illustrates in a normal subject the incorporation of a radioactive precursor of heme into circulating red cells (interrupted line) and into "early" and "late" bilirubin, the latter corresponding to completion of the life span of the labeled erythrocytes. Early bilirubin originates from both bone marrow and hepatic heme. It is markedly increased in conditions associated with ineffective erythropoiesis.

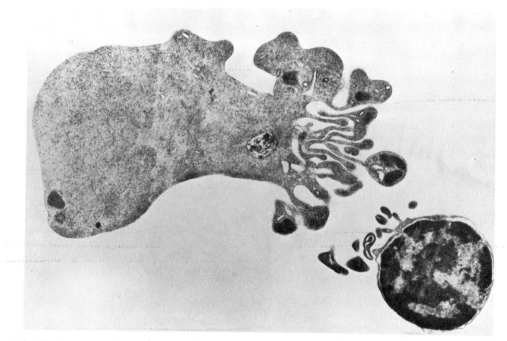

Figure 2–86 The extrusion from an erythyroid precursor of a nucleus covered with a shroud of hemoglobin, leaving behind a reticulocyte containing mitochondria and ribosomes. (Reproduced from the Sandoz-Monograph, The Life Cycle of the Erythrocyte. M. Bessis, Basel, Switzerland, 1966.)

2–85). The hepatic contribution may be increased in porphyria of hepatic origin or following the administration of certain drugs, as phenobarbital, which stimulate the endoplasmic reticulum along with heme synthesis. The bone marrow also produces heme that never reaches the safe haven of the circulating erythrocyte. This marrow heme, destined for early degradation, consists partly of hemoglobin shrouds that veil normoblast nuclei after their extrusion (Fig. 2–86), partly of defective normoblasts destroyed before they gain access to the circulation as mature erythrocytes, and possibly partly of heme that is never incorporated into hemoglobin but is "shunted" into an early catabolic demise. From the foregoing, it is apparent that hepatic or marrow defects can markedly affect the net pattern of heme degradation. The process of intramedullary hemolysis (i.e., ineffective erythropoiesis), so prominent in megaloblastic anemia and in homozygous β-thalassemia, may be the major contributor to heme catabolism and thus to the increased production of carbon monoxide and bilirubin associated with these disorders.

The measurement of red cell survival time would appear to be the most direct approach to the diagnosis of hemolytic disorders, but this measurement presents a number of difficulties from practical as well as theoretical points of view. Not the least of these is the rather long time required, during which the patient should be in the steady state with regard to the maintenance of a constant red cell mass as well as to absence of significant loss of blood by hemorrhage. There are two basic approaches, both of which follow the behavior in the circulation of a tag on the erythrocytes. The first, called the cohort label, employs the use of a radioisotope that is administered and is then incorporated into a cohort of newly formed cells. Examples are isotopes of iron (e.g., ^{59}Fe) and of amino acids (e.g., glycine-2-^{14}C, ^{75}Se selenomethionine). Normally, the cohort tag will appear in the peripheral blood erythrocytes and then rise to a plateau in about 10 days. This plateau is maintained until about 100 days, and at 120 days it reaches a maximum rate of decline as the cohort dies off (Fig. 2–85). Mean erythrocyte survival time can be estimated from such curves, but this method is difficult to carry out and may be hampered by reutilization of these biologically active tags.

The second method, the population or random label, uses a nonphysiologic marker of a representative sample of the entire erythrocyte population. The sample should be uniformly tagged without difference or discrimination as to cell age, pathologic state, or any other cell variable, so that when it is reintroduced into the circulation, a clear picture is obtained of the rate of removal of the population of erythrocytes it represents. Normally, a fixed number of erythrocytes reaches senescence and dies each day; the tag will represent this by a straight-line decline intercepting zero at 120 days, when the last of the tagged cells will have died off. This is an age-dependent pattern of cell destruction. Many hemolytic states are characterized by random destruction of erythrocytes, without regard to their age. A fixed percentage of the remaining cells are destroyed per day; the tag disappears from the circulation at an exponential rate according to first-order kinetics. The time required for disappearance of half the tag (the half-time, or T/2) is the most conventional method of expressing erythrocyte survival time as measured with a population label.

No tags are ideal, but two of the best are diisopropylfluorophosphate ($DF^{32}P$) and sodium chromate ($Na_2^{51}CrO_4$). $DF^{32}P$ attaches to red cell cholinesterase to form a tight bond that lasts for the duration of the erythrocyte's life span; its disappearance rate from the circulation yields a value quite close to the true life span, but the method is inconvenient. $Na_2^{51}CrO_4$ penetrates the red cell membrane and is reduced to the chromic state, and then the chromium tag forms a chelate with the β chain of hemoglobin. Its bond to proteins is not nearly so tight, and it elutes from red cells at a rate of about 1 percent per day, with significant differences in various disease states. Consequently, its disappearance rate from the circulation does not give a true measure of erythrocyte survival but rather a composite of this function minus the elution rate of the chromium. The normal half-time of ^{51}Cr-labeled erythrocytes is 25 to 35 days, a value considerably shorter than the physiologic half disappearance time of 60 days. Despite these patent disadvantages, ^{51}Cr has practical virtues and has gained widespread acceptance as a convenient method for the clinical assessment of erythrokinetics. Since ^{51}Cr is a strong gamma emitter, the accumulation of chromium-labeled red cells can be detected by body surface scanners to determine the degree of splenic participation in excessive red cell destruction.

MEMBRANE FUNCTION AND ENERGY METABOLISM

The biochemistry of the erythrocyte has long been a subject of practical interest in the development of satisfactory methods of pre-serving shed blood intended for transfusion therapy. This deceptively simple cell has also served as a model system in the basic investigation of glycolysis and of the structure and function of cell membranes. Along with the elucidation of the biochemical clockworks of the erythrocyte has come the definition in precise biochemical terms of a large number of different hemolytic states.

The membrane skeleton, clad with approximately equal amounts of protein and lipid, has an important voice in the governance of red cell shape. In comparison with the minimal surface/volume ratio that characterizes a spherical shape, the red cell has excess surface area. The cell uses this excess surface area to become dimpled into a biconcave disk with most of the hemoglobin squeezed into a doughnut-like ring. The preservation of this shape depends on energy expenditure. The extent of the surface area is subject to change; it normally decreases as the cell ages. However, mature erythrocytes, no longer able to synthesize lipid, may undergo volume changes through membrane interaction with the external environment. Rapid passive exchange of free cholesterol (but not esterified cholesterol) takes place between the membrane and the plasma. Phos-

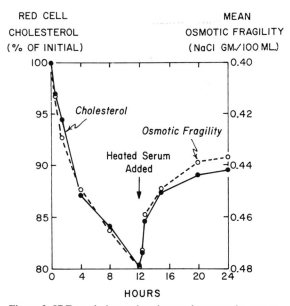

Figure 2–87 Free cholesterol exchanges between the serum and the erythrocyte membrane. After initial incubation with free cholesterol-poor serum, heated serum replete with free cholesterol was added. As the red cell cholesterol decreases, loss of membrane decreases the surface/volume ratio of the cell along with its osmotic resistance. Repletion of the red cell cholesterol reverses this change as the surface/volume ratio returns toward normal. (Redrawn from Cooper. R. A., and Jandl, J. H.: J. Clin. Invest., 48:906, 1969.)

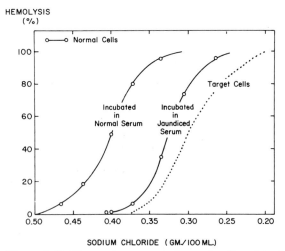

HEMOLYSIS
(%)

Figure 2–88 The erythrocyte membrane is affected by changes in its serum milieu. Osmotic resistance of normal erythrocytes increases when they are incubated in high free cholesterol serum from a patient with obstructive jaundice as compared with incubation in normal serum. The osmotic resistance of the patient's erythrocytes, which showed target cell formation, was likewise increased (dotted line). (Redrawn from Cooper, R. A., and Jandl, J. H.: J. Clin. Invest., *47*:809, 1968.)

pholipid exchange also occurs, but at a much slower rate. One can manipulate the quantity of membrane free cholesterol by varying the free cholesterol content of the surrounding medium (Fig. 2–87). A high level will cause free cholesterol to accumulate in the membrane, thereby increasing its surface area. The increased surface/volume ratio confers upon the erythrocytes a greater distensibility in hypotonic media—that is, their osmotic resistance is increased (Fig. 2–88). The redundant membrane of such cholesterol-replete cells produces a targeted appearance; the area of central pallor has a "bull's-eye" of hemoglobin deposited within. Conversely, suspension of erythrocytes in plasma or serum poor in free cholesterol will cause cholesterol loss from the membrane along with decreased osmotic resistance. Cooper (1980) has reported that other important factors such as the serum lipoproteins modify the plasma-membrane exchange.

A busy traffic hums through the pores of the erythrocyte membrane. Gas transport is high on the priority list in fulfillment of the cell's chief function. An active uptake of glucose is required to power the metabolic machinery. Of great interest—and still considerably a mystery—is the movement of electrolytes across the membrane. The pores, seemingly guarded by positively charged sentries, freely allow anions to pass rapidly into the cell. Permeability to cations is quite another matter; cations diffuse across the membrane much more slowly (Sweadner and Goldin, 1980). To oppose this slow, passive diffusion of cations, an active pumping mechanism in the membrane maintains concentration gradients of sodium and

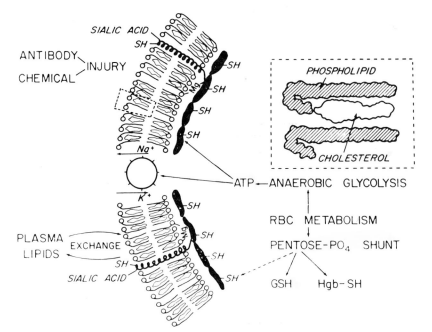

Figure 2–89 Diagrammatic representation of the erythrocyte membrane. (From Weed, R. I., and Reed, C. F.: Am. J. Med., *41*:681, 1966.)

potassium (Fig. 2–89). Sodium is actively extruded from the cell against a concentration gradient of 10 mEq. per liter inside the cell to 145 mEq. per liter in the extracellular plasma. Potassium is pumped into the cell against a concentration gradient from 4.5 mEq. per liter in the plasma to 100 mEq. per liter inside the cell.

The sodium and potassium pumps are linked to preserve a constant intracellular cation concentration. Intracellular cation concentration in turn regulates cell water content and cell volume. Cation loss from excessive egress of potassium causes water loss and cell shrinkage. Cation gain by intrusion of excess sodium brings on water gain and cell swelling. The red cell is also equipped with a calcium pump to maintain low intracellular calcium concentra-

tions against a concentration gradient. The active transport of cations requires ATP as an energy source; it consumes about 15 percent of the erythrocyte ATP production. The membrane contains an ATPase to mediate its utilization there. Energy deprivation may therefore lead to a breakdown of the pumping mechanism, with serious consequences to the osmotic equilibrium of the cell.

The erythrocyte is the principal transporter of oxygen as fuel for the entire body. In addition to the high-energy phosphate bonds of ATP, it requires energy to perform biochemical reductions to protect its own parts from oxidative denaturation by this fuel. There are two major reducing systems. One, utilizing NADH, maintains the iron atoms of hemoglobin in the reduced state, a need imposed by

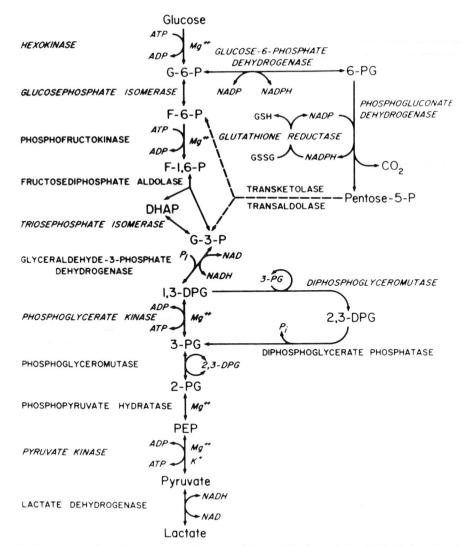

Figure 2–90 Glycolytic pathways in mature erythrocytes. (From Valentine, W. N.: Calif. Med., *108*:280, 1968.)

the continuous slow conversion of hemoglobin to methemoglobin. The reduction is mediated by an enzyme, methemoglobin reductase (Jaffé, 1981). The other reducing system assumes responsibility for maintaining the cell's thiol groups—those of the membrane, the enzymes, and the hemoglobin—in the reduced state. This pathway is mediated through NADPH, which in turn ultimately works through maintaining glutathione in the reduced state.

Glucose is the sole source of energy. The mature erythrocyte consumes 90 percent of its glucose through the anaerobic Embden-Meyerhof pathway, with conversion to lactate as the end product and the net production of two moles of ATP and the reduction of two moles of NAD to NADH per mole of glucose (Fig. 2–90). Normally, about 10 percent of the glucose is consumed through the pentose phosphate pathway with the reduction of two moles of NADP to NADPH per mole of glucose. Under the influence of certain redox compounds (e.g., methylene blue) the amount of glucose processed through this route is markedly increased, a factor of considerable importance in the pathophysiology of hemolysis in patients lacking key enzymes in this pathway.

Reticulocytes possess mitochondria and therefore have an active Krebs cycle for the oxidative metabolism of glucose, but this apparatus is lost as the reticulocyte matures.

A third pathway of glucose metabolism in the erythrocyte does not participate in energy generation, but rather sacrifices energy production to the cause of an important adaptive mechanism for changing hemoglobin oxygen affinity. This pathway, the Rapoport-Luebering shunt, is controlled by diphosphoglycerate mutase (DPGM) and generates 2,3-DPG, which binds to deoxyhemoglobin and reduces its affinity for oxygen. As more 2,3-DPG becomes bound, the free unbound pool is depleted, coaxing DPGM into detouring triose intermediates to replenish the pool. This detour costs the cell a loss of 2 moles of ATP per mole of glucose, but this loss does not appear to have any significant effect on fulfilling total energy requirements.

CLASSIFICATION OF HEMOLYTIC STATES

The seeds of premature erythrocyte destruction may lie either within the erythrocyte or outside in a hostile environment. Hemolytic states are thus readily categorized as *intrinsic* or *extrinsic* disorders, although some represent combinations of both. Most intrinsic defects are inherited; most extrinsic disorders are acquired. A classic experimental approach, no longer in common use, applied cross-transfusion techniques between the patient and a normal individual with compatible blood type. Erythrocytes from a patient with an intrinsic defect will exhibit a shortened survival time not only in the patient's own circulation but also in that of the normal recipient. Erythrocytes from a normal subject will survive as well in the patient's circulation as in his own. However, normal compatible erythrocytes will suffer a shortened survival time in the circulation of a patient with an extrinsic hemolytic disorder. Variations of this approach have also been applied to the study of combined disorders. Thus, tagged erythrocytes from a patient with glucose-6-phosphate dehydrogenase deficiency, an intrinsic drug-sensitive state, will survive quite normally in the circulation of a normal compatible recipient until the offending drug is administered, which will cause hemolysis of the tagged abnormal erythrocytes but not of the normal person's own erythrocytes. The interaction of the intrinsically defective red cells of hereditary spherocytosis with the extrinsic splenic environment has been demonstrated by the observation that such erythrocytes, appropriately labeled, will exhibit a shortened survival in the bloodstream of a normal recipient with intact spleen (Fig. 2–91) but a normal survival time in a normal person lacking a spleen.

To establish that a hemolytic state exists,

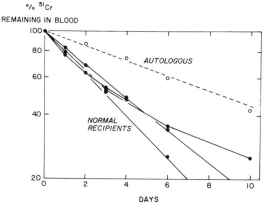

Figure 2–91 The survival of intrinsically defective ^{51}Cr-labeled erythrocytes from a patient with hereditary spherocytosis with intact spleen is even shorter in normal compatible recipients with intact spleen than in the patient. Survival time is normal in the absence of the spleen. (T/2 25 to 35 days.) (Redrawn from Wiley, J. S.: J. Clin. Invest., *49*:666, 1970.)

measurements of the reticulocyte count, the conjugated and unconjugated serum bilirubin, the serum haptoglobin, the serum lactic dehydrogenase and its isozymes, the plasma and urine hemoglobin, and the urine hemosiderin, along with careful morphologic examination of the peripheral blood and bone marrow, should indicate its severity and point to the diagnosis. A second echelon of hemolytic tests may then pinpoint the precise cellular or extracellular defect. These tests include osmotic fragility measured in a graded series of hypotonic NaCl solutions; the autohemolysis of erythrocytes incubated in vitro under sterile conditions; screening for enzyme defects; hemoglobin analysis; tests for immunologic factors, such as the Coombs' antiglobulin, cold agglutinin, and cold hemolysin tests; and tests for the complement-sensitive erythrocytes of paroxysmal nocturnal hemoglobinuria (sucrose hemolysis and acid hemolysin tests). The morphology of the red cells or the clinical circumstances (such as the fact that the patient has cirrhosis or uremia) may alone readily yield the pathophysiologic classification.

Intrinsic Hemolytic Disorders

Membrane Defects. The erythrocyte membrane skeleton preserves the cell's shape and integrity. Inherited defects in the cell's skeletal structure are associated with disorders of erythrocyte shape and survival time (Shohet and Lux, 1984). One rare but intriguing acquired membrane disorder causes exquisite complement sensitivity.

Hereditary spherocytosis (HS) is a disorder of the membrane, but in most cases the biochemical defect remains unknown. In some instances membrane skeletal defects have been found (Palek and Lux, 1983). One of these is defective association of spectrin with protein 4.1 (Fig. 2–3). Another is deficiency in the amount of spectrin. It may turn out that, as in the case of thalassemia, a variety of genetic defects will ultimately be discovered.

The inheritance is usually autosomal dominant, and multiple cases are often found in the same family. In some instances neither parent appears to have the defect. The clinical expression is variable. It may be so mild that discovery is first made incidentally during old age. At the other extreme, it may produce neonatal jaundice or severe hemolytic anemia during childhood. Many affected adults maintain a state of completely compensated hemolysis without significant anemia, but they are sus-

ceptible to a rapid drop in hemoglobin concentration if marrow production is arrested by a minor viral infection or by nutritional deficiency. Viral infections such as infectious mononucleosis may exacerbate anemia by further enlarging the spleen and increasing the hemolytic rate. As with any chronic hemolytic disorder, the development of pigment gallstones is common. The enlarged spleen is the site of trapping and destruction of the rigid spherocytic cells and its removal predictably restores the red cell survival time to normal or nearly normal values, even though the intrinsic red cell defect remains unchanged.

The diagnosis is suspected on the basis of observation of spherocytosis with polychromasia on the stained blood film. Tests for immunohemolytic anemia are negative. The autohemolysis and osmotic fragility tests are abnormal.

The weak membrane structure of the abnormal erythrocyte allows sodium to enter the cell at an increased rate. Osmotic balance can be maintained as long as there is enough glucose to provide sufficient ATP to power the cation pump. Then sodium can be moved out of the cell at a rate equal to its inflow. In a glucose-deprived environment, this need cannot be met and the erythrocyte undergoes osmotic swelling and eventually lysis. This principle is demonstrated by the autohemolysis test. Sterile whole blood is incubated at 37° C for 48 hours. The glucose supply is sufficient to keep normal erythrocytes from hemolyzing significantly, and less than 5 percent hemolysis is observed. The HS erythrocytes consume glucose at a more rapid rate. The glucose supply runs low, and then as much as 20 to 40 percent hemolysis may occur. The addition of extra glucose decreases hemolysis. The presence in the plasma of osmotically active but impermeable molecules, such as sucrose or ATP, will also decrease hemolysis by maintaining better osmotic balance.

The membrane skeleton defect also predisposes a cell to the loss of small membrane fragments. The decrease in membrane surface area without commensurate loss of cell volume forces the erythrocyte to assume a shape that can accommodate a minimal surface/volume ratio—that of a sphere. The spherocytes that form are smaller than normal erythrocytes and are called *microspherocytes* (Fig. 2–92). In stained blood films they are small, round, darkly stained cells lacking in central pallor (Fig. 2–93). They contain hemoglobin at a higher than normal concentration; that is, the mean corpuscular hemoglobin concentration is

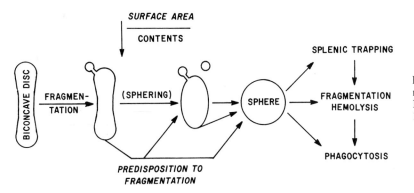

Figure 2–92 Microspherocyte formation. (From Weed, R. I., and Reed, C. F.: Am. J. Med., *41*:681, 1966.)

above the upper limit of normal, 36 gm. per 100 ml. Macrospherocytes are produced in vitro by simple cell swelling, although micro-spherocytes are the hallmark of the spherocytic hemolytic anemias. However, spherocytes of any size will be exquisitely sensitive to osmotic lysis, since they can undergo no further volume increase without membrane rupture.

The diagnosis of hereditary spherocytosis is confirmed by the osmotic fragility test, a measure of the degree of hemolysis of erythrocytes suspended in a graded series of hypotonic NaCl solutions (see Fig. 2–88). Typically, the sigmoid curve is shifted toward a greater osmotic fragility of the erythrocyte population. The microspherocytes show up as a "fragile tail,"

a subpopulation lysing even at slight reductions of the NaCl concentrations below isotonicity. If a normal osmotic fragility curve is obtained, it may be necessary to bring out the abnormality by first incubating the blood for 24 hours. The entire cell population will swell somewhat because of the aforementioned energy crisis in the autohemolysis test and become more osmotically fragile than normal erythrocyte similarly incubated. Thus, the definitive confirmatory procedure for HS should be the osmotic fragility test performed on incubated blood.

The precarious position of the HS erythrocyte in the incubated test tube without added glucose resembles its circumstance in the

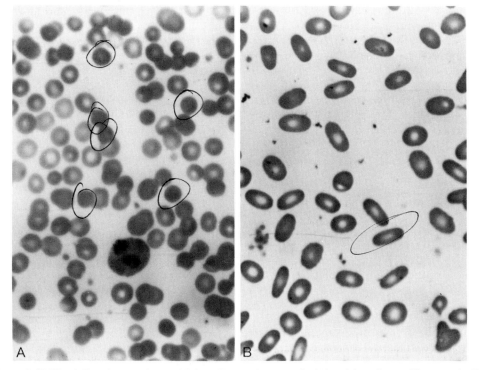

Figure 2–93 Blood films from patients with hereditary spherocytosis *(A)* and hereditary elliptocytosis *(B)*.

spleen. The spleen is an organ of erythrostasis with relatively low glucose concentration and a low pH that impedes glycolysis. The first pass through the spleen may not be fatal to the erythrocyte, but the damage that occurs with repeated passes results in microspherocyte formation. These small round cells lack the elasticity of the normal discoid cells and they ultimately become entrapped by their inability to traverse the small fenestrations between the splenic cords and sinusoids (see Fig. 1–14). No other vascular bed is so deleterious to the survival of the HS erythrocytes. When the spleen is removed, their survival time becomes virtually normal.

Hereditary elliptocytosis is a membrane disorder in which the most commonly described abnormality is defective assembly of spectrin dimers in the formation of the skeletal lattice (see Fig. 2–3). Inheritance is autosomal dominant. In some families, the defect is linked to the genes for the Rh blood factors. It is only about one fifth as frequent as HS. The diagnosis is made from an examination of the peripheral blood film. More than 20 percent of the erythrocytes have an elliptocytic rather than a round shape (Fig. 2–93). Apparently, the erythrocytes are round when they emerge from the marrow as reticulocytes, but they cannot be restored to a normal shape after they are squeezed into elliptocytic shapes during passage through small blood vessels (Fig 2–94). Smaller numbers of elliptocytes are often present in the deficiency anemias, thalassemias, and myeloproliferative syndromes. About 80 percent of patients show little or no hemolysis. The remainder have a condition that clinically resembles HS. They have splenomegaly, and hemolysis is corrected by splenectomy.

Hereditary pyropoikilocytosis is a disorder genetically and biochemically related to hereditary elliptocytosis. In hereditary pyropoikilocytosis, defective assembly of spectrin dimers is even more pronounced and membrane structure is more unstable than in hereditary elliptocytosis. The name of the disorder stems from the susceptibility of the abnormal erythrocytes to heat damage at 45° C. They fragment at this temperature, whereas normal erythrocytes resist heating up to 49° C. One subtype of the disorder is characterized by severe hemolytic anemia during the first year of life, with gradual abatement of the hemolysis as the condition spontaneously converts to typical hereditary elliptocytosis.

Paroxysmal nocturnal hemoglobinuria (PNH) is an acquired defect of the red cell membrane that renders it pathologically sensitive to destruction by the complement system. The onset may occur at any age, and the disease usually has a chronic protracted course. Its name is derived from the fact that intravascular hemolysis occurs at night, causing the first voided morning urine to be darkly colored by its hemoglobin content. In many cases, however, the nocturnal character is not prominent. Periods of exacerbation of the hemoglobinuria may follow infections, exercise, surgery, or other physical stresses. Morbidity and mortality stem from a high incidence of intravascular thrombosis, chiefly venous and often involving the mesenteric and portal venous systems. Some patients become dependent on blood transfusion. Fortunately for them, normal compatible erythrocytes survive normally in their circulation.

The etiology of PNH is unknown, but the disorder is thought to arise as a result of a somatic mutation of the multipotential stem

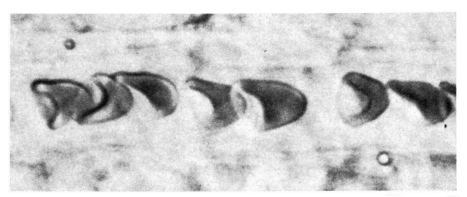

Figure 2–94 Elliptocytic distortion of normal erythrocytes as they move through small capillaries. (From Skalak, R., and Brånemark, P. I.: Science, *164*:717, 1969. Copyright 1969 by the American Association for the Advancement of Science.)

cell (Dessypris et al., 1983). Along with the anemia and the elevated reticulocyte count and signs of intravascular hemolysis, the white cell and platelet counts are commonly reduced. PNH bears an obscure relationship to aplastic anemia, both idiopathic and drug-induced. Interconversions from one syndrome to the other have been well documented. A few patients with PNH have developed acute leukemia. Some exceptional cases have undergone complete and permanent remission.

Although the red cell life span is shortened, the life span of the platelets is normal. Several cellular enzyme deficiencies are associated with PNH, including deficiency of granulocyte alkaline phosphatase and erythrocyte acetylcholinesterase, with unknown pathophysiologic significance.

The diagnosis usually is established by a positive stain of the urinary sediment for hemosiderin and a positive sucrose hemolysis test. The hemosiderinuria is a reflection of the predominantly intravascular nature of the hemolysis. Indeed, urinary losses of iron, up to 20 mg. per day, frequently lead to iron deficiency, otherwise an uncommon complication of hemolytic anemia. The sucrose hemolysis test relies on the promotion of complement fixation to the PNH erythrocyte under the conditions of lowered ionic strength obtained when the cell-plasma suspension is diluted in an aqueous sucrose solution. The reason for using sucrose is to maintain osmotic balance, since the erythrocyte membrane is impermeable to it. Another simple screening test is the observation that gross hemolysis is present in the serum surrounding the retracted clot of freshly drawn PNH blood after 2 hours' incubation at 37° C.; autologous complement lyses the erythrocytes in vitro. The diagnosis of PNH is confirmed by finding a positive acid hemolysin (Ham) test. This test utilizes still another property of complement activation, namely, its optimum at an acid pH of about 6.4. PNH erythrocytes suspended in fresh compatible complement-containing serum properly acidified will show lysis, absent when the serum is heated to 56° C. to inactivate complement. The hemolysis may be enhanced by the addition of crude bovine thrombin preparations (Crosby test), possibly because their heterophile antibody content promotes complement fixation.

There are two or three erythrocyte populations of varying complement sensitivity (Fig. 2–95). Complement activation occurs either by the classical or alternate pathway (Müller-Eberhard, 1977). The molecular defect in PNH

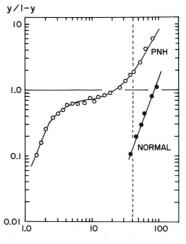

Figure 2–95 Complement sensitivity of normal and PNH erythrocytes. Two cell populations are evident. In some patients, a third population of intermediate sensitivity can be demonstrated. Complement concentration is shown on the horizontal axis, and the proportion of lysed to unlysed erythrocytes is demonstrated on the vertical axis. (Redrawn from Rosse, W. F., et al.: J. Exper. Med., *123*:969, 1966.)

appears to be a lack of specific protein that regulates the quantity of C3b present on the membrane of normal erythrocytes. This cellular deficiency causes accumulation of excessive C3b on the cell surface, activation of C5, and the formation of the cytolytic membrane attack unit C5–9 (Pangburn et al., 1983; Nicholson-Weller et al., 1983; Rosse, 1979).

Enzyme Defects. These disorders may cause either overt hemolysis or hemolytic susceptibility under adverse environmental circumstances. Dacie and his associates (1953) recognized that a group of hereditary hemolytic disorders could be set apart from hereditary spherocytosis, which they otherwise resembled clinically. Their distinguishing features were the presence of few, if any, spherocytes in the peripheral blood and either a less favorable or absent response to splenectomy. They also soon recognized that the "hereditary nonspherocytic hemolytic anemias" did not form a homogeneous group, and they classified them as Type I or Type II, according to the results of the autohemolysis test. Type I showed a modestly positive test with correction by the addition of glucose. Type II showed marked autohemolysis without correction by the addition of glucose. The subsequent development of methods for the assay of red cell enzymes has led to the discovery of a large number of deficiencies which appear to explain the etiology of many of the hereditary nonspherocytic hemolytic anemias (Valentine and Paglia, 1984). Hemolysis has been attributed to deficiency of hexokinase, glucose phosphate isomerase, triose phosphate isomerase, diphosphoglyceromutase, phosphoglycerate kinase, glutathione reductase, pyruvate kinase, and glucose-6-phosphate dehydrogenase, among others. Only the two most common—pyruvate kinase and glucose-6-phosphate dehydrogenase deficiency—will be discussed here.

Pyruvate kinase deficiency, itself a rare disorder, ranks second only to G-6-PD deficiency in frequency among the red cell enzymopathies (Miwa, 1981). The clinical severity is extremely variable, even within a given family. Inherited as an autosomal recessive, the disorder produces hemolysis only in the homozygous state. The heterozygote is hematologically normal, but demonstrates about half the normal enzyme activity. Most patients have splenomegaly. Splenectomy may produce some improvement if the anemia is severe, but the benefit is neither nearly as predictable nor as great as it is in hereditary spherocytosis. The postsplenectomy changes in the peripheral blood also contrast with those in HS. In the latter, the reticulocyte count promptly declines to near-normal levels within a week as the hemolysis is halted, whereas patients with PK deficiency often demonstrate a paradoxical rise in reticulocyte count along with the rise in hemoglobin concentration after splenectomy. This clinical observation has suggested that, as in paroxysmal nocturnal hemoglobinuria, the young erythrocyte population is particularly susceptible to hemolysis. In PK deficiency, the destruction of reticulocytes is in the spleen, whereas in PNH it is primarily intravascular.

Pyruvate kinase stands astride an important ATP-generating step, the conversion of phosphoenol pyruvate to pyruvate. Deficiency thus leads to impairment of the erythrocyte's ability to provide an adequate supply of energy in the form of ATP necessary to power the membrane cation pump as well as other glycolytic reactions. PK-deficient erythrocytes exhibit a positive autohemolysis test of the Type II variety; adding glucose does not correct the positive test because of failure to utilize glucose. The reason for the inordinate susceptibility of reticulocytes to PK deficiency is not entirely clear, but their high energy requirement presumably narrows their margin for survival in the circulation of the spleen. Reticulocytes derive their energy primarily through the high ATP-generating capacity of the oxidative Krebs cycle, which is lost as the reticulocyte matures. The conditions in the spleen—low glucose concentration, low pH, hemoconcentration, plus the delay of the passage of reticulocytes due to their excessive stickiness in comparison with mature erythrocytes—all lead to a lower safety factor, especially when the mitochondria are in the process of being lost. Although, as with many enzymes, PK concentrations are higher in young than in old red cells, the activity is not high enough to prevent the cell damage that then leads to cell destruction in both the liver and spleen.

PK deficiency can be caused by a variety of different molecular defects, as is the rule in hereditary disorders. Some represent qualitative structural defects of the enzyme that lead to low activity; others presumably are a quantitative lack of a structurally normal enzyme. In either circumstance, the result is a lack in enzyme function.

2) *Glucose-6-phosphate dehydrogenase (G-6-PD) deficiency* is by far the most common red cell enzyme abnormality (Motulsky, 1972). A sex-linked condition, it affects 11 percent of American black males. In Mediterranean regions it affects about 1 in 1000, but in certain isolated populations it has higher frequencies, affecting up to 50 percent of male Kurdish Jews, for example. Over 100 genetic variants have already been discovered. From the clinical point of view, three major categories are recognized:

1. Chronic hereditary nonspherocytic hemolytic anemia is rare, occurs sporadically among various ethnic groups (including Northern European populations), and represents a variety of differing molecular genetic defects of the enzyme.

2. The "Mediterranean" variety is one in which the loss of enzyme activity is profound (about 1 percent of normal) but does not produce clinically significant hemolysis until the erythrocyte is exposed to an extrinsic stress, usually of an oxidative nature, to which the erythrocyte, unable to regenerate reduced glutathione, cannot respond in self-defense. The extrinsic stresses include certain drugs as well as such acquired illness as hepatitis and other infections, acidosis, and uremia. Certain deficient individuals in this group are sensitive to fava beans, a sensitivity that may be so severe that it can lead to fatal hemolysis. Genetic factors apparently set these fava bean–susceptible patients apart from the others.

3. The "Negro" variety resembles the Mediterranean type but is less severe, with deficient males having about 10 to 15 percent of the

normal G-6-PD activity. The affected individual also is hematologically normal until exposed to one of the extrinsic stresses mentioned previously (with the exception of fava beans).

Inheritance is sex-linked, and significant hemolytic episodes are thus observed among affected males and the relatively rare homozygous females. The identification of heterozygous females is not always possible because of the wide range of enzyme levels found in this group, with many falling within the normal range, and hemolytic reactions are usually so mild that they pass unnoticed. Beutler and coworkers (1962) showed that random inactivation of the X chromosome in the female leads to a dual red cell population, with some erythrocytes carrying the normal X chromosome and others in the affected heterozygote carrying the G-6-PD–deficient one. The mean enzyme level will depend on the relative proportions of normal and deficient erythrocytes. Tests that utilize intact erythrocytes rather than cell lysates may thus be more successful in detecting female heterozygotes.

The two most common types—the "Mediterranean" and the "Negro"—form relatively homogeneous genetic groupings. In the normal black population there are two electrophoretic types of G-6-PD that differ in only one amino acid site on the molecule. The faster migrating type is designated A and the slower B. Thus, nondeficient normal black males possess either A or B (approximately 18 percent carry A), whereas the female may be homozygous AA or BB or heterozygous AB. The deficient enzyme in blacks has the same electrophoretic mobility as the A type and is therefore called A^-. Whites, including Mediterraneans, have only the B type of G-6-PD, and the Mediterranean type of G-6-PD deficiency is called B^- (Fig. 2–96).

The clinical severity of the drug-induced hemolysis varies from a clinically inapparent episode to a life-threatening event in an individual who may experience flank and abdominal pains, faintness from shock, and dark-colored urine from massive intravascular hemolysis. The antimalarials such as primaquine, pamaquine, and quinine are the best-known offenders, but sulfonamides, nitrofurans, analgesics, sulfones, and vitamin K derivatives are also frequently implicated. The hemolysis begins within 1 to 3 days of drug exposure, preferentially affecting the more aged erythrocytes because their level of enzyme is lower than that in the young cells. The initial change is a rapid drop in hemoglobin concentration in

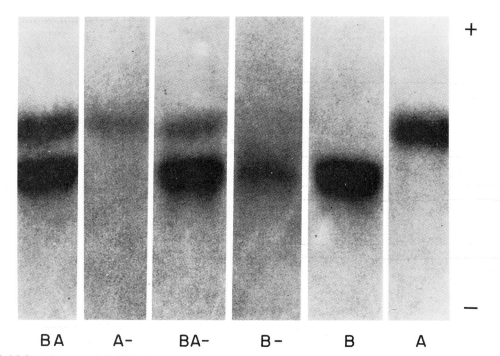

Figure 2–96 Genetic types of G-6-PD deficiency identified by electrophoresis. BA is a normal black female heterozygote and BA − is a deficient black female heterozygote. The other patterns demonstrate normal and deficient male phenotypes. (From Giblett, E. R.: Genetic Markers in Humans Blood. Oxford, Blackwell Scientific Publications Ltd., 1969.)

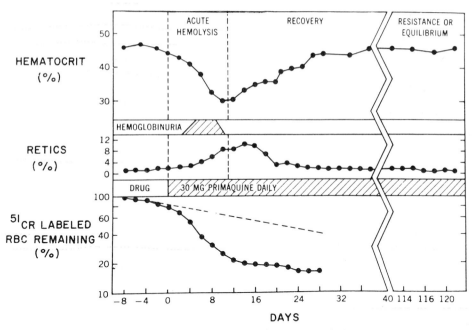

Figure 2–97 Drug-induced hemolysis in a male with G-6-PD deficiency. A period of hemolytic anemia is followed by compensation at higher hematocrit and relative drug resistance due to higher enzyme levels in the young population of erythrocytes. (Redrawn from Alving, A. S., et al.: Bull. WHO, *22*:621, 1960.)

the peripheral blood. A reticulocyte elevation is observed 4 to 5 days later. After 7 to 10 days, the patient enters into a phase of "drug resistance" during which the anemia becomes less pronounced and the patient appears to develop a tolerance to the drug (Fig. 2–97). The explanation for this apparent tolerance is that the younger erythrocytes have a higher enzyme level than the older ones and thus are somewhat better able to cope with the oxidative stress.

Some drugs act directly as oxidants, but most of the chemical agents that provoke oxidative hemolysis do so by interacting with oxyhemoglobin to cause the release of peroxide and other active states of oxygen. The normal erythrocyte meets this oxidative challenge by increasing the rate of glycolysis though the pentose phosphate pathway to maintain NADPH and glutathione in the reduced form. Reduced glutathione, through the good offices of glutathione peroxidase, rapidly detoxifies peroxide. The G-6-PD–deficient erythrocyte cannot respond in this fashion. Its hemoglobin is denatured into insoluble Heinz bodies attached to the inner membrane (Fig. 2–98). Between the increased rigidity caused by these inclusions and the direct oxidative damage wrought on the membrane and other cell constituents, hemolysis ensues. Some chemical agents, phenylhydrazine for example, are so

potent they cause oxidative hemolysis in normal people. In addition to the potency of the agent and its dose, the genetic type of G-6-PD deficiency helps determine the severity of the hemolysis. Pharmacogenetic differences in the population are sometimes important in determining whether or not oxidative hemolysis occurs (Magon et al., 1981). One person may metabolize a drug to a harmless intermediate, whereas another may convert the same agent to a byproduct with toxic oxidative properties.

Direct enzyme assay is commonly used to establish the diagnosis of the G-6-PD–deficient state, but the result is affected by the average age of the red cell population. Thus, immediately following a hemolytic episode, the levels may be nearly normal unless a correction is made for the mean cell age by the simultaneous measurement of another nonaffected enzyme, such as hexokinase, that also has a higher concentration in young than in old red cells. A number of simple screening tests have been devised, with two of the more common in clinical use being the methemoglobin reduction test and the fluorescent spot test. The methemoglobin reduction test takes advantage of the fact that methylene blue establishes a redox bridge between the pentose phosphate pathway and methemoglobin reduction with NADPH as hydrogen donor. Intracellular hemoglobin is first converted to methemoglo-

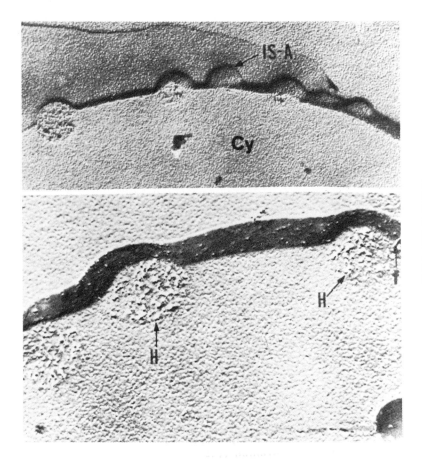

Figure 2–98 Heinz bodies (H) attached to the erythrocyte membrane demonstrated by freeze-etching electron microscopy. Cy = cytoplasm; IS-A = intramembrane surface A. (From Lessin, L. S., et al.: Arch. Intern. Med., *129*:306, 1972. Copyright 1972 by the American Medical Association.)

bin by incubation with sodium nitrite. After addition of methylene blue, normal erythrocytes rapidly reduce the methemoglobin and change color from brown to red. G-6-PD–deficient erythrocytes, unable to increase glycolysis through the pentose phosphate pathway, remain the chocolate-brown color of methemoglobin. The fluorescent spot test is based on the reduction by lysate of NADP to NADPH, which fluoresces under ultraviolet light. G-6-PD–deficient erythrocytes, unable to accomplish this reduction, fail to produce fluorescence in the spot.

Hemoglobin Defects. The role of abnormal hemoglobin in causing erythrocyte damage and premature destruction has already been discussed in a previous section. Some abnormal hemoglobins are so unstable to oxidative stresses that they undergo spontaneous precipitation into insoluble deposits in the red cell, even in the presence of a normal enzymatic machinery. Some are drug-sensitive and in this respect resemble G-6-PD deficiency. The selective destruction of newly formed erythroid cells in homozygous β-thalassemia is reminiscent of a similar preferential susceptibility of

young cells in paroxysmal nocturnal hemoglobinuria and in pyruvate kinase deficiency, but the pathogenetic mechanism is quite distinctive for each of these disorders. Sickle cell anemia, the most common of the hemoglobin diseases, results from a physicochemical alteration of the hemoglobin that produces rigid erythrocytes. The final common pathway in the intrinsic hemoglobin disorders is membrane damage and reduction in cell pliability to the point of entrapment and destruction.

Extrinsic Hemolytic Disorders

Hemolytic conditions are caused by a wide variety of extrinsic physical and chemical factors. Extensive burns cause thermal damage to the erythrocyte membrane, with fragmentation, spherocytosis, and acute hemolysis. Acute poisoning with arsenate or copper and drowning (with hypotonic hemolysis) are other examples of acute hemolytic syndromes in patients suffering severe medical emergencies. Infections produce hemolysis indirectly, as in hypersplenism secondary to miliary tuberculosis or subacute bacterial endocarditis, or directly via invasion of the erythrocyte, as in malaria and bartonellosis. In *Clostridium welchii* septicemia, the organism secretes a phospholipase that attacks the phospholipid backbone of the red cell membrane. The high oxygen tensions used in hyperbaric therapy cause hemolysis by peroxidation of membrane lipids. Chemical hemolysis by phenylhydrazine was once used therapeutically to reduce the red cell mass in patients with polycythemia. This agent, still commonly used to produce hemolytic anemia experimentally in animals, causes a "Heinz body anemia" in normal erythrocytes quite similar to that observed in G-6-PD–deficient individuals given drugs to which they are sensitive.

The types of extrinsic hemolysis of greatest clinical interest from the pathogenetic point of view are those that are caused by mechanical damage and those that are the result of nonimmune or immune plasma factors.

Mechanical Damage. Mechanical hemolysis is vividly illustrated by *march hemoglobinuria,* so called because it was observed in soldiers after their completion of a long march. The hemolysis is intravascular but benign and self-limited. The mechanical damage to the red cells occurs during the physical impact of the soles of the feet on hard surfaces. Ingeniously simple experiments have shown that it can be prevented among track athletes by placing shock absorbing material in the footwear or by running on soft grass instead of hard asphalt or concrete. The syndrome has even been seen in karate fighters, with the damage in these individuals resulting from impact on the palms of the hands as well as the soles of the feet.

Mechanical hemolysis also occurs because of damage to erythrocytes from physical impacts within the circulation. High-pressure turbulence behind a stenotic aortic valve may cause mild cardiac hemolysis even in the patient who has not been operated on. Modern cardiovascular surgery has contributed an important iatrogenic variety of *traumatic hemolysis* from red cell damage in the heart after insertion of prosthetic devices (Marsh and Lewis, 1969). Its presence indicates an abnormal turbulence of blood or an exposed plastic surface not yet covered with endothelium. Examples of underlying causes are a loosened stitch at the base of a valve prosthesis through which a high-pressure jet of blood squirts; a bare Teflon patch used to close a septal defect upon which a regurgitant jet of blood strikes; and "ball variance," a late cause of postoperative hemolysis due to improper valve closure

from slow swelling and distortion of the plastic ball. Technical improvements such as the use of a metal ball or a porcine valve have reduced the frequency of postoperative traumatic hemolysis. Cardiac hemolysis is intravascular. When it is severe, the loss of iron in the urine from the chronic hemoglobinuria and hemosiderinuria leads to iron deficiency and compromises the ability of the bone marrow to compensate for the reduced red cell life span.

Traumatic cardiac hemolysis has been aptly called the *Waring blender syndrome* because the morphologic alterations of the red cells suggest that they have been chopped by the whirling blades of this kitchen apparatus. They are sheared into bits and pieces, and they display pointed and triangular forms, "helmet" shapes, and other distorted contours. Microspherocytes and polychromasia are also present.

These morphologic changes are also a characteristic feature of another group of hemolytic disorders that have in common an occlusive process of the microvasculature and hence have been called the *microangiopathic hemolytic anemias* (Fig. 2–99). The fragmentation has been reproduced experimentally in vitro by forcing red cells through a fibrin meshwork and in vivo by inducing intravascular coagulation in animals with injections of endotoxin or thrombin (Fig. 2–100). The clinical counterparts of these experiments are those conditions characterized by a thrombo-occlusive process in the small vessels, including the various disseminated intravascular coagulation syndromes, hemolytic uremic syndromes, vasculitis, and thrombotic thrombocytopenic purpura (Bukowski, 1982). Fragmentation hemolysis has also been encountered in patients with malignant hypertension or disseminated carcinoma. Since platelets are often consumed in the process, thrombocytopenia is commonly seen together with the signs of mechanical hemolysis.

Nonimmune Plasma Factors. Plasma factors that adversely affect the erythrocyte survival time may be classified as nonimmune and immune. Of the nonimmune factors, the role of the plasma lipids and lipoproteins in the hemolytic anemia associated with liver disease deserves special emphasis.

Anemia in cirrhosis is the result of a combination of factors—blood loss, iron and/or folate lack, and hypersplenism. Even in the absence of these complicating factors, the erythrocyte life span is slightly to moderately reduced. Macrocytosis is a common feature of

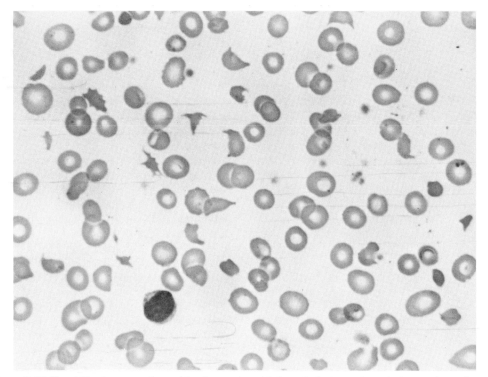

Figure 2–99 Blood film from a patient with microangiopathic hemolysis due to hemolytic uremic syndrome.

hepatocellular disease, often in association with target cells (Fig. 2–101). The increased erythrocyte volume comes from accumulation of excessive lipid in the erythrocyte membrane, free cholesterol to a greater degree than phospholipid (Cooper, 1980). The passive exchange between plasma and red cell membrane favors

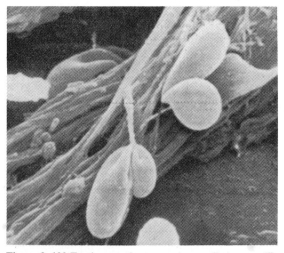

Figure 2–100 Erythrocyte fragmentation on fibrin strands. (From Bull, B. S., and Kuhn, I. N.: Blood, *35*:104, 1970. By permission of Grune & Stratton, Inc., New York.)

uptake into the latter because impairment of cholesterol esterification in liver disease leads to a relative increase in plasma free cholesterol at the expense of cholesterol esters. Indeed, inherited deficiency of the cholesterol esterifying enzyme, lecithyl cholesterol acyl transferase (LCAT), also causes macrocytosis with target cells. The increased levels of plasma free cholesterol secondary to obstruction of the biliary tract affect erythrocytes in a similar way. Marked hemolysis is not a feature of these forms of target cell anemia.

The *spur cell anemia of cirrhosis* is a more severe form of hemolysis. Its name is derived from the pointed thorny projections that protrude from the red cells (Fig. 2–101). This hemolytic disorder is seen in association with fulminating hepatocellular disease and is apparently a more extreme form of membrane accumulation of free cholesterol in excess of phospholipid. Plasma lipoproteins with abnormally high ratios of free cholesterol to phospholipid are important in its pathogenesis. The spur cells are susceptible to entrapment in the enlarged spleen commonly present in cirrhosis. Normal compatible erythrocytes transfused into affected patients soon acquire the membrane defect. Serum from patients with these disorders when added in vitro to normal com-

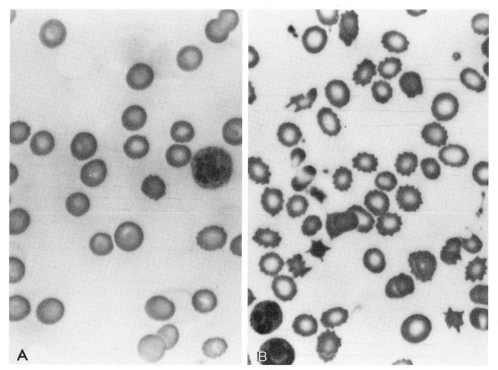

Figure 2–101 Blood films from patients with macrocytosis of cirrhosis, showing some target cells *(A)* and spur cell anemia of cirrhosis *(B)*.

patible erythrocytes will produce macrocytosis and targeting or spur cell formation, as the case may be.

Hereditary acanthocytosis is characterized by absence of plasma β-lipopoteins together with hypolipidemia and abnormal erythrocytes that closely resemble spur cells but are called *acanthocytes*. The degree of hemolysis is mild. Acanthocytosis is occasionally seen in individuals after splenectomy who are otherwise hematologically normal. Spiculated erythrocytes are also seen. The pathogenesis of the erythrocyte shape change under these circumstances remains unexplained.

Immune Plasma Factors. *Immune hemolysis* may take place when antibodies present in the circulation react with antigens on the red cell surface. Hidden behind this deceptively simple theme lie the countless complexities of antigens, antibodies, and complement. *Isoimmune hemolysis* is the result of immunologic reactions between antibodies and antigens that reflect differences between individuals. Examples of isoimmune hemolysis include hemolytic transfusion reactions and immunohemolytic disease of the newborn (i.e., erythroblastosis fetalis). ABO incompatible erythrocytes are destroyed by "natural" isoantibodies normally present in the plasma.

"Irregular" isoantibodies are produced only as a result of previous antigenic exposure, usually from transfusion or pregnancy. An autoantibody produced within a given individual with specificity directed against the individual's own autologous erythrocyte antigens may cause *autoimmune hemolytic anemia*.

The "natural" isoantibodies of the ABO system are predominantly IgM immunoglobulins with potent complement-fixing ability. Isoimmune hemolytic reactions due to accidental transfusion of ABO incompatible erythrocytes are abrupt and life-threatening. The degree of complement fixation is extensive and provokes prompt intravascular hemolysis with hemoglobinemia and hemoglobinuria. Hypotension, disseminated intravascular coagulation, and acute renal failure are common complications.

"Irregular" antibodies directed against other red cell antigens, such as those of the Rh locus (CcDEe), are usually IgG immunoglobulins with a lesser propensity to fix complement. Their activity is maximal at 37°C. Demonstration of their presence requires the Coombs test. They are "warm," "incomplete" antibodies, distinct from the isoantibodies of the ABO system, which agglutinate erythrocytes in saline suspension at room temperature and therefore are "complete." Hemolysis secondary to irregular antibodies is less brisk and may be relatively more extravascular (Conrad, 1981).

The Coombs test is central to the evaluation of immunohemolytic states. It is designed to detect either immunoglobulin or complement components coated on the erythrocyte surface. Coombs reagent, or "antiglobulin serum," is an antiserum raised in animals injected with these human plasma protein constituents. This antiserum, when incubated with erythrocytes coated with immunoglobulin or with complement, causes them to clump together. In general, antiglobulin serum of broad specificity is used, sensitive to the presence of either immunoglobulin or complement. Antiglobulin serum of more restricted specificity will distinguish immunoglobulin from complement on the erythrocyte surface. Antiglobulin serum of even greater specificity permits identification of immunoglobulin subclasses. The "direct" Coombs test is performed on washed erythrocytes suspected of being coated in the circulation. The "indirect" test detects antibodies present in serum by first reacting the serum in vitro with erythrocytes and then testing these washed erythrocytes as described.

Isoimmune hemolytic disease of the newborn is caused by the passage of 7S IgG antibodies across the placental barrier from the maternal circulation into the fetal, where they proceed to combine with antigens present on fetal erythrocytes. Although most of the natural isoantibodies of the ABO system are IgM antibodies too large to cross the placenta, some natural ABO isoantibodies are IgG and can cause erythroblastosis even during the first pregnancy. The usual incompatibility pairing is maternal type O and fetal type A or B. The hemolysis is generally mild and often requires no treatment. The antibody coating on the fetal erythrocyte may be so sparse that the Coombs test is negative.

Transplacental hemorrhage of fetal erythrocytes containing an antigen absent on the maternal red cell surface may raise the production of an irregular isoantibody in the maternal circulation, harmless to the mother but potentially detrimental to fetal erythrocytes once it crosses the placental barrier. Most significant is the D antigen of the Rh locus, although other antigens are occasionally responsible. (Rh positive indicates presence of the D antigen, Rh negative denotes its absence.) Erythroblastosis fetalis due to Rh incompatibility causes severe hemolysis. Intra-

uterine diagnosis is based on observation of an elevated amniotic fluid bilirubin concentration. The direct Coombs test on fetal erythrocytes is always positive. Hemorrhage of fetal erythrocytes into the maternal circulation is an event that most often occurs near term or at the time of labor and delivery. They can be demonstrated by a simple slide elution test that depends on the resistance of fetal hemoglobin to acid elution. Because of this requirement for prior immunization, first-borns are usually spared, assuming that the mother has not been accidentally sensitized by previous transfusion of Rh-incompatible cells.

A number of natural factors operate to reduce the incidence of Rh-incompatibility neonatal hemolytic disease. One of these is the dependence on prior occurrence of fetomaternal hemorrhage. Another is "ABO cancellation." If incompatibility within the ABO system coexists with Rh incompatibility, the rapid removal of the fetal erythrocytes by the natural isoantibodies anti–A and/or anti–B prevents active maternal immunization to the foreign Rh antigen on the fetal erythrocyte.

Following on this observation, it was reasoned that rapid removal of Rh-incompatible fetal erythrocytes from the maternal circulation by the passive administration to the mother of a human gamma globulin preparation, hyperimmune with respect to its anti–D

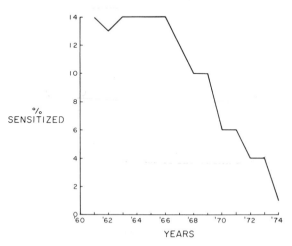

Figure 2–102 Following the routine prophylactic administration of anti Rh hyperimmune gamma globulin to mothers at risk, there has been a dramatic decrease in the incidence of erythroblastosis fetalis due to Rh incompatibility. The vertical axis represents the proportion of the Rh negative mothers sensitized to Rh. Clinical trials began in 1964, and routine use started in 1968. (Redrawn, by permission, from Freda, V. J., et al.: New England Journal of Medicine, *292*:1014, 1975.)

titer, would prevent active maternal sensitization. This has indeed proved the case, and current practice calls for the routine prophylactic use of such gamma globulin preparations shortly after delivery in all Rh negative mothers at risk. Since this form of preventive therapy has been introduced, the incidence of Rh-incompatibility neonatal hemolytic disease has decreased dramatically (Fig. 2–102).

Kernicterus is the most dreaded complication of neonatal hemolytic disease, provided the infant survives the initial crisis. Lipid-soluble unconjugated bilirubin, present in excess of the plasma albumin–binding capacity, is taken up into the nervous tissue, causing toxic damage. Therapeutic strategy is aimed at preventing the build-up of unconjugated bilirubin. This has traditionally been accomplished by exchange transfusion. Other measures include the use of albumin infusion, of pharmacologic agents such as phenobarbital to stimulate the hepatic enzymes to increase the rate of bilirubin conjugation in the immature fetal liver, and exposure to light that appears to convert the bilirubin to less toxic derivatives (McDonagh et al., 1980).

The *autoimmune hemolytic anemias* are classified as *warm antibody* or *cold antibody* types. Warm antibody is an IgG immunoglobulin with maximal activity at 37°C (Petz and Garrity, 1980; Zweiman and Patten, 1982). Its presence on the red cell is demonstrated by a positive Coombs test. It may or may not fix complement. Many of the warm antibodies have a specificity for the "core" antigen of the Rh locus. They react with all Rh phenotypes but not with the rare type Rh null, presumably a genetic deletion of the entire Rh locus.

Cold-reactive autoantibody has increased activity as the temperature is reduced; the highest titer is at 4°C. It is demonstrated by the cold agglutinin test. In this simple procedure, dilutions of the patient's serum are mixed with normal type-compatible erythrocytes and incubated overnight at 4°C. The greatest dilution at which agglutination occurs is recorded. Titers greater than 1:64 are abnormal. Clinical hemolysis is associated with titers in excess of 1:1000, and they usually are considerably

higher, sometimes as high as several million. The cold antibody, with one exception noted further on, is an IgM immunoglobulin. It usually has specificity for the I antigen, present on most adult erythrocytes but absent on fetal erythrocytes, which have the i antigen. Cord blood erythrocytes are thus usually not agglutinated by cold reactive antibody. A few cold antibodies have specificity for the i rather than the I antigen. Curiously, the reason for the cold reactivity of this class of antibodies does not appear to be a function of the antibody but rather of the Ii antigens. These presumably move to more accessible positions at the membrane surface as the temperature is reduced. Conversely, as the temperature is again increased the antigen sinks down into the more fluid lipid membrane, the immune complex is broken, and the antibody is released (Pruzanski and Shumak, 1977). However, the complement component, fixed by the cold antibodies to the membrane surface, remains and is responsible for the positive direct Coombs test usually observed in cold antibody hemolytic anemia (Table 2–18).

Warm antibody autoimmune hemolytic anemia is the most common of the immunohemolytic anemias. It affects all age groups. The onset may be insidious or acute, with fever, weakness, and flank and abdominal pain. The spleen is commonly enlarged, and the patient slightly jaundiced. The peripheral blood film shows microspherocytes mixed together with polychromatophilic macrocytes. It is distinguished from hereditary spherocytosis by the positive Coombs test. The autohemolysis test gives variable results. Osmotic fragility testing may show a "fragile tail" because of the population of osmotically susceptible microspherocytes.

Cold antibody autoimmune hemolytic anemia is almost always of the cold agglutinin type. It may occur in acute and self-limited form during the recovery phase of certain infections, most notably mycoplasma pneumonia and infectious mononucleosis. A chronic variety occurring in older patients is associated with a monoclonal autoantibody—and often with a monoclonal M-com-

Table 2–18 LABORATORY DIAGNOSIS OF AUTOIMMUNE HEMOLYTIC ANEMIA

	Broad-spectrum Coombs Test	IgG Coombs Test	Complement Coombs Test	Cold Agglutinin Test
Warm type	+	+	+ or −	−
Cold agglutinin type	+	−	+	+

ponent on serum protein electrophoresis. This "idiopathic" condition is presumably "para-neoplastic" and closely related to the lympho-proliferative diseases. The degree of hemolysis is often mild in chronic cold agglutinin disease, even when the titer is very high. Exposed parts of the body—the fingers, toes, ears, and nose—may suffer the consequences of reduced temperatures, demonstrating vaso-occlusive signs such as Raynaud-like symptoms and local tissue necrosis. The *thermal amplitude* refers to antibody activity as a function of tempera-ture. The activity decreases as the temperature increases, and usually no activity is present above 32°C. Spontaneous agglutination of an-ticoagulated blood at room temperature may cause technical errors in the laboratory unless precautions are taken to maintain the blood at temperatures above 32°C. Autoagglutination, along with spherocytosis, is a dominant feature of the peripheral blood film. The marrow is often infiltrated with lymphocytes in the idi-opathic chronic variety.

Paroxysmal cold hemoglobinuria is a very rare acquired immunohemolytic anemia caused by an IgG cold-reactive autoantibody demonstrated by the Donath-Landsteiner test. The antibody is bound at 4°C, and complement is fixed. Agglutination is not present, but as the sample is warmed complement-induced hemolysis takes place. Acute hemolytic epi-sodes are provoked by exposure to cold. Signs of intravascular hemolysis are marked. Some cases are idiopathic, whereas others are related to infections, especially syphilis.

The pathogenesis of the hemolysis in au-toimmune hemolytic anemia has posed appar-ent paradoxes. For example, a strongly posi-tive Coombs test may be associated with an absence of clinical hemolysis on the one hand, whereas on the other an occasional case of acquired autoimmune hemolytic anemia may be discovered with a negative Coombs test. Some explanations for these apparent contra-dictions between laboratory tests and clinical events have in large measure been provided by new information about the subclasses of immunoglobulins and their relationships to complement fixation and to specific receptors on the surface of macrophages.

It stands to reason that the density of the antibody coating on the red cell is a major determinant of the severity of hemolysis (Fig. 2–103). About 500 IgG molecules per eryth-rocyte are necessary to produce a positive Coombs test. For a given antibody, the greater this number, the shorter the red cell life span.

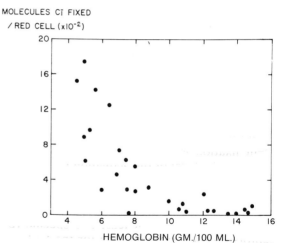

MOLECULES C̄1 FIXED / RED CELL (×10⁻²)

HEMOGLOBIN (GM./100 ML.)

Figure 2–103 The relation between IgG density on the erythrocyte membrane and the degree of anemia in non-splenectomized patients with warm antibody autoimmune hemolytic anemia. The measurement of membrane anti-body density employs a sensitive technique of first reacting the coated erythrocytes with antihuman gamma globulin and then measuring complement fixation on the doubly coated cells. (Redrawn from Rosse, W. F.: J. Clin. Invest., *50*:734, 1971.)

However, reduced erythrocyte life span may also be present at values less than 500.

The process of complement fixation is a direct function of the density of antibodies on the red cell surface. In order for the first component of complement to be fixed, two IgG molecules must achieve a certain critical distance apart from each other (250 to 400 Å). Low-density IgG coatings are thus not likely to fix complement. However, the pentameric IgM contains within its intrinsic structure five potential immunoglobulin-binding sites. Since these five "feet" fall within the critical dis-tance, IgM on the cell surface invariably fixes complement. If the antigenic sites on the red cell surface are spaced too far apart to permit the corresponding IgG antibodies to be placed within the critical distance, then complement fixation cannot take place. Such is the case with the Rh antigens; immunohemolytic dis-ease due to Rh antibodies lacks complement on the cell surface.

The immunoglobulin subclasses do not fix complement equally well. In addition to IgM, IgG3 and IgG1 are active. IgG2 has only weak activity. IgG4, IgA, and IgE do not fix com-plement at all. Thus, the specific subclass to which the autoantibody belongs, along with its concentration, is important as a hemolytic de-terminant (Logue and Rosse, 1976).

The specific details of the complement system have been clearly depicted by Müller-Eberhard. The _recognition unit_ (C1qrs) is followed by the _activation unit_ (C4, 2, 3), which in turn may develop a _membrane attack unit_ (C5–9). An immense amount of C1 must be fixed to bring on the membrane attack unit to punch holes through the cell surface and cause direct hemolysis. This usually does not occur in autoimmune hemolytic anemia. If complement fixation is achieved, it ordinarily is arrested at the level of the activation unit, which leaves C3b on the cell surface. However, this component can also bring about cell damage by interaction with macrophages.

Macrophages have at least two specific receptors on their surfaces, one for the Fc fragment of IgG and the other for the C3b component of complement (Fig. 2–104). Once again, the subclasses of IgG are important; receptor activity is greatest for IgG3 and IgG1 and absent for IgG4 and IgA, parallel to the complement-fixing activity of these immunoglobulin types. The presence of immunoglobulin or C3b or both on the erythrocyte surface brings the coated erythrocyte into close juxtaposition to macrophages at these receptor sites. At the interface, the macrophage proceeds with its work, gnawing bits and pieces

away from the cell surface (Fig. 2–105). Lost surface causes spherocytosis, culminating in the eventual entrapment and engulfment of the entire erythrocyte.

Other variables also affect the severity of the hemolytic anemia (Conley et al., 1982). One of these is the state of activation of macrophages. Another is C3 inactivator. This ingredient of the complement system cleaves C3b on the erythrocyte surface, leaving behind a fragment called C3d. This is still detectable in the Coombs test, but its presence on the cell surface protects against further phagocytosis, thus limiting hemolysis. In fact, C3 inactivator appears to be able to release the C3b coated erythrocyte from the grasp of the hepatic macrophage and allow it once again to circulate without further damage (Fig. 2–104).

Thus the lack of correlation between the results of routine clinical tests and clinical phenomena has become more understandable. The reason that IgG4 and IgA do not produce hemolysis is clear; neither fix complement and neither bind to macrophages. Conversely, an erythrocyte coated with both IgG3 and C3b is rapidly destroyed, since both moieties bring about lethal contacts with macrophage receptors.

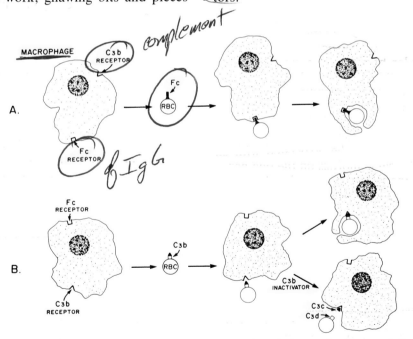

Figure 2–104 The role of macrophage surface receptors in immune hemolytic anemia, illustrated diagrammatically. Macrophages have separate receptors for immunoglobulins and for complement. The immunoglobulin receptors have a restricted specificity for the Fc fragment of the subclasses IgG1 and IgG3. The other immunoglobulins do not bind to macrophages. The complement receptor is specific for the C_3b component. _A,_ An IgG-coated erythrocyte is attached to a macrophage. Erythrocyte fragmentation and/or outright engulfment follows. _B,_ A C3b-coated erythrocyte is attached to a macrophage. Phagocytosis may follow, as in _A,_ or C3b inactivator may cleave C3b and cause release of the erythrocyte from the clutches of the macrophage. C3d is left behind on the erythrocyte. This surface coating renders the erythrocyte resistant to further phagocytic damage.

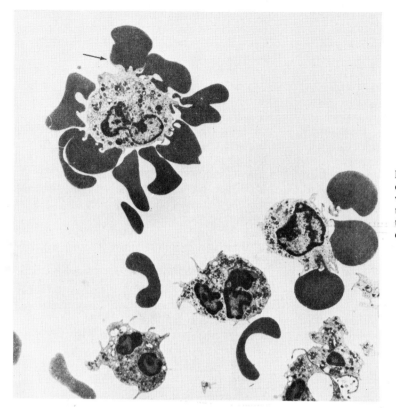

Figure 2–105 The adherence of IgG-coated erythrocytes to macrophages, with fragmentation of small pieces of the erythrocyte membrane at the cell-to-cell interface. (From Abramson, N., et al.: J. Exper. Med., *132*:1191, 1970.)

What determines splenic as opposed to hepatic hemolysis? In warm antibody hemolytic disease, the IgG coating on the erythrocyte is often unaccompanied by complement, and splenic macrophages are the preferred site of destruction. Hence, splenectomy is often successful as a definitive means of therapy if glucocorticoids cannot adequately control the hemolysis. However, cold agglutinin hemolytic disease is predominantly hepatic, probably because C3b on the erythrocyte surface favors interaction with the hepatic Kupffer cells. Splenectomy is usually unsuccessful and glucocorticoids are of less benefit than in warm antibody hemolytic disease. By similar reasoning, resistance of warm antibody hemolytic anemia to these therapeutic measures may be related to class and concentration of antibody and to complement fixation.

Glucocorticoids act primarily by blocking macrophage-erythrocyte interactions and inhibiting phagocytosis. Only later do they cause autoantibody concentrations to fall. Other immunosuppressive modalities have also been used in the treatment of resistant cases.

Administration of red cell transfusion to patients with immunohemolytic anemia is complicated by the difficulty in finding blood that can be cross-matched. The endogenous antibodies present in the patient's serum are "nonspecific" in the sense that they react with all donor types. After transfusion, the donor red cells are not distinguished by the hemolytic process from the patient's own erythrocytes. Thus, transfusion is best avoided unless warranted by the severity of the anemia or by life-threatening cardiovascular complications.

How does an autoantibody come to be produced in violation of the principle of immune self-recognition and tolerance to autologous antigens? Hypotheses for this phenomenon as a pathogenetic factor in a variety of disease states have been put forth:

1. There is a shared antigenicity between an exogenous inciting antigen and an autologous antigen that brings on the immune attack against the autologous tissue.

2. "Forbidden clones" of immunocytes emerge, perhaps owing to lack of proper immunologic "suppressor" or "surveillance" activity, and these produce antibodies against autologous antigen.

3. A subtle change takes place in autologous antigen, rendering it immunogenic.

What is clear is that a large proportion of autoimmune hemolytic anemias occur in association with altered states of immunity. Acute self-limited syndromes appear in the recovery phase from certain infections while the immune response is taking place. Others occur in association with immune deficiency syndromes, such as agammaglobulinemia and a variety of chronic lymphoproliferative disorders, especially chronic lymphocytic leukemia, lymphocytic lymphoma, and Hodgkin's disease. They also complicate the course of other autoimmune disorders, such as disseminated lupus erythematosus and ulcerative colitis. Many, however, remain unexplained and are designated *idiopathic*.

Immunohemolytic anemias that are Coombs positive also occur as adverse reactions to certain medications, and a consideration of these may provide some further insight into pathogenetic mechanisms. They fall into three classes:

1. The haptene, or penicillin, type. The serum of the patient contains antipenicillin antibodies of the 7S type. Penicillin, if given in very high doses, is soaked up into the erythrocyte membrane. The antipenicillin antibodies are not directed against red cell antigens but do bind to the penicillin in the membrane, giving rise to a positive Coombs test and to hemolysis.

2. The immune complex, or "innocent bystander," type. IgM antibody is formed to the drug (quinidine, quinine, stibophen) which is associated with an unidentified serum protein as carrier. The antibody then reacts with the antigen to form an immune complex, which attaches to the red cell membrane and fixes complement. The antibody may then be detached, leaving complement behind. The Coombs test is positive because of the complement coat. The red cell is the innocent bystander. The mechanism is the same as that of quinidine thrombocytopenia, except that the latter is characterized by the production of a 7S IgG antibody.

3. The true autoimmune, or alphamethyldopa, type. In a time- and dose-dependent manner, the drug induces the formation of an antibody specifically directed against a normal red cell antigen, usually of the Rh complex. The autoimmune state persists for months after discontinuation of the drug, gradually subsiding without additional treatment. This drug-related form of autoimmunity may be a prototype for other types of autoimmune states by undefined exogenous agents.

Some medications, notably the cephalosporin antibiotics, occasionally cause nonspecific adherence of plasma proteins to the red cell membrane. The Coombs test becomes positive, but significant hemolysis usually does not occur.

THE SPLEEN

From the foregoing discussion it is evident that the spleen plays an important role in the pathogenesis of hemolysis both in certain intrinsic disorders, such as hereditary spherocytosis, and in some extrinsic disorders, such as warm antibody immunohemolytic anemia. However, marked splenomegaly of whatever cause can produce hemolytic anemia even in the absence of any other intra- or extracorpuscular factor. Examples of conditions that might become complicated by splenomegalic hemolysis include chronic lymphocytic leukemia, lymphoma, myelofibrosis with myeloid metaplasia, and hairy cell leukemia. The adverse effects of splenic erythrostasis on red cell viability were discussed in the second part of Chapter 1.

References

Beutler, E., Yeh, M., and Fairbanks, V. F.: The normal human female as a mosaic of X-chromosome activity. Studies using the gene for G-6-PD deficiency as a marker. Proc. Natl. Acad. Sci. U.S.A., *48*:9, 1962.

Bukowski, R. M.: Thrombotic thrombocytopenic purpura: a review. Progr. Hemostas. Thromb., *6*:287, 1982.

Conley, C. L., Lippman, S. M., Ness, P. M., et al.: Autoimmune hemolytic anemia with reticulocytopenia and erythroid marrow. N. Engl. J. Med., *306*:281, 1982.

Conrad, M. E.: Blood transfusion: uses, abuses, and practices. Semin. Hematol., *18*:81, 1981.

Cooper, R. A.: Hemolytic syndromes and red cell membrane abnormalities in liver disease. Semin. Hematol. *17*:103, 1980.

Dacie, J. V., Mollison, P. L., Richardson, N., et al.: Atypical congenital hemolytic anemia. Quart. J. Med., *22*:79, 1953.

Dessypris, E. N., Clark, D. A., McKee, L. C., Jr., and Krantz, S. B.: Increased sensitivity to complement of erythroid and myeloid progenitors in paroxysmal nocturnal hemoglobinuria. N. Engl. J. Med., *309*:690, 1983.

Gemsa, D., Woo, C. H., Fudenberg, H. H., and Schmid, R.: Erythrocyte catabolism by macrophages in vitro. The effect of hydrocortisone on erythrophagocytosis and on induction of heme oxygenase. J. Clin Invest., *52*:812, 1973.

Jaffe, C. J., Atkinson, J. P., and Frank, M. M.: The role of complement in the clearance of cold agglutinin sensitized erythrocytes in man. J. Clin. Invest., *58*:942, 1976.

Jaffé, E. R.: Methemoglobinemia. Clin. Haematol., *10*:99, 1981.

Logue, G., and Rosse, W.: Immunologic mechanisms in autoimmune hemolytic disease. Semin. Hematol., *13*:277, 1976.

Magon, A. M., Leipzig, R. M., Zannoni, V. G., and

Brewer, G. J.: Interactions of glucose 6 phosphate dehydrogenase deficiency with drug acetylation and hydroxylation relations. J. Lab. Clin. Med., *97*:764, 1981.

Marsh, G. W., and Lewis, S. M.: Cardiac hemolytic anemia. Semin. Hematol., *6*:133, 1969.

McDonagh, A. F., Palma, L. A., and Lightner, D. A.: Blue light and bilirubin excretion. Science, *208*:145, 1980.

Miwa, S.: Pyruvate kinase deficiency and other enzymopathies of the Embden-Meyerhof pathway. Clin. Haematol., *10*:57, 1981.

Motulsky, A. G.: Hemolysis in glucose-6-phosphate dehydrogenase deficiency. Fed. Proc., *31*:1286, 1972.

Müller-Eberhard, H. J.: Chemistry and function of the complement system. Hosp. Pract., *12(8)*:33, 1977.

Nicholson-Weller, A., March, J. P., Rosenfeld, S. I., and Austen, K. F.: Affected erythrocytes of patients, with paroxysmal nocturnal hemoglobinuria are deficient in the complement regulatory protein, decay accelerating factor. Proc. Natl. Acad. Sci. U.S.A., *80*:5066, 1983.

Palek, J., and Lux, S. E.: Red cell membrane skeletal defects in hereditary and acquired hemolytic anemias. Semin. Hematol., *20*:189, 1983.

Pangburn, M. K., Schreiber, R. D., and Müller-Eberhard, H. J.: Deficiency of an erythrocyte membrane protein with complement regulatory activity in paroxysmal nocturnal hemoglobinuria. Proc. Natl. Acad. Sci. U.S.A., *80*:5430, 1983.

Petz, L. D., and Garrity, G.: Acquired Immune Hemolytic Anemias. London, Churchill-Livingstone, 1980.

Pruzanski, W., and Shumak, K. H.: Biologic activity of cold reacting autoantibodies. N. Engl. J. Med., *297*:538, 1977.

Rosse, W. F.: Interaction of complement with the red cell membrane. Semin. Hematol., *16*:128, 1979.

Shohet, S. B., and Lux, S. E.: The erythrocyte membrane skeleton: pathophysiology. Hosp. Pract., *19*(11):89, 1984.

Sweadner, K. J., and Goldin, S. M.: Active transport of sodium and potassium ions. Mechanism, function, regulation. N. Engl. J. Med., *302*:777, 1980.

Valentine, W. N., and Paglia, D. E.: Erythrocyte enzymopathies, hemolytic anemia, and multi system disease: an annotated review. Blood, *64*:583, 1984.

Zweiman, B., and Patten, E.: Immunohematologic diseases. J.A.M.A., *248*:2677, 1982.

3

Leukocytes

Phagocytes

STRUCTURE

The two major families of leukocytes, the phagocytes and the immunocytes, are derived from a common marrow stem cell. Morphologically and functionally, however, they are quite different and will be discussed in separate sections.

The phagocytes are divided into granulocytes and monocyte-macrophages. They share a common progenitor cell identifiable in cell culture and designated as a CFU-GM (colony-forming unit—granulocyte-monocyte). In response to one or several colony-stimulating factors, this cell will undergo transformation to a precursor cell, either a myeloblast or myelomonoblast.

Like all blast cells, the myeloblast has evenly dispersed nuclear chromatin, scant cytoplasm, and no cytoplasmic granulation. It is smaller than a proerythroblast, has no perinuclear halo, and both nucleus and cytoplasm are far less basophilic. It can be distinguished from a lymphoblast by its prominent nucleoli and indistinct nuclear membrane.

After one of several mitotic divisions, the myeloblast enlarges to form a promyelocyte characterized by large reddish-purple granules, some of them overlying the nucleus. These granules are lysosomes, containing large amounts of myeloperoxidase as well as lysozymes and bactericidal cationic proteins. The nucleus is still blastic with nucleoli, but after further divisions nuclear chromatin condenses into distinct blocks, and the capacity for mitotic division ceases. At this myelocytic state, new species of lysosomal granules appear, giving the mature granulocytes their characteristic morphologic appearance. The neutrophilic granules are small and pink and contain bactericidal lactoferrin and lysozymes as well as an alkaline phosphatase. The eosinophilic granules are large and round and contain red-staining basic mucopolysaccharides. The basic granules are coarse, often concealing the nucleus, and contain histamine, heparin, and acid mucopolysaccharides. The background cytoplasm of all three cell types is pink and stays unchanged, whereas the nucleus becomes indented and segmented during subsequent maturation to a metamyelocyte and a mature granulocyte. The segmented granulocyte has a nucleus consisting of three to five lobes connected by thin strands (Fig. 1–10). In blood, granulocytes circulate as spherical bodies with a mean diameter of about 12 μ and a mean volume of about 500 to 600 μ^3. When attached to an object, a granulocyte assumes a triangular shape with a veil-like hyaline moving edge and a tapered uropod attached temporarily to a surface like the tail of an inchworm (Fig. 3–1).

The differentiation from myelomonoblast to mature monocytes is undoubtedly also a process of integrated proliferation and maturation, but distinct stages are difficult to recognize. The mature monocyte is a large cell with a diameter of about 20 to 30 μ and a prominent multishaped nucleus. The chromatin structure is less clumped than that of the mature granulocyte or lymphocyte and appears lacelike, with small chromatin particles tied together by fine strands. The cytoplasm is grayish-blue and contains many fine lysosomes stained pink with Wright's stain. Even on fixed smears, the cytoplasm gives an impression of being "free

135

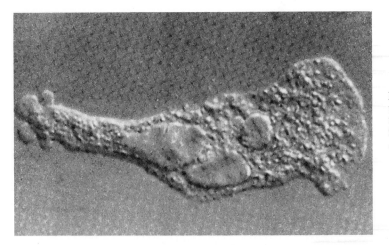

Figure 3–1 Crawling granulocyte with uropod on the left and moving edge on the right. (Reproduced with permission from Wade, B. H., and Mandell, G. L.: Am. J. Med., *74*:686, 1983.)

flowing," reflecting active ameboid motions right up to the time the cell becomes permanently fixed to the glass slide. The clear cytoplasmic vacuoles frequently observed may be artifactual and caused by the smearing technique.

After the monocyte leaves blood it is transformed into a lysosome-filled macrophage. Cline (1978) has reviewed the sequence of this transformation, which involves a sudden burst in metabolic activities (Fig. 3–2). Energy production is increased, synthesis of hydrolytic enzymes by the endoplasmic reticulum and their subsequent packing by the Golgi apparatus into lysosomes are enhanced, and the cell enlarges until it has taken on the appearance of the large mobile macrophage found in pulmonary alveoli, peritoneal cavities, and inflammatory exudates. These cells reach a diameter of 50 μ or more and send out far-reaching cytoplasmic tentacles. The cytoplasm may contain lipid droplets and lysosomes—with incompletely digested material such as

carbon particles—and hemosiderin granules. The oval nucleus, off to one side, is relatively small in proportion to the cytoplasm, and has an open, lacy chromatin network (Fig. 3–3). Although the mobile macrophages retain common phagocytic properties, they develop characteristics of the organ to which they belong. For example, alveolar macrophages depend on oxidative phosphorylation for their energy production, whereas most other macrophages depend on glycolysis. The fixed macrophage in the liver, spleen, and marrow appears to exist in a dynamic equilibrium with the mobile macrophage, and the characteristic foreign body giant cell, or Langerhans cell, may represent fusion of a number of mobile macrophages. The term *reticuloendothelial system* is traditionally used to describe this large system of mobile and fixed macrophages. Since neither reticular nor endothelial cells are phagocytic, a better but still not widely used term is *mononuclear phagocyte system,* as suggested by Meuret in 1977.

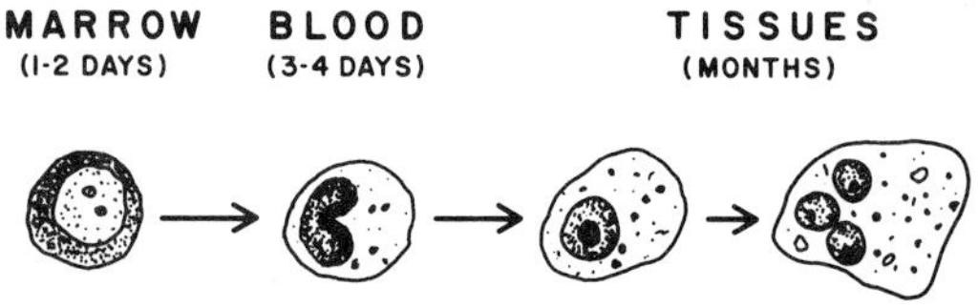

	MARROW (1-2 DAYS)	**BLOOD** (3-4 DAYS)	**TISSUES** (MONTHS)	
	PROMONOCYTE	MONOCYTE	IMMATURE MACROPHAGE	MATURE MACROPHAGE
PROLIFERATION	++++	+ to +++	++	o
PHAGOCYTOSIS	±	+	+++	++++
GLASS ADHERENCE	+	++	+++	+++
LYSOSOMES	+	++	++++	++++
IgG RECEPTORS	+	++	+++	+++
LYMPHOCYTE INTERACTION	?	++	++++	++++

Figure 3–2 Cellular kinetics and functional properties of the monocyte-macrophages. The mature macrophage is represented by a multinucleated epithelial giant cell, but other types include the alveolar macrophages, Kupffer cells, brain microglia, and the macrophages of the spleen, lymph nodes, marrow, and other tissues. (From Cline, M. J.: Ann. Int. Med., *88*:78, 1978.)

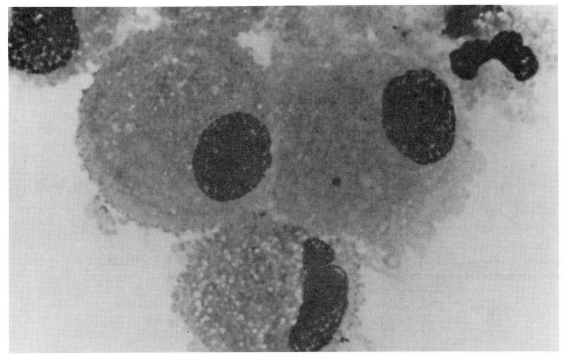

Figure 3–3 Alveolar macrophages. These macrophages live in aerobic circumstances, and, in contrast to other phagocytic cells, they utilize aerobic metabolism for energy. (From Golde, D. W., Finley, T. N., and Cline, M. J.: N. Engl. J. Med., *290*:875, 1974.)

FUNCTION

Although the functions of the granulocytes and the monocyte-macrophages overlap, it seems reasonable to suggest that granulocytes function primarily as the first line of defense against microbial organisms, whereas the monocyte-macrophages provide final removal of such organisms and also clear the body of its own aged and damaged cells. In order to accomplish this, the phagocytes must (1) accumulate in sufficient numbers at the right place, (2) become attached to the foreign or nonviable material, (3) engulf, (4) dissolve, and (5) dispose of it (Stossel, 1974).

Under normal conditions, granulocytes spend less than a day in the circulation before they migrate through the endothelial wall at random and are disposed of in the tissues. Infectious or inflammatory tissue injury will direct this migration by causing the release of a variety of vasoactive and chemotactic factors. The vasoactive factors increase capillary permeability and induce local migration of the granulocytes. The chemotactic factors combine with surface receptors on the granulocytes, and the resulting ligand-receptor complexes will direct locomotion of granulocytes toward the inflammatory focus, where they will envelop and engulf the foreign or nonviable material by endocytosis (Fig. 3–4).

The responsible chemotactic factors range from endogenous products such as activated complement (especially C3b and C5a) and secretions from transformed lymphocytes and macrophages to bacterial products such as endotoxins and leukotrienes. The leukotrienes

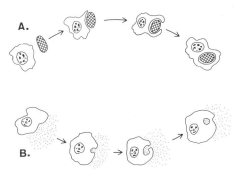

Figure 3–4 Endocytosis: the process of engulfing a portion of the cell's exterior into its interior. *A,* Phagocytosis. This refers to the inclusion of relatively large particles. The phagocyte membrane sends out pseudopodia to grasp the particle, utilizing a propulsive mechanism biochemically similar to that of muscle. *B,* Pinocytosis. This refers to the cellular interiorization of smaller particles included as a droplet of the fluid exterior into an interior membrane-lined vesicle.

are by far the most potent chemotactic factors known and, like the prostaglandins, are derived from membrane phospholipids via arachidonic acid (see Fig. 4–5). Some of these chemotactic factors, especially C3b, also function as opsonins, coating microbes and enhancing their recognition by phagocytes. Antibody coating will also cause opsonization, primarily attracting monocytes and macrophages that have numerous binding sites for the Fc region of IgG.

Granulocyte mobility and endocytosis appear to be caused by changes in the molecular structure of actin. Actin is the most abundant element of the granulocyte cytoplasm, representing almost 10 percent of total protein. It is present as a "sol" of globular monomers in a dynamic equilibrium with a "gel" of filamentous polymers. This equilibrium is maintained by a "treadmill," with monomers continuously being added to one end of the polymers and split off from the other end. A number of actin-binding proteins, including the calcium-dependent gelsolin, support this equilibrium. The induction of directed motion toward an inflammatory focus appears to be accomplished by a change in this equilibrium initiated by the formation of complexes between receptors and chemotactic factors in the lipid membrane. These complexes aggregate in one area, which becomes the uropod tail of the granulocyte (Fig. 3–1). They also cause depletion of intracellular calcium, and Southwick and Stossel (1983) have suggested that it is this loss of calcium that upsets the actin equilibrium by inactivating gelsolin. Actin monomers become trapped on polymers with remodeling of the actin filament network and contraction in response to the ATP-ase activity of small amounts of cytoplasmic myosin. This contraction results in cellular motion and cytoplasmic envelopment of opsonized material.

Inside the cytoplasm the enveloped material is covered by internalized surface membrane, forming distinct phagosomes. Activated lysosomal granules become attached and empty their cargo of hydrolytic enzymes into the phagosomes, killing and/or dissolving their content (Fig. 3–5) and morphologically degranulating the phagocytes. This lysosomal activation and attachment are initiated by a still elusive enzyme (Badwey et al., 1979). In macrophages, certain bacteria and parasites fail to trigger this enzyme. Such organisms (*Mycobacterium, Brucella, Legionella, Rikettsia, Leishmania, Toxoplasma,* and *Trypanosoma*) will be phagocytized by macrophages but not killed.

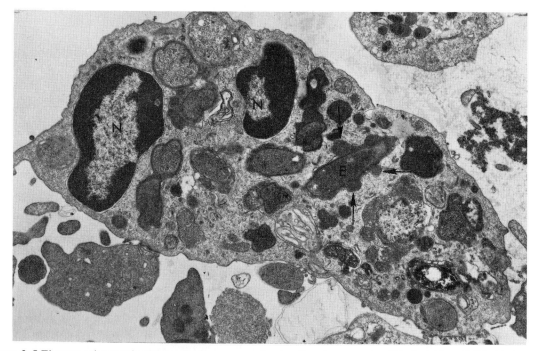

Figure 3–5 Electron microscopic picture of a human granulocyte after phagocytosis of E*scherichia coli (E).* Coalescence of lysosomes with the phagocytic vacuoles is seen at arrows. *N* = nucleus. (From Zucker-Franklin, D., Elsbach, E., and Simon, P. J.: Lab Invest., *25*:415, 1971. U.S.–Canadian Division of the International Academy of Pathology. The Williams and Wilkins Company [Agent].)

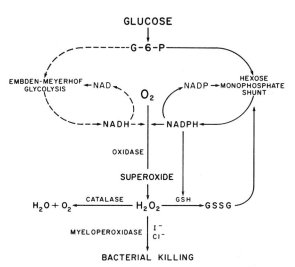

Figure 3–6 Generation of superoxide and hydrogen peroxide by an oxidase that transfers electrons from reduced pyridine nucleotides to molecular oxygen. The reduced pyridine nucleotides are primarily but not exclusively generated via the hexose monophosphate shunt. The H_2O_2 can be used for bacterial killing via a myeloperoxidase pathway utilizing the halides, iodide and chloride. Excess H_2O_2 is destroyed by catalase or by reduced glutathione (GSH), which in its oxidized state further activates the monophosphate shunt. (Adapted from Karnofsky, et al., 1970, and Stossel, 1974.)

Final bacterial killing occurs via processes that are both oxygen-dependent and oxygen-independent. Molecular oxygen is reduced by an oxidase to superoxide and hydrogen peroxide with reduced pyridine nucleotides as electron donors (Fig. 3–6) (Babior, 1984). Hydrogen peroxide kills bacteria in the phagosomes by peroxidation with the assistance of the enzyme myeloperoxidase, using halides as cofactors. These processes are associated with a rapid increase in energy demand, and, because the granulocytes have few mitochondria, this demand is met primarily by glycolysis via the Embden-Meyerhof pathway and the hexose monophosphate shunt. Oxygen-independent bacterial killing is accomplished by hydrogen ions, lysozymes, and bactericidal proteins present in the phagosome.

The final release of the degradation products amplifies the inflammatory response. Released lysosomal enzymes injure surrounding tissues, endogenous pyrogens cause fever, thromboplastic products cause fibrinous obstruction of vessels, and cationic proteins cause vasodilatation.

In addition to participating in the phagocytic inflammatory response to foreign antigens, the tissue macrophages play a key role in the important process of antigen-induced blast transformation of lymphocytes. This process depends on a preliminary processing or digestion of antigens by the macrophages, followed by secretion of a lymphocyte-activating factor, interleukin-1, and "presentation" of the antigens on specific surface sites. Compatible lymphocytes are attracted to these sites, initiating the cellular reactions necessary for the immune response (Fig. 3–7).

The tissue macrophages are also responsible for the daily destruction of aged blood cells, denatured plasma proteins, and plasma lipids. This large and somewhat unappreciated function is accomplished through phagocytosis of whole cells and pinocytosis of small droplets

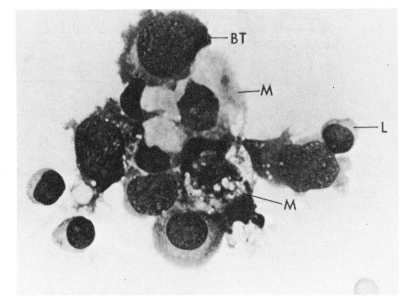

Figure 3–7 An "immunologic island" composed of central macrophages *(M)*, surrounding lymphocytes undergoing blast transformation *(BT)* and untransformed lymphocytes *(L)*. (From Cline, M. J.: Ann. Int. Med., *88*:78, 1978.)

containing plasma proteins and lipid microcolloids (Fig. 3–4). There still is no clear explanation of the process by which the macrophage recognizes nonviable blood cells or plasma constituents. Studies of red blood cells have revealed that aging is associated with a decreased membrane content of sialic acid resulting in a decreased negative change, but whether it is this or another subtle membrane change that is responsible for the fatal interaction with macrophages is unknown. The avidity of the tissue macrophage to slightly altered cells, to denatured proteins, or to macrocolloids has been used diagnostically to measure the size and blood flow of organs containing many macrophages—such as the liver, spleen, and bone marrow. The technique has been to label a cell or protein with a radioactive tracer, expose the labeled material to heat or chemicals, and use scanning techniques to determine the tissue transit or deposit of the isotopes. Similarly, certain isotopes of gold and technetium can be prepared in a colloidal form, and the clearance rate from blood and the uptake in the tissues can be used in the diagnostic evaluation of the size and function of mononuclear phagocyte organs (Fig. 3–8).

Macrophages are also placed in the mainstream of iron metabolism. A variety of tissue macrophages possess inducible heme oxidase activity, enabling them to break down red cell hemoglobin. The released iron is incorporated into ferritin and subsequently into insoluble hemosiderin. Macrophages of the liver, spleen, and bone marrow can again return iron to transferrin for transport back to the erythroid marrow. Alveolar macrophages are lacking in the ability to provide reutilization of iron, and, indeed, in pulmonary hemosiderosis, abundant iron-laden alveolar macrophages are demonstrable even in the face of iron-deficiency anemia and an absence of storage iron elsewhere.

The macrophage has been increasingly recognized as one of the most important effector cells in the body (Nathan et al., 1980). The ever-growing list of its secretory products shows an involvement in most inflammatory events, including the secretion of interleukin-1 (Il-1), of growth promoters of granulocytes, lymphocytes, erythrocytes, and platelets and of regulators of complement, coagulation, and kinin cascades.

Tissue macrophages presented with a phagocytic load may show a temporary decrease in efficiency, a phenomenon that Wagner and Iio called *blockade.* There is a degree of specificity, however, since blockade induced by one injected material does not necessarily block the subsequent clearance of a different particle. Nevertheless, blockage produced by excessive hemolysis may cause impaired removal of foreign antigens. Fortunately, a chronic challenge to macrophage function causes *overwork hyperplasia* with an appropriate compensating increase in the mass of the mononuclear phagocyte system.

The pathophysiologic relationship of eosinophils and basophils to allergic reactions is extremely complex. The basophils and their

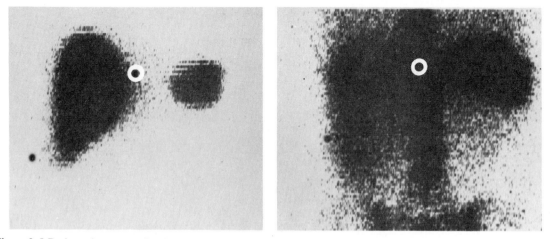

Figure 3–8 Body surface scans after intravenous injection of technetium (^{99m}Tc) sulfur colloid. Anterior views are shown. The position of the xiphoid is shown by the white circle. *Left,* In a normal individual 85 to 95 percent of the colloid is taken up by the macrophages of the liver because of the large hepatic blood flow, but the spleen is also well visualized. *Right,* In a patient with cirrhosis, hepatic uptake is reduced. The enlarged spleen is shown with increased colloid uptake, and the bone marrow macrophages now participate in the clearance, as shown by uptake over the vertebral column and pelvis. The clearance rate from the circulation is also slowed, leaving a heavy "background." (Kindly provided by Dr. M. Croll, Division of Nuclear Medicine, Lankenau Hospital, Philadelphia, PA.)

tissue descendants, the mast cells, have been shown to contain sites of attachment for IgE antibody, and their degranulation is associated with the release of a great number of vascular reactants, including heparin and histamine (Kaliner, 1979). However, the eosinophils, which are much more closely identified with allergy than the basophils, have not as yet been found to interact specifically with antigen-antibody complexes (Beeson and Bass, 1977).

KINETICS

Because of the relatively long tissue phase prior to and following the brief appearance of the granulocyte in the bloodstream, information about the rate and control of production and destruction has been difficult to obtain. However, reliable labeling techniques have been developed, both cohort labeling of DNA with ^{32}P or with tritiated thymidine and random labeling with radioactive diisopropyl fluorophosphate, ^{51}Cr-chromate, or ^{111}In-indium oxine. With such techniques it has been possible to construct a model for granulocyte kinetics similar to models developed for erythrocytes and thrombocytes (see Fig. 1–7).

Granulocyte renewal and control appear to be executed at the level of a stem cell progenitor pool. As described in the bone marrow section, this pool is divided morphologically or functionally into a multipotential stem cell pool and several unipotential progenitor cell pools committed to specific cell lines. The culturing of bone marrow on soft agar has disclosed the existence of a colony-forming cell, CFU-GM, which, when stimulated by a colony-stimulating factor (CSF), will grow colonies containing thousands of granulocytes and monocytes. The CFU-GM is believed to be the unipotential progenitor cell committed to the granulocyte-monocytic cell line. After blast transformation, the myeloblasts divide about three to five times while they mature into myelocytes. Warner and Athens have proposed that the number of divisions is not predetermined but actively regulated and that skipped divisions or additional divisions may adjust the responsiveness of granulocytic production to peripheral demands. After the myelocytes mature into metamyelocytes and become mitotically inactive, maturing cells accumulate as a marrow granulocyte reserve. This reserve is under normal conditions made up by about 5 days' worth of granulocytes. Following their final release from the bone marrow, the granulocytes spend

Table 3–1 GRANULOCYTIC POOLS

Cell Types	Number of Cells in 10^9 per kg. Body Weight
Proliferating cells	2.1
Marrow granulocytic reserve	5.6
Circulating granulocytes	0.3
Marginated granulocytes	0.2
Daily production and destruction	0.9

less than 1 day in the bloodstream, establishing two pools of about equal size—a circulating pool and a marginated pool. From the bloodstream they migrate into the tissue in which they will be destroyed either randomly in defense actions or by senescence about 2 to 3 days later (Boggs, 1967; Robinson and Mangalik, 1975).

Table 3–1 gives some approximations of the size of the various granulocytic pools. The combined size of the marrow pools is almost 1.5 times that calculated for the nucleated red blood cell pools, despite the fact that the daily production of red cells is about twice the daily production of granulocytes. This, of course, is due to the fact that the marrow contains a large reserve of maturing and mature granulocytes.

In peripheral blood, the normal granulocyte count should always be considered a range rather than a value. The fluctuating equilibrium between circulating and marginated cells precludes a completely stable granulocyte count, and the existence of an extensive granulocyte reserve in the bone marrow permits the granulocyte count to adjust temporarily to the demands for phagocytic cells.

The exact mechanism regulating granulocyte production is still unknown, although it undoubtedly involves a feedback between circulating granulocytes and the bone marrow. In support of the existence of a feedback mechanism is the observation that the granulocyte count in some patients with depleted bone marrow reserves exhibits an oscillatory pattern (Fig. 3–9). The reason for not observing such oscillations more often probably is the fact that under normal conditions the large bone marrow reserve pool will dampen or obliterate the amplitude of oscillations.

Various factors have been claimed to be responsible for maintaining the feedback adjustment between the peripheral demands for granulocytes and the bone marrow supply of granulocytes. Several granulocyte-mobilizing factors have been described, including endo-

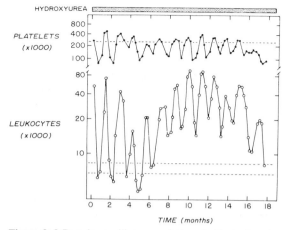

Figure 3–9 Regular oscillatory variations in the leukocyte and platelet count in a patient with chronic granulocytic leukemia receiving hydroxyurea therapy. (From Kennedy, B. J.: Blood, *35*:751, 1970, by permission of Grune & Stratton, Inc., New York.)

toxin, etiocholanolone, Menkin's tissue leukotaxines, and a leukocyte-mobilizing factor, but, as emphasized by Craddock and coworkers, it seems unlikely that any of these are involved in the physiologic regulation of granulocyte production. Other factors released by mature circulating granulocytes have been claimed to act as inhibitors or chalones of mitotic divisions within the myelocyte pool. Studies summarized by Burgess and Metcalf suggest that the true granulopoietin is a glycoprotein derived from monocytes, macrophages, and T lymphocytes and named *colony-stimulating factor,* or *CSF.* This glycoprotein, which is present in both plasma and urine, is necessary for the induction of clonal growth of

granulocyte precursors in vitro. Consequently, it is tempting to construct a feedback model for the control of granulocyte production, as outlined in Figure 3–10. This model, however, is quite hypothetical, since the existence of a granulopoietin and its identification with CSF are based primarily on in vitro data. Nevertheless, Richard and co-workers have shown that CSF is present in higher concentrations in leukopenic individuals than in normals, and Metcalf and Stanley have shown that it may increase granulocyte production when injected into mice. Furthermore, the apparently well-established existence of a circulating eosinophilopoietin in mice (Mahmoud et al., 1977) and men (Slungaard et al., 1983) gives support to the operation of granulocytic feedback systems based on the release and action of specific poietins.

The kinetics and regulation of the monocyte-macrophage complex are even less understood than those of the granulocyte complex (Burgess and Metcalf, 1980). The monocytes are derived from the bipotential progenitor cell CFU-C or CFU-GM. It is not known at what level of differentiation the monocyte precursors separate clearly from the myeloid precursors. It has been assumed that this separation occurs at an early level, possibly induced by a specific CSF, but studies by Perussia and coworkers suggest that even differentiated myelocytes or metamyelocytes may become monocytes if appropriately stimulated. The monocytes appear to have a shorter intramedullary life span than the granulocytic precursors, since they tend to emerge earlier than the granulocytes after a temporary bone marrow suppression. The life span of the monocyte in the circulation is probably about 36 hours, or two to three times longer than that of the granulocyte. The extravascular life span after it has been transformed to mobile or fixed macrophages is undoubtedly long and may be counted in months if not years.

PATHOPHYSIOLOGY

Granulocyte Disorders

Classification and General Considerations

Disorders of the granulocytes are traditionally classified according to the number of circulating granulocytes into granulocytopenias and granulocytoses. However, a classification based on function and kinetics is of more

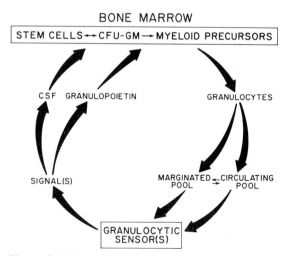

Figure 3–10 Hypothetical feedback circuit controlling granulocyte homeostasis.

Table 3–2 CLASSIFICATION OF GRANULOCYTE DISORDERS

I. *Quantitative abnormalities*
  Granulocytopenia
  Granulocytosis

II. *Qualitative abnormalities*
  Defective delivery
  Defective phagocytic activity
  Defective bactericidal activity

III. *Myeloproliferative disorders*
  Chronic: Polycythemia vera
       Chronic myelogenous leukemia
       Agnogenic myeloid metaplasia
       Essential thrombocythemia
       Chronic erythremia
  Subacute: Dyshemopoietic (preleukemic) syndrome
  Acute: Acute myelogenous leukemia

contemporary importance. On the basis of such criteria, the following classes of disorders can be recognized: quantitative abnormalities, qualitative abnormalities, and myeloproliferative disorders (Table 3–2).

The pathophysiologic effect of quantitative disorders is determined by the size of the actual and potential granulocyte pools. In granulocytopenia, the lack of defense against microorganisms and other foreign invaders dominates the clinical picture, whereas in granulocytosis the problems are more subtle. Although much larger and stickier than the red cells, the viscosity of blood with a high granulocyte count is about the same as for normal blood with the same total hematocrit (white cell crit plus red cell crit), and hyperviscosity due to granulocytosis is rare. However, if the white blood cell count measures in the hundreds of thousands and if the cells are composed primarily of blasts with large nuclei, there may be areas of symptomatic and even life-threatening leukostasis in the brain or lungs. More common is bone tenderness caused by expansion of the bone marrow and uric acid arthropathy or nephropathy caused by destruction of granulocytes. The qualitative disorders are characterized by impaired granulocyte defense despite a normal number of circulating neutrophils. Finally, the clinical manifestations of myeloproliferative disorders are related to the extent and character of cellular proliferation and cellular replacement.

Quantitative Abnormalities

Granulocytopenia. When the absolute granulocyte count is less than 3000 per mm.[3], the term *granulocytopenia* is used, but even at this level there are adequate numbers of granulocytes for normal defense activities. When the absolute number reaches 1000 per mm.[3], the patient becomes vulnerable to microbial attacks, but serious risk is usually first experienced at absolute counts of less than 500 per mm.[3] When playing this "numbers game," one must remember to take into account the presence of monocytes, which, although not as readily phagocytic as granulocytes, do contribute to the defense. The term *agranulocytosis* is usually reserved for the serious granulocytopenias in which both the marginated pool and the bone marrow reserve have been depleted. A depletion of the marrow reserve leaves the proliferating immature cells as the only myeloid cells present in the marrow and has given rise to the erroneous expression "maturation arrest." The immature cells are not arrested at all, but as soon as they reach maturity they are swept out of the marrow to shore up peripheral defenses.

The granulocytopenias may be caused by decreased production, ineffective production, or increased destruction. Decreased production is responsible for the granulocytopenia observed in patients with disorders causing marrow replacement or marrow aplasia. It is most acutely present after exposure to radiation or to radiomimetic drugs. The granulocytopenia here is part of a general suppression of cellular proliferation in the marrow, but because of the short granulocyte life span and the limited reserves, granulocytopenia is observed earlier than thrombocytopenia or anemia. Pisciotta has described a similar suppression of the marrow of certain susceptible individuals after the use of phenothiazine-type drugs. These appear to have a predominant effect on the myeloid cells, with less suppression of the erythroid cells and almost complete sparing of the megakaryocytic elements. A similar idiosyncratic granulocytopenia has been observed occasionally after the use of phenylbutazone, indomethacin, captopril, and a few other drugs. Underproduction of granulocytes has also been found to be responsible for a number of hereditary and acquired granulocytopenias. Of special interest is *cyclic neutropenia,* a disorder in which at regular intervals patients develop granulocytopenia, fever, mouth ulcerations, and infections. The pathogenesis has been linked to hormonal cycles, but other studies indicate that the recurrent granulocytopenia may be caused by an undampened feedback between the peripheral granulocyte pool and granulocytic committed progenitor cells.

Ineffective granulocytopoiesis is undoubtedly responsible for the granulocytopenia observed in *megaloblastic anemias* as well as in some of the *dyshemopoietic syndromes.* Blume and coworkers have suggested that the granulocytopenia observed in *Chediak-Higashi's syndrome* may be caused by intramedullary autodestruction by the large abnormal lysosomes that characterize the cells in this interesting disease.

Increased peripheral destruction is caused by increased utilization, antibody-coating of the granulocytes, or hypersplenism. As in patients with ineffective granulocytopoiesis, the granulocytopenia is associated with a striking granulocytic hyperplasia in the bone marrow. Increased removal or destruction is an appropriate physiologic response to inflammation. An early transient granulocytopenia actually precedes the leukocytosis of bacterial infection. When the infection is particularly severe, as in septicemia, the marrow reserves of mature granulocytes may be used up, with granulocytopenia ensuing. Granulocytopenia is also commonly observed during and after viral infections, especially hepatitis and infectious mononucleosis, but the mechanism is not known. Transient granulocytopenia is a feature of procedures involving exposure of large volumes of blood to foreign surfaces, such as hemodialysis coils and filtration leukapheresis columns. The surfaces presumably activate complement, which in turn causes granulocyte aggregation and transient granulocytopenia (Jacob et al., 1980).

Antibody-mediated destruction of circulating granulocytes is dramatically expressed in the much-feared syndrome of *drug-induced agranulocytosis.* After a varying period of drug exposure—usually ranging from a week to several months but occasionally lasting as long as several years—the neutrophilic granulocytes vanish from blood and marrow, leaving the patient extremely vulnerable to infection and sepsis. It the drug is discontinued, recovery usually occurs within a week or two. Although every drug the patient is taking must be suspected, some of the more common offenders in this fortunately rare type of adverse drug reaction are sulfonamides, phenylbutazone, and propylthiouracil. The cellular destruction is believed to be caused by attachment on the granulocyte surface of circulating antigen-antibody complexes, the "innocent bystander" concept (see Fig. 4–10), with subsequent engulfment by splenic and marrow macrophages.

Chronic benign neutropenia is an asymptomatic condition of unknown cause. Although occasionally severe, infectious complications are rare, presumably owing to the fact that the marrow pool of mature granulocytes is preserved and can be mobilized when needed. Chronic neutropenia is also a feature of most collagen vascular diseases, especially *Felty's syndrome,* but attempts to identify antigranulocyte antibodies have been inconclusive. The term *immune neutropenia* is warranted for the few patients in whom antigranulocyte antibodies are demonstrable in the plasma (Minchintou and Waters, 1984). Studies by Bagby and coworkers have suggested that neutropenia may be caused by cellular rather than humoral mechanisms, specifically by T lymphocytes inhibitory to the growth of CFU-GM.

Hypersplenism or *splenic neutropenia* is observed in patients without overt antibody production but with splenomegaly. Despite many studies of the pathogenesis of the hypersplenic syndrome, we still do not understand why a large spleen should destroy otherwise healthy granulocytes. It may be a question of sequestration rather than destruction similar to hypersplenic thrombocytopenia or it may involve antibodies or hemopoietic inhibitory T cells too few to be detected by current techniques.

Granulocytosis. Granulocytosis is present when the granulocyte count exceeds 10,000 per mm.^{3} When the count is over 30,000 per mm.^{3}, the term *leukemoid reaction* is often used. Although a nonleukemic granulocytosis may reach levels of 50,000 per mm.^{3} or higher, counts in excess of 100,000 per mm.^{3} are extremely rare. Furthermore, leukemoid reactions are characterized by lack of myeloid precursors in blood and by elevations in the concentration of leukocyte alkaline phosphatase.

An acute granulocytosis of moderate degree can be caused by a mere shift of granulocytes from the marginal pool and the bone marrow reserve pool into the circulation. It is frequently observed after exposure to acute infections, trauma, or emotional or physical stress and after the administration of epinephrine, adrenal steroids, and endotoxin. Chronic granulocytosis is observed under conditions of sustained overproduction of granulocytes. The most common causes are bacterial infections and tissue injury. Neoplasias presumably cause granulocytosis by inducing tissue necrosis with the release of hypothetical bone marrow–stimulating substances.

Eosinophilic granulocytosis is observed primarily in conditions characterized by the sustained presence of antigen-antibody complexes, such as in patients with chronic parasitic invasion or with dermatologic or allergic manifestations. Eosinophilia also occurs in association with neoplasias and in the *hypereosinophilic syndrome,* a condition having unknown etiology but involving potentially destructive tissue infiltration of eosinophils. An increase in the number of basophils may be a sign of myeloproliferative disease.

Qualitative Abnormalities

A decreased resistance to infection may occur despite normal granulocyte counts if the functional competence of the granulocytes is impaired. In the so-called *lazy leukocyte syndrome* described by Miller and coworkers, the granulocytes do not respond appropriately to chemotactic factors, and the granulocytes fail to accumulate and produce an inflammatory focus. Similar dysfunction of chemotaxis and migration is also present if the classic or alternate activation of C3 is impaired. Defective attachment and phagocytosis of foreign bodies are usually caused by impaired antibody production and complement function.

Impaired killing of ingested microorganisms causes recurrent and chronic infections and may lead to massive granuloma formation. Despite its rarity, *chronic granulomatous disease,* discussed by Gallin and colleagues, has provided considerable insight into normal and abnormal bactericidal function. Morphologic and metabolic studies have shown that the granulocytes are capable of phagocytosis of microorganisms but incapable of their subsequent killing and disposal. The lysosomes, present in normal number, discharge their enzymatic cargo into the phagosomes, but the enzymes apparently are not bactericidal. The usual acceleration of glycolysis and hexose monophosphate shunt activity does not occur, and the production of H_2O_2 is decreased. It has been proposed that in the absence of H_2O_2, the iodination of the microbial membrane cannot take place, and the organisms remain unharmed inside the phagosomes. Support for this hypothesis has been obtained from the fact that some hydrogen peroxide–producing organisms such as *Lactobacillus* are killed by the granulocytes from patients with chronic granulomatous disease. Furthermore, phagocytosis of latex particles coated with a hydrogen peroxide–producing oxidase will restore killing of simultaneously phagocytized bacteria. Chronic granulomatous disease encompas-

ses both sex-linked and autosomal variants. Although an inherited deficiency of an NADH oxidase could explain both the lack of H_2O_2 production and hexose monophosphate shunt acceleration (Fig. 3–6), such deficiency has not been definitely established (Newburger et al., 1980).

A distinct disorder of lysosomal morphology is characteristic of the *Chediak-Higashi syndrome,* in which giant lysosomes can be observed in granulocytes, melanocytes, fibroblasts, and other cellular elements. As suggested by White and Clawson (1980), abnormal membrane function may lead to uncontrolled granule fusion with the production of potentially autodestructive giant lysosomes, eventually resulting in granulocytopenia. Whether phagocytosis and lysosomal killing also are abnormal is not known, since the decreased resistance to infection exhibited by patients with this syndrome could be accounted for by their granulocytopenia. The abnormal melanocytic lysosomes may in some way be responsible for the hypopigmentation observed in patients with Chediak-Higashi syndrome and in the closely related lysosomal disorders of the Aleutian mink and the beige mouse.

Myeloproliferative Disorders

In 1951, Dameshek, with characteristic abandon, lumped all the disorders that involve uncontrolled proliferation of bone marrow cells into one syndrome, *the myeloproliferative syndrome.* Some investigators have objected to this blatant oversimplification of a difficult problem and have marshalled impressive evidence of basic differences among the diseases included. However, so far the similarities are more numerous than the differences, and the unified myeloproliferative concept has been useful in our pathophysiologic and clinical approach to these diseases.

The prototype for the myeloproliferative diseases is *polycythemia vera* (see p. 51), with its uncontrolled proliferation of erythrocytic, granulocytic, and megakaryocytic elements and its frequent termination in myelofibrosis. The cellular proliferation characterizing the other members of the syndrome involves predominantly single cell lines.

Chronic Myelogenous Leukemia. This dramatic disease was undoubtedly the disorder observed by Rudolf Virchow in 1845 and reported under the catching title *Weisses Blut,* or, in Greek terminology, *leukemia.* Even today we occasionally see untreated patients in whom the white cell crit exceeds the red cell crit, the blood appears pale, and the bone marrow looks whitish green, as in Virchow's original case.

The characteristic of early chronic myelogenous leukemia is an expansion of all granulocytic pools overflowing into peripheral blood and spleen. Since the proportional sizes of the pools closely approximate those of normal bone marrow, it has been tempting to consider this disease as being caused by an impaired cellular control with autonomy of the granulocytic stem cells. However, the manifestations cannot be explained solely on the basis of uncontrolled normal stem cell function; they also indicate dysfunction of abnormal committed and multipotential stem cells.

In 1960, Nowell and Hungerford described a specific chromosomal abnormality in the myeloid cells of patients with chronic myelogenous leukemia, an abnormality that subsequently has been found to be present in about 90 percent of cases. It consists of a deletion of part of the long arm of chromosome 22, leaving a tiny structure named the *Philadelphia chromosome (Ph[1])* (Fig. 3–11). A simultaneous lengthening of chromosome 9 suggested that the alteration is not a deletion but a translocation.

Subsequent studies have extended the bio-logic and diagnostic importance of this fortunate discovery. It was first established that erythroid cells and megakaryocytes in patients with chronic myelogenous leukemia also are Ph[1] positive, whereas fibroblasts are Ph[1] negative, suggesting that the former cells are derived from the same altered multipotential stem cell as the granulocytes, whereas fibroblasts are normal. These findings were supported by Fialkow and coworkers in their studies of women, heterozygous for the X-linked gene for glucose-6-phosphate dehydrogenase (G-6-PD), who also suffered from chronic myelogenous leukemia. According to the X-chromosome inactivation hypothesis (Fig. 2–24), all cells derived from a single abnormal stem cell will have the same G-6-PD enzyme, whereas reactive normal cells will have a mosaic of the two G-6-PD enzymes. In the women studied, all granulocytes, erythrocytes, and megakaryocytes had the same enzyme, whereas the fibroblasts demonstrated a 50:50 mixture of the two enzymes. Furthermore, it was found that B lymphocytes in some patients also were clonal, suggesting that the mutagenic event must have occurred in a slightly earlier cell than the multipotential marrow stem cell. Studies of the cellular characteristic of blast cells in the final acute phase of

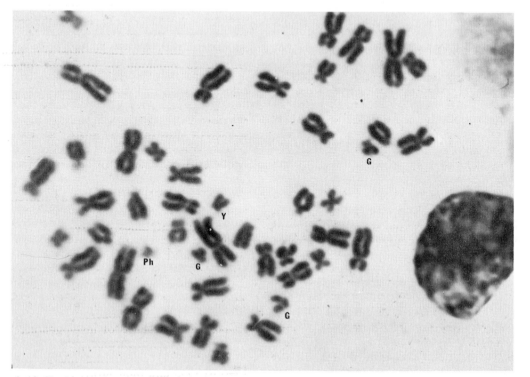

Figure 3–11 Chromosomal pattern of a male (Y chromosome) with chronic granulocytic leukemia (three normal G chromosomes and one tiny Ph[1] chromosome). (Courtesy of Dr. L. Jackson, The Thomas Jefferson University, Philadelphia, PA.)

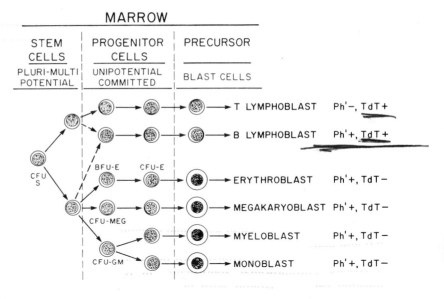

MARROW

STEM CELLS	PROGENITOR CELLS	PRECURSOR
PLURI-MULTI POTENTIAL	UNIPOTENTIAL COMMITTED	BLAST CELLS

T LYMPHOBLAST Ph'−, TdT+

B LYMPHOBLAST Ph'+, TdT+

ERYTHROBLAST Ph'+, TdT−

MEGAKARYOBLAST Ph'+, TdT−

MYELOBLAST Ph'+, TdT−

MONOBLAST Ph'+, TdT−

Figure 3–12 Blastic evolution from pluri- and multipotential stem cells and unipotential progenitor cells in acute leukemia as suggested by the determination of the presence or absence of the Philadelphia chromosome (Ph[1]) and terminal deoxynucleotidyl transferase (TdT). (Redrawn from Griffin, J. D., et al.: Blood, *61*:85, 1983.)

chronic myelogenous leukemia further support a pluripotential origin of the leukemia. In some patients, these blast cells look morphologically more like lymphoblasts than myeloblasts, and the demonstration of terminal desoxynucleotidyl transferase (TdT) in such cells has identified them as lymphoid-derived. Since monoclonal antibodies show that they are B lymphocytes, these studies have suggested that at least in patients with chronic myelogenous leukemia the differentiation pattern of pluripotential stem cells distinguishes T lymphocytes from other circulating blood cells (Fig. 3–12).

Another offshoot of the Ph[1] discovery is related to the effect of gene translocation. The transfer of a large piece of chromosome 22 to chromosome 9 provides an important visual clue in the differential diagnosis of leukocytosis. However, this translocation is reciprocal, and a small piece of chromosome 9 can be identified on chromosome 22. Since this piece contains the normal cellular homologue (c-abp) of a recognized oncogene, the Abelson murine leukemia virus, and since chromosome 22 encodes for immunoglobulin λ light chains, it seems possible that the new microenvironment for c-abp has altered its expression and in turn contributed to the pathogenesis of chronic myelogenous leukemia (Chaganti, 1983).

Although present in almost all patients with chronic myelogenous leukemia, the Ph[1] chromosome is absent in about 10 percent. Members of this small subgroup of Ph[1] negative patients have similar physical and laboratory findings but apparently a more aggressive

course and poorer prognosis. The Ph[1] positive patients rarely change to Ph[1] negativity, even during prolonged asymptomatic remissions. However, some normal stem cell clones must be present, at least early in the disease, since Smalley and coworkers have shown that intensive, ablative chemotherapy occasionally and temporarily transforms a Ph[1] positive marrow to a Ph[1] negative one.

In most patients with chronic myelogenous leukemia there is no inkling as to the character of the insult that has caused such a somatic mutation. In a few cases, however, past exposure to radiation or to drugs suggests a cause-effect relationship. For many years, radiation has been recognized to be leukemogenic in certain strains of mice, but its potential for inducing leukemia in humans was not appreciated until the early 1940s. At that time, statistical studies of the incidence of leukemia in physicians showed an overall incidence of 1.7 times that in the general population, and more importantly the studies by March indicated that the incidence of leukemia in radiologists was nine times that of physicians with little personal radiation exposure. This startling finding was accentuated by the finding of a high incidence of leukemia among the Japanese survivors from the atomic bomb explosions in Hiroshima and Nagasaki. Here, as summarized by Bizzozero and coworkers (1966), the incidence of myelogenous leukemia, either acute or chronic, increased to about three times normal during the period from 1946 to 1955 and then slowly returned toward normal again. Studies of patients receiving therapeutic radiation have indicated that this form of radiation exposure also may be leukemogenic, but at present there are no convincing data showing that diagnostic radiation will cause leukemia. The obvious issue is whether or not the leukemogenic effect of radiation has a threshold. Some feel that any amount of radiation is potentially dangerous and should be avoided at all costs, whereas others feel that the leukemogenic risk of diagnostic radiation or radiation from natural sources or atomic bomb fallout is too small to be of public health concern.

The clinical and laboratory features of chronic myelogenous leukemia are predominantly caused by the increased body load of myeloid cells. This load may be increased up to 150 times normal and causes bone marrow expansion with sternal tenderness, anemia, splenomegaly, and granulocytosis. The nutritional demands made by the overproduction of myeloid cells may cause an increased metabolic rate, with fever and weight loss, and the final breakdown of these cells may cause uricemia, gouty arthritis, and renal stones. The red cell production is usually decreased in unrestrained cases of chronic myelogenous leukemia, probably owing to decreased "Lebensraum" in the marrow. The same may be true for platelet production. When granulocyte production has become controlled by adequate therapy, the red cell and platelet mass will return to normal. The differential count of the granulocytes of peripheral blood is similar to that of the myeloid cells in normal bone marrow and is distinctly different from that of patients with leukemoid reactions in whom the cells are predominantly mature. These cells also have a normal or high content of alkaline phosphatase, whereas the cells of chronic myelogenous leukemia even during remission have a reduced content. Despite this biochemical abnormality, the phagocytic and bactericidal functions of the leukemic granulocytes appear normal. The number of basophils is usually increased and may even dominate the granulocytic picture, an unexplained but prognostically ominous sign. Serum vitamin B_{12} levels are high, as is the concentration of one of the main B_{12} binders, transcobalamin I. The latter appears to be derived from broken-down granulocytes, but its role in the symptomatology of chronic granulocytic leukemia is unknown.

Chronic myelogenous leukemia is usually well managed with the use of alkylating agents such as busulfan. Unmaintained remissions may last for months, even years. Incipient relapses are readily recognized by the rising granulocyte count, often accompanied by a return of splenic enlargement. Because of the leukemogenic potentials of busulfan and other alkylating agents (Calabresi, 1983), a myelotoxic antimetabolite, hydroxyurea, is being employed increasingly despite its brief effect and inability to induce unmaintained remissions. Radiation therapy delivered to the spleen also successfully produces hematologic and clinical remission but currently is considered less satisfactory than chemotherapy.

After about 2 to 5 years, the disease in most patients begins to assume a more aggressive character. Myeloblasts appear in the peripheral blood, anemia becomes more severe, and thrombocytopenia develops. The spleen increases in size, and the response to treatment becomes increasingly unsatisfactory. Blast cells take over the marrow, and the patient eventually succumbs to the metabolic and cellular effects of an acute refractory leukemia, the so-called "blast crisis." Some patients enter the aggressive phase by developing rapidly progressive myelofibrosis. The blast cells are usually Ph^1 positive, and they also display the chromosomal breaks and duplications seen frequently in acute myelogenous leukemia (Pedersen, 1973). Nevertheless, as mentioned before, some of these terminal blast cell leukemias are of lymphatic origin and respond temporarily to vincristine and prednisone. The rest, although of myeloid origin, usually fail to respond to regimens successfully used in the treatment of acute myelogenous leukemia. This may be due either to the unique character of the blast cells or, more likely, to an absence of normal clones to replace leukemic clones damaged by intensive chemotherapy. As in patients with polycythemia vera, the question has been raised as to the pathogenetic role of treatment in the final development of acute leukemia. No definite answer can be given, since in the past patients with untreated chronic myelogenous leukemia usually died from the effects of their chronic leukemia and only a few lived long enough to reach the stage in which contemporary patients develop their blast crisis.

Agnogenic Myeloid Metaplasia. Bone marrow fibrosis with distortion and obliteration of marrow cavities occurs as an independent disease, agnogenic myeloid metaplasia. However, it also occurs in response to tissue destruction and necrosis, as in patients with marrow invasion by tuberculosis, Hodgkin's disease, or carcinomatosis or as a complication of polycythemia vera and chronic myelogenous leukemia. Because of this latter relationship, agnogenic myeloid metaplasia has been considered a member of the myeloproliferative family. Studies by Jacobson and coworkers on women with agnogenic myeloid metaplasia who also were heterozygous for glucose-6-phosphate dehydrogenase isoenzymes (see Fig. 2–24) have supported this relationship. These studies showed that, as in polycythemia vera and chronic myelogenous leukemia, all marrow-derived blood cells are the progeny of a single abnormal clone while the fibroblasts are polyclonal and reactive. What the fibroblasts are reacting to is not certain, but it may be a growth factor released by the abnormal megakaryocytes.

The characteristic splenomegaly of this disorder has been attributed to compensatory extramedullary hemopoiesis. However, the adult spleen appears to have lost most of its fetal capacity as a primary hemopoietic organ, and compensatory extramedullary hemopoiesis is rarely found in older people who develop an increased requirement for extra blood cell production. When foci of extramedullary hemopoiesis in the spleen are found, they are probably made up of clones of bone marrow cells originating from immature cells prematurely released from the marrow and trapped in the sinusoids of the spleen. In agnogenic myeloid metaplasia, the spleen is packed with hemopoietic tissue. Since this may occur at a time when the bone marrow is only minimally replaced by fibrous tissue and is in no need of supplementary extramedullary support, it seems more likely that the splenomegaly is caused by a pathologic myeloid metaplasia rather than by a physiologic extramedullary hemopoiesis. Foci of myeloid metaplasia are also observed in the liver but rarely elsewhere.

The most striking laboratory finding is an abnormal blood smear. The red blood cells show distorted and fragmented forms, and immature blood cells such as late erythroblasts, metamyelocytes, and myelocytes are present. It is usually assumed but has not been proved that such abnormalities are caused by cells being produced in and released from a microenvironment with less organized and regulated architecture than normal bone marrow. Progressive anemia is part of the disease, but the platelet count behaves erratically, and thrombocytosis may be as common as thrombocytopenia. Marrow aspiration is usually "dry," and marrow biopsy late in the disease merely shows islands of megakaryocytes in a sea of fibrous tissue. As the disease progresses

anemia becomes more severe, necessitating androgen administration, with often excellent but temporary effects. Eventually, the patient becomes transfusion-dependent, and the question must be raised whether the large spleen destroys more cells than it produces. Erythrokinetic studies, including organ-scanning, have been of only limited help in answering this question. However, experience from splenectomy first performed to relieve physical discomfort, indicates that this procedure often is of hematologic benefit, resulting in reduction or elimination of transfusion requirements. Nevertheless, splenectomy provides only a temporary lull in the slow but relentless progress of the disease. Occasionally, the progress is rapid, with early marrow replacement by fibrous tissue and immature megakaryocytes justifying the terms *acute myelofibrosis* or *acute megakaryocytic leukemia.*

Essential Thrombocythemia. Essential thrombocythemia is another of the clonal myeloproliferative disorders and is identified by a predominance of megakaryocytic proliferation. Large numbers of viable but ineffective platelets are produced, causing a characteristic but unexplained mixture of bleeding and clotting problems. It is a chronic disorder, readily corrected but not cured by appropriate myelosuppressive therapy.

Chronic Erythroleukemia. Chronic erythroleukemia is a rare disorder characterized by the presence of macrocytosis, megaloblastic nucleated red cells in peripheral blood and bone marrow, ineffective erythropoiesis, and gradual progression into acute granulocytic leukemia. In the early stages, it can be difficult to distinguish from chronic sideroblastic anemia, since marrow examination may also disclose ringed sideroblasts. However, granulocytopoiesis and thrombopoiesis in erythroleukemia are almost always abnormal and ineffective.

Dyshemopoietic Syndrome. The dyshemopoietic syndrome encompasses a family of subacute and chronic marrow disorders characterized by ineffective cellular production. They are believed to be caused by a lesion in a member of the marrow stem cell pool leading to increased proliferation and inadequate maturation of its progeny. Since this lesion may be in any of the many stem and progenitor cells, the manifestations are protean and range from refractory anemia to refractory pancytopenia (Table 3–3). The red cells are often macrocytic and show evidence of a mixed clonal origin (double population). The marrow

Table 3–3 DYSHEMOPOIETIC SYNDROMES: FAB CLASSIFICATION (French-American-British)

Refractory anemia (RA)
RA with ringed sideroblasts
RA with excess of blasts (RAEB)
RAEB in transformation
Chronic myelomonocytic leukemia (CMML)

may or may not contain ringed sideroblasts, and the terms *with excess blasts* and *in transformation* are added to indicate the degree of potential malignancy.

In general, these disorders behave like benign tumors with controlled cellular dysplasia, but at any time they may transform into the uncontrolled neoplastic growth of acute myelogenous leukemia. Because of this propensity, they are often termed *preleukemias,* but it should be remembered that many patients never go beyond the subacute or chronic dysplastic stage, and it is always risky to use a term that implies an element of inevitability.

Acute Myelogenous Leukemia. Acute myelogenous leukemia is a rapidly progressive disease characterized by the replacement of the bone marrow with immature and poorly differentiated myelogenous cells. At present, we relate the acute myelogenous leukemia to the myeloproliferative syndrome on the one hand and to acute lymphocytic leukemia on the other, relationships that, although tenuous, are useful in the clinical approach to this frustrating and discouraging disorder.

About 50 percent of all leukemias are of the acute variety. There appears to be a slow but definite increase in this percentage—possibly due to growing diagnostic skills of physicians, and possibly due to increased exposure to leukemogenic agents.

The acute leukemias can be divided into two major groups: the *acute myelogenous* and the *acute lymphocytic.* This subdivision of a rapidly progressive and uniformly fatal disease was initially felt to be a wasteful exercise in morphologic hair-splitting. However, at present we recognize a fundamental difference between these two groups with regard to incidence, etilogy, course, treatment, and prognosis. Acute myelogenous leukemia is a disease of adulthood, occasionally related to past exposure to radiation or chemicals, frequently with a long preleukemic phase and somewhat resistant to chemotherapeutic agents. Acute lymphocytic leukemia is the predominant leukemia of childhood, rarely preceded by chemical exposure or preleukemic

symptoms and highly responsive to chemotherapeutic agents.

Because of its many morphologic manifestations, acute myelogenous leukemia is often designated *acute nonlymphocytic leukemia* and is subclassified as shown in Table 3–4. M-1 is a blast cell leukemia that is considered myelogenous because of lack of lymphoid cytochemical and surface markers. M-2 contains enough promyelocytes to identify it as a myelogenous leukemia. In M-3, the promyelocyte is the predominant cell. This third type is often associated with the occurrence of disseminated intravascular coagulation. However, owing to the high content of thromboplastic material in myeloid cells, this syndrome also occurs in other acute myelogenous leukemias. M-4 and M-5 comprise the conditions in which the progeny of the leukemic clone have both myeloid and monocytic characteristics. Finally, M-6 is the rare but dramatic acute erythroleukemia, also called *Di Guglielmo's syndrome.* Here, the marrow in the early stages is dominated by a profusion of abnormal, often multinucleated, but always ineffective erythroblasts (Fig. 3–13).

The important classification of the acute leukemias first into myelogenous and lymphocytic types and then into their subtypes is usually not too difficult for experienced hematologists relying on blood and marrow smears stained by Wright's or Giemsa stain. Occasionally, diagnosis is facilitated by observation of an eosinophilic rod known as an *Auer body* in the cytoplasm of the leukemic blast cells. The Auer body is probably a giant lysosome and is never present in lymphoblasts, a useful diagnostic tidbit.

Various cytoplasmic stains and surface markers are being used in order to sharpen diagnostic accuracy. Myeloperoxidase, Sudan black, and chloroacetate esterase stain myeloid cytoplasm; nonspecific esterases react best with monocytic cytoplasm; and periodic acid–Schiff (PAS) often stains specifically with the cytoplasm of abnormal erythroblasts (Table 3–5). Terminal desoxynucleotidyl transferase (TdT)

Table 3–4 MORPHOLOGIC CLASSIFICATION OF ACUTE MYELOGENOUS LEUKEMIA (FAB)

M-1: Acute undifferentiated leukemia
M-2: Acute myeloid leukemia with some promyelocytes
M-3: Acute promyelocytic leukemia with many hypergranular promyelocytes
M-4: Acute myelomonocytic leukemia
M-5: Acute monocytic leukemia
M-6: Acute erythroleukemia

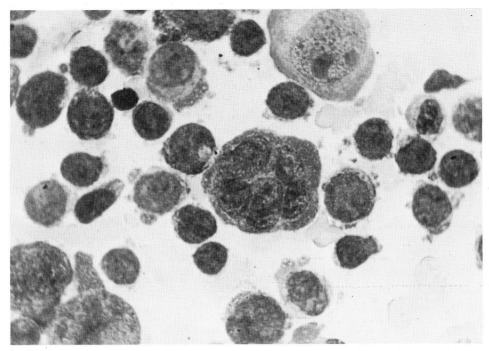

Figure 3–13 Multinucleated erythroblasts in bone marrow from patient with acute granulocytic leukemia of the Di Guglielmo variety.

is much more characteristic of the cytoplasm of lymphoid cells. Monoclonal antibodies to surface antigens have begun to be used in the diagnostic work-up of acute leukemias and should eventually provide specific identification of leukemic blast cells.

The etiology of acute leukemias is not known, but there is mounting evidence for the hypothesis that leukemia is caused by the action of a leukemogenic virus on stem cells rendered susceptible by genetic predisposition or chemical alteration. The presence of a genetic or chromosomal susceptibility is supported by statistical studies that indicate that the chance of developing acute leukemia is about 1 in 5 if one's identical twin has leukemia, 1 in 60 if one's nonidentical twin has leukemia, 1 in 700 if one's sibling has leukemia, and 1 in 3000 if no one else in the family has leukemia (Zuelzer and Cox, 1969). However, these data also tend to rule out an inborn mutation as the sole etiologic mechanism, since only 20 percent of individuals with a leukemic identical twin develop the disease. Certain chromosomal defects, both congenital and acquired, appear to predispose to acute leukemia. Children with inborn chromosomal defects such as *Down's syndrome, Fanconi's anemia,* and *Bloom's syndrome* all have an increased incidence of acute leukemia, and leukemogenic chemicals and radiation have the capacity to cause chromosomal changes. Such changes, especially chromosomal translocations, may provide silent proto-oncogenes with a new, more stimulating environment. This challenging possibility has renewed interest in chromosome mapping in patients with preleukemia and acute leukemia (Sparkes, 1984).

The potential leukemogenic effect of ionizing radiation was mentioned in the section on chronic myelogenous leukemia. Radiation and radiomimetic, chemotherapeutic agents are potentially leukemogenic, and the incidence of acute leukemia in patients previously treated successfully for a neoplasm has reached disturbing proportions (Calabresi, 1983). Of the chemotherapeutic agents, the alkylating components capable of cross-linking DNA molecules and preventing DNA repair even in

Table 3–5 CYTOPLASMIC MARKERS FOR THE BLASTS OF ACUTE MYELOGENOUS LEUKEMIA

	M-1	M-2	M-3	M-4	M-5	M-6
Peroxidase	+/−	+	+	+	+	−
Sudan black	+/−	+	+	+	+	−
Chloroacetate esterase	+/−	+	+	+	+	−
Nonspecific esterase	−	−	+/−	+	+	−
PAS	−	−	−	−	−	+

resting cells appear to be most dangerous, especially when given continuously over prolonged periods. Although these agents could cause a chromosomal mutation with the production of autonomous leukemic blast cells, the possibility that they provide a latent leukemogenic virus with the opportunity for unchecked multiplication appears equally good. It has been known for about 75 years that avian leukemia is caused and transmitted by a virus, and studies by Gross in 1965 provided strong evidence for the existence of a similar etiologic mechanism for murine leukemias. The murine leukemogenic viruses are RNA viruses, and their mechanism of replication has been clarified by the discovery of a reverse transcriptase, an enzyme capable of incorporating the information coded in viral RNA into DNA of the host. Such an enzyme has been found in human leukemic cells, but its presence there is of questionable significance, since it has also been found in human nonleukemic embryonic cells. Direct demonstration of viral particles in and around leukemic cells is difficult to achieve, and, when found, their pathogenic importance is difficult to interpret (Jarrett, 1973).

Epidemiologic data suggesting direct transmission of leukemia are scant, but strong indirect evidence for the presence of an infective agent has been provided by Fialkow and coworkers, who reported the course of leukemia in a girl who had received a bone marrow transplant from her brother. After some months the leukemia recurred, but this time the leukemic blast cells were cytogenetically XY cells. This unique case has generated considerable speculation and has even raised the possibility that leukemic relapses after prolonged remission are caused by reinfection rather than by the survival of a few leukemic cells, a most unorthodox view.

The conventional view of cellular kinetics in acute leukemia is based on data obtained by Skipper and coworkers and suggests that the relapses and remissions of the disease are determined by the size of the leukemic mass. Manifest leukemia with the presence of leukemic cells in the bloodstream and with considerable leukemic bone marrow replacement is present when the leukemic mass is about 1 kg. in weight or 10^{12} cells in number. The reduction in mass to about 1 gm. will cause a morphologic and symptomatic remission but will still leave about 10^9 leukemic cells at large. Further therapy will reduce the body load and prolong the remission, but only total cell kill

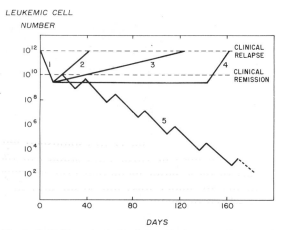

Figure 3–14 Hypothetical relationship between therapy of acute leukemia, leukemic cell number, and remission or relapse: *(1)* The effect of a successful induction therapy on cell count; *(2)* the immediate relapse that occurs after unmaintained therapy; (3) the slow relapse after partially effective maintenance therapy; (4) the prolonged remission on effective maintenance therapy; and (5) the hoped-for effect of repeated course of reinduction therapy on leukemic cell number. (Redrawn from Spiers, A. S. D.: Clin. Haematol., *1*:127, 1972.)

will provide a cure (Fig. 3–14). This latter assumption is derived from data in rodents in which the transplantation of a single leukemic cell into an inbred recipient will result in leukemia. However, immunologic assistance in outbred species such as humans may make it less mandatory to aim for total cell kill, a goal that probably could not be accomplished without irreparable damage to normal tissues.

By now, it has been shown convincingly that leukemic blast cells do not proliferate as actively as normal bone marrow cells (Killmann, 1968). The mitotic index and the tritiated thymidine labeling index are lower for leukemic blast cells than for normal blast cells. Even without the help of sophisticated quantitative techniques, it is evident from looking at leukemic bone marrow smears that mitotic figures are relatively rare. This paradox—that a rapidly growing tumor such as acute leukemia should consist of sluggishly proliferating cells—has been difficult to accept. However, the therapeutic use of cytotoxic agents is based on the fact that normal bone marrow cells recover early, while there is a much more delayed recovery of leukemic blast cells; in other words, leukemic cells must have a longer generation time than normal cells. It is possible that the leukemic cell mass is made up of several cellular populations, with the majority of the cells being inert, long-lived, and slowly proliferating and the minority having a rapid cellular turnover. It is the activity of this latter population that presumably accounts for the abrupt changes that occur in the bone marrow and peripheral blood during relapse.

Various studies have shown that leukemic blast cells, when specifically stimulated, are capable of normal maturation. This startling observation has been made after the addition of phorbol esters or metabolites of vitamin A (retinoids) and vitamin D to established leukemic cell lines in vitro. Pilot studies of the effect of these latter metabolites on leukemic patients are under way, but so far they have not shown dramatic in vivo effects (Koeffler, 1983).

The signs and symptoms of acute myelogenous leukemia usually can be attributed to mechanical or metabolic interference with the normal function of a number of organs. The leukemic cells will amass in great numbers in the bone marrow, spleen, liver, lymph nodes, and blood. Bone marrow function is first and most seriously threatened, either because the finite marrow volume precludes compensatory expansion or because blast cells exert a suppressive effect on the remaining normal cells. The liver, spleen, and lymph nodes can expand considerably without functional impairment, but a liver extensively infiltrated with leukemic cells may show signs of failure, an enlarged spleen may cause sequestration and injury to normal blood cells, and lymphatic tissue with architectural displacement may be immunologically less effective. Leukostasis either in the lungs with pulmonary failure or in the brain with cerebral hemorrhage may occur if the white cell count is extremely high. The effect of leukemic cells on the function of blood is less clear. Whole blood viscosity is probably not changed significantly, since an increase in the white blood cell mass usually is offset by a decrease in the red blood cell mass.

Anemia is almost invariably present at the time of diagnosis. Hypersplenic and febrile red cell destruction may contribute, but the cause is usually suppressed or ineffective erythropoiesis. The anemia is best managed by judicious transfusions of packed red blood cells.

Hemorrhages and petechiae are most often the features that bring the patient to a physician. With few exceptions, they are caused by thrombocytopenia and are ameliorated by transfusion of concentrated platelet preparations. The critical level of platelet count below which spontaneous bleeding occurs is hard to define, since the effect of thrombocytopenia may be aggravated by platelet dysfunction or even disseminated intravascular coagulation. In general, platelet counts below 30,000 per mm.³ should cause concern, and platelet counts below 10,000 per mm.³ are associated with spontaneous hemorrhages and petechiae. Infections and fever are common and are most often caused by granulocytopenic impairment of host defenses. Although it has been claimed that an infection is always present when a leukemic patient develops fever, tissue necrosis and endogenous pyogens undoubtedly contribute. Nevertheless, fever in a granulocytopenic patient in whom defenses often are reduced even further by steroids and immunosuppressive drugs should always be treated as if an infection were present. During the last decades important changes have occurred in the ecology of the infecting microorganisms. Bacteria and fungi of low virulence and high antibiotic resistance have emerged as major offenders and contribute to the chilling statistics that show that about 70 percent of all leukemic patients die from infections. The preventive use of absorbable antibiotics has had little or no effect on infectious morbidity or mortality, and even the use of careful reverse isolation techniques, laminar air flow chambers, and nonabsorbable oral anibiotics has been of little help. Complete isolation in life islands tends to isolate patients from good nursing care and compassionate personal attention. The transfusion of normal granulocytes harvested by centrifugation or filtration leukopheresis is coming of age, but its efficacy remains to be proved.

The triad of anemia, hemorrhage, and infection will respond to effective treatment of the leukemia. Unfortunately, this treatment is not specific, and normal hemopoietic elements are wiped out together with the leukemic cells. If the patient survives the initial weeks of severe bone marrow failure first brought on by the disease and then temporarily aggravated by the treatment, complete remission may be achieved with the restoration of a normal bone marrow picture and peripheral blood counts. Without treatment, survival is about 3 to 6 months. Modern multiagent treatment induces a complete remission in about 40 to 60 percent of patients, but the median survival is still only about 1 year. The selection of treatment programs remains quite empiric. Some drugs shown to be quite effective in animal studies, such as hydroxyurea, are relatively inactive. Other agents known to be very effective in acute lymphatic leukemia, such as vincristine and prednisone, are far less effective in acute

Table 3–6 CHEMOTHERAPEUTIC AGENTS CURRENTLY USED IN TREATMENT OF LEUKEMIA

Drug	Drug Category	Mechanisms of Action
Cytosine arabinoside	Pyrimidine antagonist	Inhibition of de novo synthesis of deoxycytidine riboside and of DNA polymerase
6-Mercaptopurine 6-Thioguanine	Purine antagonists	Inhibition of de novo purine synthesis
Hydroxyurea	Antimetabolite	Inhibition of ribonucleotide reductase
Nitrogen mustard Cyclophosphamide Chlorambucil Busulfan Melphalan	Polyfunctional alkylating agents	Cross-linkage of DNA
Methotrexate	Folic acid antagonist	Inhibition of dihydrofolate reductase. Inhibition of DNA synthesis
Daunorubicin Doxorubicin	Antitumor antibiotics isolated from *Streptomyces peucetius*	Inhibition of DNA and RNA synthesis
Bleomycin	Antitumor antibiotics isolated from *Streptomyces verticillus*	Inhibition of DNA synthesis
Prednisone	Synthetic adrenocorticosteroid	Direct lysis of lymphocytes and lymphoblasts. Inhibition of cell cycle. Inhibition of DNA synthesis and/or DNA-directed RNA synthesis.
Vincristine	Alkaloid of periwinkle plant	Metaphase arrest resulting from inhibition of mitotic spindle (microtubule) formation
L-Asparaginase	Enzyme, catalyzing the hydrolysis of L-asparaginase	Depletion of exogenous L-asparagine needed for the metabolism of malignant cells incapable of synthesizing this amino acid

myelogenous leukemia. Table 3–6 lists some of the agents used currently in the treatment of leukemia, along with their presumed modes of action. The goal of contemporary chemotherapy is obviously to eliminate leukemic stem cells and their progeny while salvaging normal clones and permitting them to repopulate the marrow. This goal seems to be met most often in children and in adults diagnosed early as having acute myelogenous leukemia. If the preleukemic phase is prolonged or if the patient is in the older age group, normal clones are scant or nonexistent, and no chemotherapy can effect a cure or even a prolonged remission. Marrow transplantation in such patients appears to be the only way by which to provide normal clones and hope for cure. Current studies in patients with compatible sibling donors suggest that marrow transplantation in young patients with acute myelogenous leukemia is the treatment of choice. In order to be of greatest benefit, however,

transplantation must be performed during the first chemotherapy-induced remission. Unfortunately, transplantation has been of much less benefit in patients in the older age group, who also demonstrate the worst response to chemotherapy.

Monocyte-Macrophage Disorders

Disorders of the monocyte-macrophage complex can be classified as quantitative, qualitative, and malignant cellular disorders (Table 3–7).

Quantitative Abnormalities

A monocytosis with an absolute increase in circulating monocytes to more than 500 per mm.[3] is frequently a nonspecific sign of some occult disease and should lead to a thorough search for a cause. Before the antibiotic era,

Table 3–7 CLASSIFICATION OF MONOCYTE-MACROPHAGE DISORDERS

Quantitative abnormalities
  Reactive monocytosis
  Reactive mononuclear phagocytic response
Qualitative abnormalities
  Gaucher's disease
  Niemann-Pick disease
Malignant disorders
  Monocytic leukemia
  Histiocytic lymphoma
  Letterer-Siwe disease
  Histiocytic medullary reticulosis
  Hand-Schüller-Christian disease
  Eosinophilic granuloma

monocytosis usually meant tuberculosis, subacute bacterial endocarditis, or some other generalized infectious disease. Now, it more often is an early "preleukemic" manifestation of a hematologic malignancy. However, it may also herald a collagen disease or a cancer.

An increase in the number of tissue macrophages may reflect an appropriate response to foreign antigens, so-called "overwork hyperplasia." It can be seen in conditions of sustained but low-grade invasion of microorganisms, such as *Whipple's disease, kala azar, malaria,* and *histoplasmosis.* In these condi-

tions, the macrophage proliferation causes splenomegaly and, to a lesser extent, lymphadenopathy. Cytopenias are frequently present, and it may be difficult to distinguish between increased blood cell destruction due to hypersplenism and decreased production due to encroachment by macrophages on available bone marrow space.

Qualitative Abnormalities

The lipid storage diseases include a number of rare autosomal recessive disorders, each characterized by a deficiency in one of the catabolic enzymes involved in the breakdown of the sphingolipids (Brady, 1972). The deficiency affects all tissues, but the macrophages, by virtue of their prominent role in the catabolism of the lipid-rich membrane, are particularly prone to accumulate undegraded lipid products. This leads to the production of lipid-laden and probably "blocked" foamy macrophages, to stimulation of further macrophage production, and eventually to a tremendous expansion of the mononuclear phagocyte system.

In *Gaucher's disease,* there is a deficiency of β-glucosidase which normally splits glucose from its parent sphingolipids, globoside and

Table 3–8 SPHINGOLIPIDS

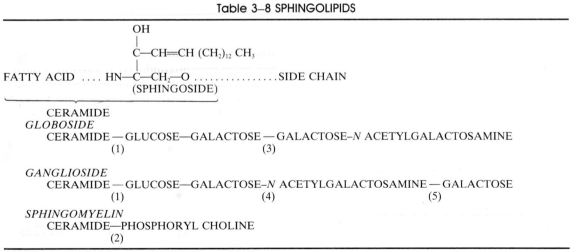

In the lysosomal degradation of glycolipids of senescent cells, the carbohydrates or the phosphorylcholine constituents of the side chains have to be removed sequentially before final hydrolysis of ceramide, the sphingosine–fatty acid complex. Absence of the following specific enzymes will lead to accumulation of their substrate in the macrophages:

1. β-Glucosidase deficiency: Gaucher's disease
2. Sphingomyelinase
     deficiency: Niemann-Pick disease
3. α-Galactosidase deficiency: Fabry's disease
4. Hexosaminidase deficiency: Tay-Sachs disease
5. β-Galactosidase deficiency: Gangliosidosis

ganglioside (Table 3–8). The accumulation of glycosphingolipids, derived chiefly from granulocytes, gives an onion-skin appearance to the pale lipid-laden macrophage cytoplasm. These cells, of course, also show a positive PAS stain for carbohydrate. In its typical form, Gaucher's disease is a slowly progressive disease in which the accumulation of Gaucher's cells causes massive splenomegaly and hepatomegaly, bone marrow expansion, and pulmonary infiltration.

In *Niemann-Pick disease*, the deficiency is in an enzyme that normally cleaves phosphoryl choline from its parent sphingolipid, sphingomyelin. The macrophages in this condition have the appearance of typical "foam cells" and do not stain with PAS. They cause a rapidly progressive hyperplasia of the mononuclear phagocyte system, and the accumulation of undegraded sphingomyelin leads to neuronal degeneration and death within a few years of life.

Cells resembling Gaucher's cells and "foam cells" can also be seen in the marrow of patients with chronic myelogenous leukemia. Here the cause lies not in a deficiency of a catabolic enzyme but rather in an increased lipid load from the sphingolipid-rich granulocyte membrane. "Foam cells" are also seen in the hyperlipidemias, demonstrating that the plasma may be a source of lipid in the macrophage cytoplasm (Ferrans et al., 1971).

Malignant Disorders

The acute monocytic or myelomonocytic leukemia is for diagnostic and therapeutic convenience treated as a myeloproliferative disorder closely related to acute myelogenous leukemia. *Chronic monocytic leukemia,* however, is logically a disorder of the monocyte-macrophage system and is usually classified as a dyshemopoietic or preleukemic disease (Table 3–3). Chronic monocytic leukemia is a rare, often slowly progressive condition with minimal lymphadenopathy and moderate splenomegaly. The blood smear shows numerous promonocytes and mature monocytes, but the morphologic identification of the cells can be quite taxing.

A number of variations have been described under designations such as *histiocytic leukemia, leukemic reticuloendotheliosis, hairy cell leukemia,* and *reticulum cell leukemia.* These conditions have traditionally been assigned to the monocyte-macrophage system, although basic phagocytic properties of the involved cells have

not always been clearly demonstrated (Katayama and Finkel, 1974). Attempts to identify cellular surface markers have raised the possibility that some or all of the involved cells synthesize immunoglobulins and that these conditions actually belong to the lymphoproliferative system. Such taxonomic questions may appear clinically unimportant today. However, our progress in designing chemotherapeutic agents tailored to the metabolic functions of malignant cells is so rapid that we can anticipate having future treatments for conditions belonging to the phagocytic system that are very different from treatments for conditions belonging to the immunocytic system.

Malignant proliferative disorders of the more differentiated macrophages may result in *histiocytic medullary reticulosis.* This is a rapidly progressive and fatal febrile disorder of adults with lymphadenopathy, hepatosplenomegaly, hemolytic anemia, thrombocytopenia, and leukopenia. Its hallmark is erythrophagocytosis, and red cell–laden macrophages are readily demonstrable in the pleomorphic cellular infiltrate. The childhood counterpart is termed *Letterer-Siwe disease,* but the phagocytic cells here are less erythrophagocytic, and hemolytic anemia is not a prominent factor. Chronic unrestrained proliferation of completely differentiated macrophages is found locally as *eosinophilic granuloma* or more diffusely as *Hand-Schüller-Christian disease.* These diseases have been lumped together under the term *histiocytosis X,* but a thorough clinical and pathologic evaluation should provide a specific diagnosis and especially should distinguish these probably malignant disorders from benign reactive hyperplasia of the mononuclear phagocyte system.

References

Babior, B. M.: The respiratory burst of phagocytes. J. Clin. Invest., *73*:599, 1984.

Badwey, J. A., Curnutte, J. T., and Karnovsky, M. L.: The enzyme of granulocytes that produces superoxide and peroxide. An elusive Pimpernel. N. Engl. J. Med., *300*:1157, 1979.

Baehner, R. L., and Nathan, D. G.: Quantitative nitroblue tetrazolium test in chronic granulomatous disease. N. Engl. J. Med., *278*:971, 1968.

Bagby, G. C., Lawrence, H. F., and Neerhout, R. C.: T-Lymphocyte–mediated granulopoietic failure. In vitro identification of prednisone-responsive patients. N. Engl. J. Med., *309*:1073, 1983.

Beeson, P. B., and Bass, D. A.: The Eosinophil. Philadelphia, W. B. Saunders Co., 1977.

Bizzozero, O. J., Johnson, K. G., and Ciocco, A.: Radiation-related leukemia in Hiroshima and Nagasaki, 1946–1964. N. Engl. J. Med., 274:1095, 1966.

Blume, R. S., Bennett, J. M., Yankee, R. A., and Wolff, S. M.: Defective granulocyte regulation in the Chediak-Higashi syndrome. N. Engl. J. Med., 279:1009, 1968.

Boggs, D. R.: The kinetics of neutrophilic leukocytes in health and disease. Semin. Hematol., 4:359, 1967.

Brady, R. O.: Biochemical and metabolic basis of familial sphingolipidosis. Semin. Hematol., 9:273, 1972.

Burgess, A. W., and Metcalf, O.: The nature and actions of granulocyte-macrophage colony stimulating factors. Blood, 56:947, 1980.

Calabresi, P.: Leukemia after cytotoxic chemotherapy—a pyrrhic victory. N. Engl. J. Med., 309:1118, 1983.

Chaganti, R. S. K.: Significance of chromosome changes to hematopoietic neoplasms. Blood, 62:515, 1983.

Cline, M. J.: Monocytes and macrophages. Functions and diseases. Ann. Int. Med., 88:78, 1978.

Craddock, C. G., Perry, S., Lawrence, J. S., et al.: Production and distribution of granulocytes and the control of granulocyte release. In Wolstenholme, G. E. W., and O'Connor, M. (Eds.): Ciba Foundation Symposium on Haemopoiesis. London, Churchill, 1960, p. 237.

Dameshek, W.: Some speculations on the myeloproliferative syndromes. Blood, 6:392, 1951.

Ferrans, V. J., Buja, M., Roberts, W. C., and Frederickson, D. S.: The spleen in Type I hyperlipoproteinemia. Am. J. Pathol., 64:67, 1971.

Fialkow, P. J., et al.: Chronic myelocytic leukemia: clonal origin in a stem cell common to the granulocytic, erythrocyte, platelet and monocyte/macrophage. Am. J. Med., 63:125, 1977.

Fialkow, P. J., Thomas, E. D., Bryant, J. J., and Neiman, P. E.: Leukaemic transformation of engrafted human marrow cells in vivo. Lancet, 1:251, 1971.

Gallin, J. J., et al.: Recent advances in chronic granulomatous disease. Ann. Int. Med., 99:657, 1983.

Golde, D. W., Finley, T. N., and Cline, M. J.: The pulmonary macrophages in acute leukemia. N. Engl. J. Med., 290:875, 1974.

Gralnick, H. R.: Classification of acute leukemia. Ann. Int. Med., 87:740, 1977.

Griffin, J. D., et al.: Differentiation pattern in the blastic phase of chronic myeloid leukemia. Blood, 61:85, 1983.

Gross, L.: Viral etiology of leukemia and lymphomas. Blood, 25:377, 1965.

Holmes, B., Quie, P. G., Windhorst, D. B., and Good, R. A.: Fatal granulomatous disease of childhood: an inborn abnormality of phagocytic function. Lancet, 1:1225, 1966.

Jacob, H. S., et al.: Complement-induced granulocyte aggregation. N. Engl. J. Med., 302:789, 1980.

Jacobson, R. S., Sale, A., and Fialkow, P. S.: Agnogenic myeloid metaplasia. A clonal proliferaton of hematopoietic stem cells with secondary myelofibrosis. Blood, 51:189, 1978.

Jarrett, W. F. H.: Viruses and leukemia. Br. J. Haematol., 25:287, 1973.

Kaliner, M. A.: The mast cell—a fascinating riddle. N. Engl. J. Med., 301:498, 1979.

Karnofsky, M. L., Noseworthy, J., Simmons, S., and Glass, E. A.: Metabolic patterns that control the functions of leukocytes. In Greenwalt, T. J., and Jamieson, G. A. (Eds.): Formation and Destruction of Blood Cells. Philadelphia, J. B. Lippincott Co., 1970, p. 207.

Katayama, T., and Finkel, H. E.: Leukemic reticuloendotheliosis. A clinicopathologic study with review of the literature. Am. J. Med., 57:115, 1974.

Kennedy, B. J.: Cyclic leukocyte oscillations in chronic myelogenous leukemia during hydroxyurea therapy. Blood, 35:751, 1970.

Killmann, S. A.: Acute leukemia: the kinetics of leukemic blast cells in man. An analytical review. Series Haematol., 1:38, 1968.

Klebanoff, S. F.: Oxygen metabolism and the toxic properties of phagocytes. Ann. Int. Med., 93:480, 1980.

Koeffler, H. P.: Induction of differentiation of human acute myelogenous leukemic cells. Therapeutic implications. Blood, 62:709, 1983.

Koeffler, H. P., and Golde, D. W.: Chronic myelogenous leukemia—new concepts. N. Engl. J. Med., 304:1201; 1269, 1981.

Mahmoud, A. A. F., Stone, M. K., and Kellermeyer, R. W.: Eosinophilopoietin: A circulating low molecular weight peptide-like substance which stimulates the production of eosinophils in mice. J. Clin. Invest., 60:675, 1977.

March, H. C.: Leukemia in radiologists, ten years later. Am. J. Med. Sci., 242:137, 1961.

Metcalf, D., and Stanley, E. R.: Haematological effects in mice of partially purified colony stimulating factor (CSF) prepared from human urine. Br. J. Haematol., 21:481, 1971.

Meuret, G.: Disorders of the mononuclear phagocyte system. An analytical review. Blut, 34:317, 1977.

Miller, M. E., Oski, F. A., and Harris, M. B.: Lazy leucocyte syndrome. Lancet, 1:665, 1971.

Minchintou, R. M., and Waters, A. H.: The occurrence and significance of neutrophil antibodies. Br. J. Haematol., 56:521, 1984.

Nathan, C. F., Murray, H. W., and Cohn, Z. A.: The macrophage as an effector cell. N. Engl. J. Med., 303:622, 1980.

Newburger, P., et al.: Chronic granulomatous disease. Expression of the metabolic defect by in vitro culture of bone marrow progenitors. J. Clin. Invest., 66:599, 1980.

Nowell, P. C., and Hungerford, D. A.: A minute chromosome in human chronic granulocytic leukemia. Science, 132:1497, 1960.

O'Riordan, M. L., Robinson, J. A., Buckton, K. E., and Evans, H. J.: Distinguishing between the chromosome involved in Down's syndrome (trisomy 21) and chronic myeloid leukemia (Ph¹) by fluorescence. Nature, 230:167, 1971.

Pederson, B.: The blast crisis of chronic myeloid leukemia. Acute transformation of a preleukemic condition? Br. J. Haematol., 25:141, 1973.

Perussia, B., et al.: Immune interferon and leukocyte-conditioned medium induce normal and leukemic myeloid cells to differentiate along the monocytic pathway. J. Exp. Med., 158:2058, 1983.

Pisciotta, A. V.: Studies on agranulocytosis X. A biochemical defect in chlorpromazine-sensitive marrow cells. J. Lab. Clin. Med., 78:435, 1971.

Pisciotta, A. V.: Immune and toxic mechanisms in drug-induced agranulocytosis. Semin. Hematol., 10:279, 1973.

Richard, K. A., Morley, A., Howard, D., and Stohlman, F., Jr.: The in vitro colony-forming cell and the response to neutropenia. Blood, 37:6, 1971.

Robinson, W. A., and Mangalik, A.: The kinetics and regulation of granulopoiesis. Semin. Hematol., 12:7, 1975.

Skipper, H. E.: Cellular kinetics associated with "curability" of experimental leukemia. In Dameshek, W., and Dutcher, R. M. (Eds.): Perspectives in Leukemia. New York, Grune and Stratton, 1968, p. 187.

Slungaard, A., et al.: Pulmonary carcinoma with eosinophilia. Demonstration of a tumor-derived eosinophilopoietic factor. N. Engl. J. Med., *309*:778, 1983.

Smalley, R. V., Vogel, J., Huguley, C. M., Jr., and Miller, D.: Chronic granulocytic leukemia: cytogenetic conversion of the bone marrow with cycle-specific chemotherapy. Blood, *50*:107, 1977.

Southwick, F. S., and Stossel, T. P.: Contractile proteins in leukocyte function. Semin. Hematol., *20*:305, 1983.

Sparkes, R. S.: Cytogenetics of leukemia. N. Engl. J. Med., *311*:848, 1984.

Spiers, A. S. D.: Chemotherapy of acute leukaemia. Clin. Haematol., *1*:127, 1972.

Stossel, T. P.: Phagocytosis. N. Engl. J. Med., *290*:717; 774; 833, 1974.

Wade, B. H., and Mandell, G. L.: Polymorphnuclear leukocytes: dedicated professional phagocytes. Am. J. Med., *74*:686, 1983.

Wagner, H. N., Jr., and Iio, M.: Studies of the reticuloendothelial system (RES). III Blockade of the RES in man. J. Clin. Invest., *43*:1525, 1964.

Ward, P. A.: Insubstantial leukotaxis. J. Lab. Clin. Med., *79*:873, 1972.

Warner, H. R., and Athens, J. W.: An analysis of granulocyte kinetics in blood and bone marrow, in leukopoiesis in health and disease. Ann. N.Y. Acad. Sci., *113*:523, 1964.

White, J. G., and Clawson, C. C.: The Chédiak-Higashi syndrome: The nature of the giant neutrophil granules and their interactions with cytoplasm and foreign particulates. Am. J. Pathol., *98*:151, 1980.

Zucker-Franklin, D., Elsbach, P., and Simon, E. J.: The effect of the morphine analog levorphanol on phagocytosing leukocytes. Lab. Invest., *25*:415, 1971.

Zuelzer, W. W., and Cox, D. E.: Genetic aspects of leukemia. Semin. Hematol., *6*:228, 1969.

Immunocytes

STRUCTURE

The cells of the immune system are morphologically quite similar but show an amazing functional diversity. This diversity is based on variations in the expression of immunoglobulin and histocompatibility genes, which in turn render the immunocytes capable of a vast number of immune interactions and immune responses.

Cellular Morphology

In stained blood and marrow films, the *small lymphocyte* is a round cell measuring approximately 9 μm. in diameter with a skimpy rim of pale blue cytoplasm that may contain a few azurophilic granules. Its nucleus has a chromatin pattern arranged in bluish-purple blocks, often with a small indentation in the nuclear membrane (Figs. 3–15 and 3–16). The *large lymphocyte* has a more generous cytoplasm that stains a deeper shade of blue. Its nucleus is also larger, with chromatin blocks spaced farther apart in a looser arrangement. Nucleoli may be seen. The lymphoblast is a large lymphocyte in which the nuclear chromatin no longer exhibits a block-like character but instead is finely divided into a grainy texture, in the midst of which are one or two nucleoli (Fig. 3–16). Cell size is related to cell division.

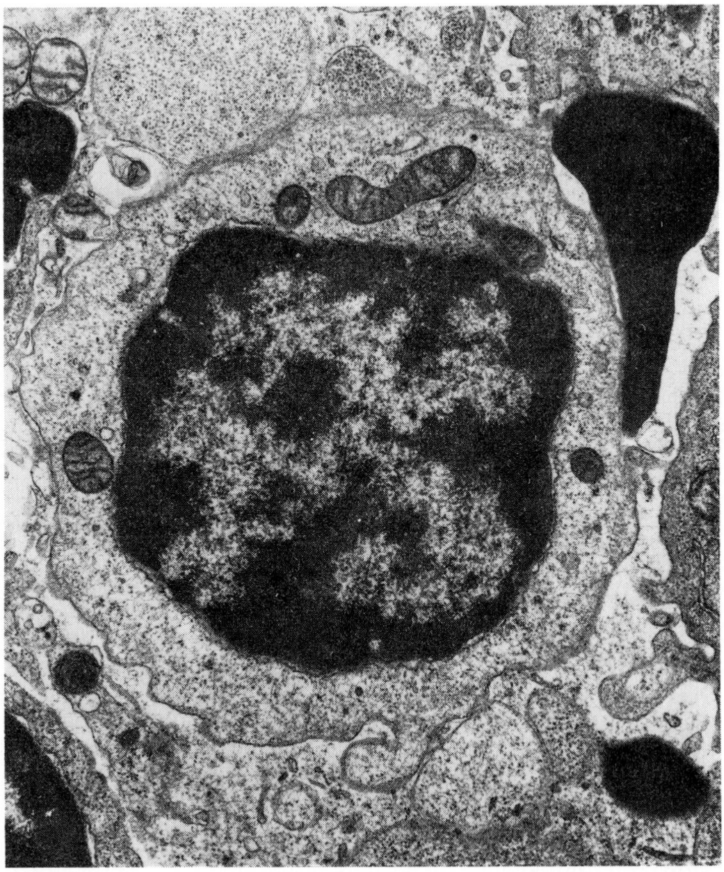

Figure 3–15 Electron microscope picture of a small mature human lymphocyte. Cytoplasm is scanty and contains mitochondria and ribosomes. Chromatin is densely packed into masses in a centrally placed nucleus. (Courtesy of Dr. A. Abraham, Lankenau Hospital, Philadelphia, PA.)

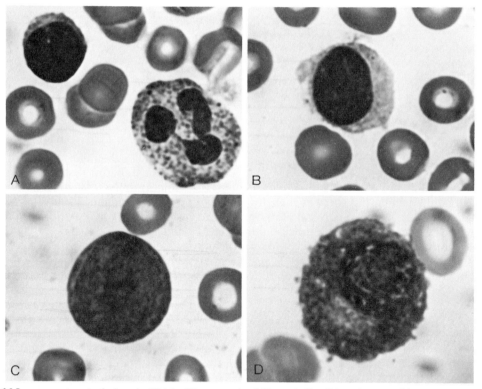

Figure 3–16 Immunocyte morphology in Wright-Giemsa–stained films. *A,* Small lymphocyte with segmented neutrophil. *B,* Large lymphocyte. *C,* Lymphoblast. *D,* Plasma cell.

Small lymphocytes are nondividing. Large lymphocytes and lymphoblasts are in a transformation associated with active cell proliferation, demonstrable by the uptake of tritiated thymidine into the DNA of cell nuclei. *Plasma cells* are identified by the eccentrically placed nucleus, with densely stained compact chromatin blocks and deep bluish-green cytoplasm indicative of a high level of secretory activity. A clear zone containing the Golgi apparatus is located adjacent to the nucleus (Figs. 3–16 and 3–17). Cytoplasmic inclusions are frequently seen, such as grapelike vacuoles and crystalline structures, also signs of active secretion. The *immunoblast (plasmablast)* contains a large blastlike nucleus along with the secretory cytoplasm of the plasma cell, although clear cell variants are described.

In fixed tissue sections, small lymphocytes are often compactly arranged, uniform and monotonous in their overall appearance, with small, round, darkly stained nuclei. Large lymphocytes and lymphoblasts vary somewhat more in size and shape and have large, vesicular nuclei. The lymphocytes in the centers of germinal follicles have irregularly shaped nuclei, often with linear cleavages. They are somewhat larger than small lymphocytes, vary

considerably in size and shape, and are more loosely arranged (Fig. 3–18). These cells have been called *follicular center cells, cleaved cells,* and *centrocytes.* Lymphoblasts found in germinal centers have been called *centroblasts.* Plasma cells in fixed sections are identified by the eccentric nucleus with densely stained chromatin blocks and by the deeply basophilic cytoplasm.

T and B Cell Markers

Although T and B lymphocytes cannot be distinguished by conventional morphology, a number of differences in surface topography permit their identification. The membrane of B lymphocytes contains intrinsic immunoglobulin, mostly as IgM and IgD, readily identified by immunofluorescent techniques. T cells lack membrane immunoglobulin but possess a receptor for sheep erythrocytes. This is identified by the formation of rosettes between sheep red blood cells and T lymphocytes (Fig. 3–19). The sum of surface immunoglobulin-positive (sIg^+) cells and E rosette–positive (ER^+) cells accounts for almost 100 percent of the peripheral blood lymphocytes. Normally, ER^+ lym-

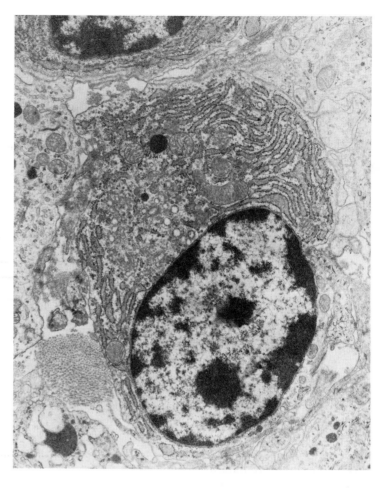

Figure 3–17 Electron microscope picture of a mature human plasma cell. Rough endoplasmic reticulum completely fills the cytoplasm of this immunoglobulin-secreting cell. The nucleus resembles that of the small lymphocyte but assumes an eccentric position. (Courtesy of Dr. A. Abraham, Lankenau Hospital, Philadelphia, PA.)

phocytes predominate, constituting approximately 65 to 80 percent of the total.

There are other ways of distinguishing T cells from B cells by differences in their surfaces (Table 3–9). They each have specific membrane antigens that can be accurately detected by monoclonal antibodies (e.g., B_1 in B cells and T_3 in T cells). T and B cells respond

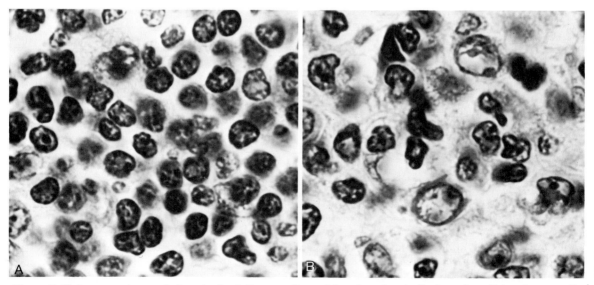

Figure 3–18 Immunocyte morphology in fixed tissue sections of lymph node. *A*, Region of small lymphocytes. *B*, Follicular center cells.

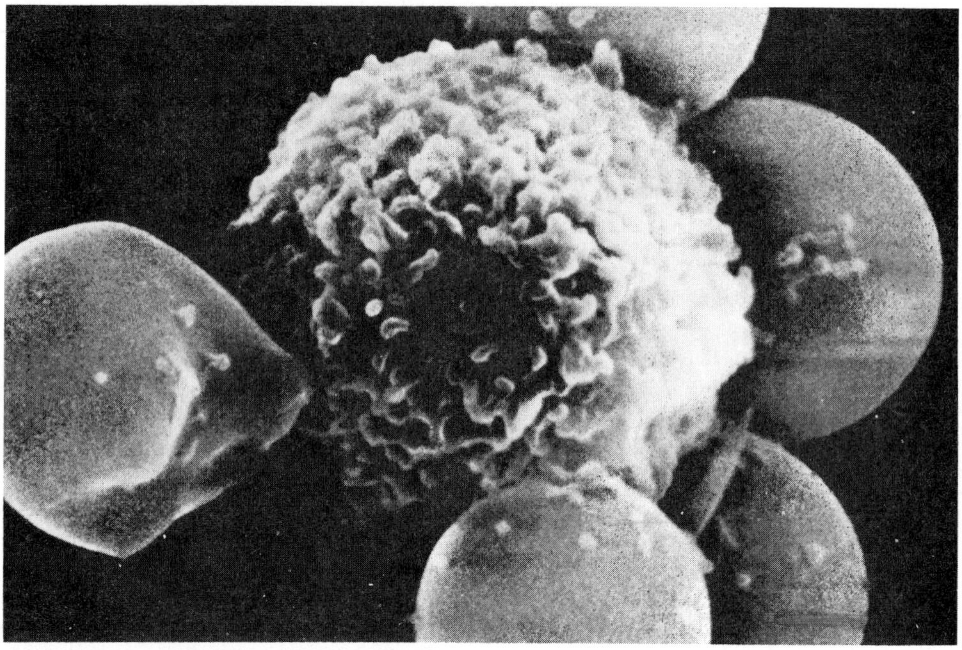

Figure 3–19 Demonstration by scanning electron microscopy of erythrocytes adhering to a lymphocyte to form a "rosette."

differently to certain lectins, such as phytohemagglutinin and pokeweed mitogen. Both cell lines carry the HLA-ABC histocompatibility antigens (class I), but only resting B cells have the HLA-D antigens (class II). However, class II antigens are expressed on activated T cells. Both B and T cells may possess receptors for complement and for Fc immunoglobulin units, and one cannot rely on these surface markers to distinguish B cells from T cells.

In attempting to identify lymphocyte subsets, one must remember that the surface characteristics of T and B cells change with their stage of differentiation. Furthermore, some of the markers mentioned above are found on other cell types. For example, macrophages, monocytes, and neutrophils also have complement and Fc receptors, and macrophages and immature erythroid and granulocytic cells express HLA-D antigens. From the technical

Table 3–9 SURFACE FEATURES OF MATURE LYMPHOCYTES

B Cells	
Surface immunoglobulin	(sIg)
Fc receptor for IgG	(FcγR)
Complement receptor	(C3R)
Epstein-Barr virus receptor	(EBV-R)
Mouse erythrocyte receptor	(ME-R)
Class I antigens	(HLA-A, HLA-B, HLA-C)
Class II antigens	(HLA-D, HLA-DR)
Pokeweed mitogen (PWM) response*	
B cell lineage antigens – specific antigen	(e.g. B_1)
T cells	
Sheep erythrocyte receptor	(ER)
Fc receptors†	(FcγR, FcμR)
Phytohemagglutinin (PHA) receptors	
Concanavalin A (ConA) receptors	
Class I antigens	(HLA-A, HLA-B, HLA-C)
T cell lineage antigens	(e.g. T_3)

*T cells also respond to PWM.
†On some subpopulations.

Table 3–10 IMMUNOGLOBULIN CLASS PROPERTIES

	IgG	IgA	IgM	IgD	IgE
Serum concentration (mg. per 100 ml.)	800–1600	140–400	50–200	0–40	.002–.05
Sedimentation constant	7S	7S, 11S	19S	7S	8S
Carbohydrate content (%)	3	8	12	13	12
Heavy chains	γ	α	μ	δ	ε

point of view, one must exercise caution to distinguish intrinsic membrane immunoglobulin from that which is merely adsorbed.

Antibody Structure

The secretion of antibodies of great diversity into plasma and extravascular fluids is the special prerogative of mature B cells. One must understand the molecular structure of antibodies to appreciate how specificity and diversity are combined in one family of proteins, the structures of which are under the control of a unique genetic mechanism that permits the production of a vast array of differently structured molecules.

There are five classes of immunoglobulins (Table 3–10). The major class present in serum, IgG, has a molecular weight of 146,000 to 170,000 daltons, a sedimentation constant of 7S, and a normal serum concentration of about 1250 mg. per 100 ml. IgA is present in monomeric form in serum, where its concentration is about 250 mg. per 100 ml. It is the major immunoglobulin of body secretions (saliva, tears, colostrum, and gastrointestinal, res-

piratory, and genitourinary tract fluids). Secretory IgA is present in dimeric form protected from the action of digestive enzymes (Fig. 3–20). IgM is the first immunoglobulin to be formed in an immune response. It is a large molecule of sedimentation constant 19S, a pentamer of 7S units well suited for agglutination and complement fixation (Fig. 3–20). Its normal serum concentration is about 120 mg. per 100 ml. IgM associated with the B cell membrane is in monomeric form. The other two classes, IgD and IgE, are present at much lower serum concentrations. IgD functions almost exclusively as a membrane-bound protein. IgE exists primarily in complex formation with mast cells, where it awaits combination with antigen, triggering mast cell release.

All immunoglobulin classes have a basic structure in common (Fig. 3–21). Two identical light (L) chains of molecular weight 23,000 daltons combine with two identical heavy (H) chains of 50,000 to 70,000 daltons. Disulfide bonds bind the H chains to each other and to the L chains. Hydrogen bonding also helps hold the molecule together. The N terminal ends of an L and H chain together form the antigen-binding site. Because there are two

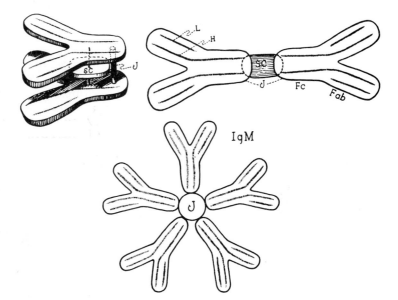

Figure 3–20 Assembly of 7S units in higher molecular weight immunoglobulins, IgA (*above*) and IgM, showing "secretory component" *(SC)* and "joining piece" *(J)*. Joining piece is necessary to form polymers. Secretory component is produced by mucosal epithelial cells and is necessary for the transport of dimeric IgA into body secretions. It appears to protect IgA from the action of digestive enzymes. (Reprinted, by permission, from Tomasi, T. B.: N. Engl. J. Med., *287*:501, 1972.)

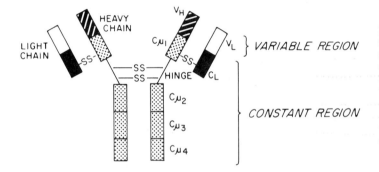

Figure 3–21 Diagram of the polypeptide structure of an IgM monomer, a general structure common to all immunoglobulin classes. C_{μ_1} through C_{μ_4} indicate constant region domains of the μ heavy chain. The N terminals are at the variable region where antibody binding occurs. The C terminals are at the opposite F_c end of the molecule. (From Vogler, L. B.: Clin. Haematol., 11:515, 1982.)

such regions, the immunoglobulin unit is divalent and can combine with two antigenic sites. Univalent antibody can be artificially produced by enzymatic cleavage of the molecule at the "hinge site," yielding one Fc fragment, which carries the C terminals of both H chains, and two Fab fragments, each of which carries an antigen-combining site. The Fc region binds to cellular Fc receptors (Turner, 1983).

There are only two different types of L chains—κ and λ, normally present in a ratio of 60:40. Only one type is present in any given molecule, but both types are represented in all immunoglobulin classes.

Class specificity goes with the H chain, of which there are five basic types: μ (in IgM), δ (in IgD), γ (in IgG), α (in IgA), and ϵ (in IgE). There are four subclasses of γ chains ($\gamma1$, $\gamma2$, $\gamma3$, $\gamma4$). IgA combines with a "secretory piece" that facilitates its transport into body fluids (Fig. 3–20).

The amino acid sequences of the L and H chains are under genetic control. However, some regions of the immunoglobulin molecule show great variability in amino acid sequence, whereas other regions are found to be remarkably constant from molecule to molecule. These have been designated as the V (variable) and C (constant) regions. The V segments consist of half the L chains and one fourth the

H chains and contain the specific antigen-binding sites. The other half of the L chains and three fourths of the H chains are the C regions (Fig. 3–21).

Inherited differences in amino acid sequence occur within the C region. These allotypic differences, however, constitute a relatively minor source of diversity.

B Cell Differentiation and Immunoglobulin Gene Rearrangements

As differentiation transforms an immature stem cell into a fully developed B cell geared to the production of specific antibody, several maturation stages can be defined (Fig. 3–22) (Calvert et al., 1984). B precursor cells show immunoglobulin gene rearrangements that can be distinguished from immunoglobulin genes that remain in the "germ line" configuration and are found in all other cells of non-B lineage. Pre–B cells are those that demonstrate the first appearance of cytoplasmic immunoglobulin (cIg) primarily as μ chains. Immature B cells begin to show membrane immunoglobulin along with some of the other membrane receptors. Mature B cells have a full complement of sIgM and sIgD and other receptors. Plasma cells are end stage cells specialized for

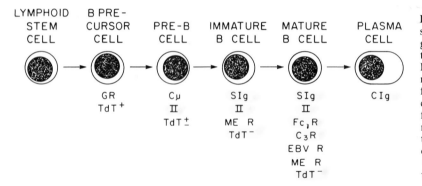

Figure 3–22 B cell differentiation stages. GR = immunoglobulin gene rearrangements; $C\mu$ = cytoplasmic μ chains; II = class II MHC antigen; SIg = surface immunoglobulin; ME R = rosette formation with mouse erythrocytes; $Fc_\gamma R$ = receptors for F_c fragments of IgG; C_3R = complement receptors; EBV R = receptors for Epstein-Barr virus; CIg = cytoplasmic immunoglobulin; TdT = terminal deoxyribonucleotidyl transferase.

the production and secretion of immunoglobulin. They lose sIg and other receptors but contain copious quantities of cIg. Class II antigens are present on very early B cells and persist throughout cell development. The marker enzyme terminal deoxynucleotidyl transferase (TdT) is present in B precursor cells but not in mature B cells. B lineage–specific surface antigens also appear during cell development and remain as the cells mature.

Major changes in DNA composition mark the transformation of an undifferentiated cell into a B lymphocyte and of the latter into a plasma cell. Each of these differentiation steps is initiated by decisive changes in the DNA structure. Widely separated segments on the DNA strand are selected for fusion, and then the intervening material is deleted. As a result of the random nature of the selection of specific segments for fusion, an enormous number of different antibody molecules are encoded in the family of B cells.

The genes for μ immunoglobulin heavy chains are the first to become activated. The following discussion will show how specific variable-region gene segments are selected from among many choices to fuse with one constant-region μ gene block to yield a rearranged differentiated gene empowered to direct the synthesis of a specific μ heavy chain in the B cell. The genetic model explains how the μ chain may be secreted or membrane-bound and why both IgM and IgD are coexpressed in the same cell.

The term *germ line DNA* refers to the DNA structure in undifferentiated, or embryonic, cells. Figure 3–23 illustrates an example of the differentiation of a B cell line in which the DNA on chromosome 14 coding for heavy chain structure changes from the germ line configuration to the differentiated structure that characterizes a B cell line. From the 5′ to the 3′ end of the DNA, arranged in the germ line configuration, there exists first a succession of gene subsegments each of which codes for different variable-region amino acid sequences. There are probably at least

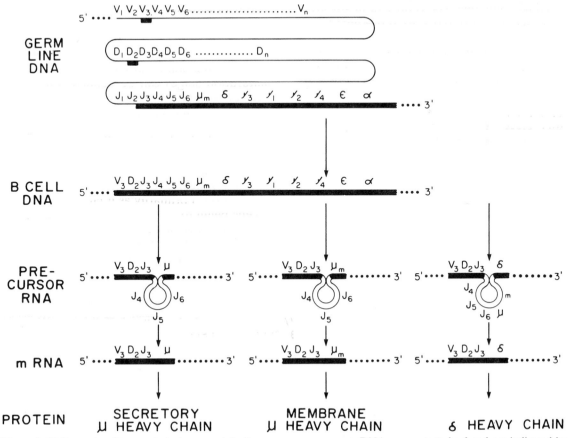

Figure 3–23 Example of heavy chain immunoglobulin gene rearrangement. DNA segments to be fused are indicated by a heavy line, and those destined for deletion are demonstrated by a light line. Unshaded loops are intron sequences spliced out during RNA processing. (Based on Leder, P.: Hosp. Pract., *18(2):*81, 1983.)

several hundred of these units, designated $V_1V_2V_3V_4V_5V_6...V_n$. At a considerable distance down the segment, there is another gene region containing a series of about 50 smaller subsegments, each coding for only approximately 10 amino acids. These are called diversity units ($D_1D_2D_3D_4D_5D_6...D_n$. Still farther down the DNA filament, there are approximately six joining units ($J_1J_2J_3J_4J_5J_6$). These units also code for only a few amino acids. Immediately beyond follow the gene blocks coding for the constant-region gene products in the μ, δ, γ, ϵ, and α heavy chains.

The first dramatic event in B cell differentiation involves the fusion of one V and one D region subsegment to one J region unit (illustrated as V_3, D_2, and J_3). The particular V, D, and J regions apparently are selected randomly, offering thousands of different possibilities. The intervening DNA sequences between the fusion points are deleted. This gene rearrangement, the earliest cellular marker of B cell differentiation, is detectable by restriction endonuclease mapping.

The genetic events that remain during the life of the B cell before its further differentiation into a plasma cell occur at the RNA level. RNA is transcribed through to the completion of constant-region μ sequences. The J units placed between the J fusion point and the μ constant-region gene block (J_4, J_5, J_6 in the example) are spliced out during the processing of precursor RNA, leaving mRNA programmed ($V_3D_2J_3$ μ in the example) for translating a specific μ heavy chain.

An alternate RNA transcription form adds a terminal set of sequences that codes for the addition of a hydrophobic polypeptide membrane anchor to the end of the μ chain, causing it to become membrane-bound.

The μ and δ constant-region DNA sequences are located one after the other on the same gene block, opening a further alternative pathway during RNA transcription and processing. This option allows RNA transcription to continue beyond the μ chain through to the end of the δ chain sequences. During RNA splicing, the μ chain sequences are removed along with the superfluous J units. The mRNA emerges programmed for δ chains that have the same variable region structure as the μ chains formed by the same cell line ($V_3D_2J_3$ δ). Because these events occur at the RNA level without a change in DNA structure, both μ and δ chains are produced in the same cell. There, they pair with the same light chain to give IgM and IgD of identical specificity. As previously noted, IgD is almost all membrane-bound.

After the differentiation of μ heavy chain genes, a similar process occurs for the light chain genes, first on chromosome 2, the locus for κ chain genes, and then—if the attempt is unsuccessful—on chromosome 22, the site of the λ genes. One of the large number of V region subsegments in the germ line DNA randomly fuses with one of the series of J units immediately preceding the single constant-region gene block. Superfluous J regions are excised during RNA processing, and a mRNA is formed that translates the synthesis of specific light chains ready for combination with completed heavy chains to form whole immunoglobulin molecules. There are no diversity units in the light chain genes.

The process of gene rearrangement is not always successful in producing a functional transcript, but several chances are available to make a "hit." In the case of the heavy chain genes, first one allele is rearranged, and, if the result is the production of a functional mRNA, further efforts at gene rearrangement on the opposite allele are blocked. However, if the first allele fails, the other is called on to make an attempt. *Allelic exclusion* means that only one allele is expressed. In the case of the light chain genes, there are four instead of two chances. First, a κ gene is called on, to be followed in the event of its failure by its allele. If neither succeeds, then one λ gene is given a chance, to be followed by its allele. Thus, the choice for light chain gene rearrangements follows the order $\kappa_a \rightarrow \kappa_b \rightarrow \lambda_a \rightarrow \lambda_b$. The expression of only one light chain in the same cell line is called *isotypic exclusion*. The relative success of κ chain gene rearrangement in humans explains why κ chains outnumber λ chains. If all opportunities for successful gene rearrangements fail, the early B cell clone is doomed to become functionally deleted.

The mature B lymphocytes have the option to remain programmed for IgM secretion or to mature into plasma cells producing IgG, IgA, and IgE. Plasma cell development is marked by another decisive step in DNA structure required for heavy chain class-switching. Beyond the gene region for μ and δ constant sequences lie additional blocks of DNA containing the remaining constant-region nucleotide sequences, those for γ, ϵ, and α chains (Fig. 3–23). To reset the switch from one set for μ or δ chains, the VDJ gene segment formed in the first fusion step described previously breaks its attachment from the μ gene block and recombines with one of the other constant-region gene blocks downstream from the μ and δ DNA sequences. The intervening strip of DNA containing these latter regions is deleted, and the superfluous J units are cut out during RNA processing. In the plasma cell that develops, the capacity for IgM and IgD synthesis is lost, and the power to secrete immunoglobulins of one of the other heavy chain classes is gained. The new heavy chains have the same VDJ sequences and share the same light chains as the μ and δ chains that preceded them. Because they share the same variable-region polypeptide structures, they also have the same antigenic specificity.

As a result of this complex process of apparently random selection of a few from many available gene sequences, B cells and their progeny have the potential of producing about 10^8 different kinds of antibodies.

T Cell Differentiation

Changes in surface antigens characterize the various stages of T cell development under the influence of the thymus. The most striking change segregates T cells into two major subsets, helper/inducer and suppressor/cytotoxic T cells. Although several systems of nomenclature are available, with the choice depending on the source of monoclonal antibodies used for T cell identification, the OK-T system has had a large measure of acceptance and will be used here. T_1 and T_{11} (the sheep red blood cell receptor) appear as early markers and are retained throughout differentiation as common

Table 3–11 OK-T CELL DIFFERENTIATION ANTIGENS AND ASSOCIATED CELLULAR FUNCTIONS

T_1 : Common T cell marker; found on some B cells
T_3 : Common T cell marker; T cell receptor
T_4 : Helper/inducer subset
T_5 : Cytotoxic/suppressor subset
T_6 : Transient marker
T_8 : Cytotoxic/suppressor subset
T_9 : Activation marker; transferrin receptor (not T cell–specific)
T_{10}: Activation marker (not T cell–specific)
T_{11}: Common T cell marker; sheep erythrocyte receptor

T cell markers (Fig. 3–24). They are joined by T_3 (the T cell receptor), another common T cell marker at the medullary stage of differentiation. T_9 (the transferrin receptor) and T_{10} appear in early maturation stages but are lost as the early T cells continue their development. However, even though they are absent on mature resting T cells, they reappear when these cells are activated to proliferate. Thus, their presence on the cell surface may be more related to cell proliferation than to cell differentiation stage. Furthermore, T_9 and T_{10} are not T cell–specific but are found on other hemopoietic cells. T_6 appears transiently early in differentiation and then is lost as T cell subsets are split off. From the foregoing, it is apparent that T_1, T_3, and T_{11} are the best markers for identifying mature T cells, regardless of subset (Table 3–11).

Early in T cell differentiation, T_4, T_5, and T_8 appear together as cell lineage markers. At the next differentiation stage, they segregate into separate populations. T_4 marks the helper/inducer subset, constituting 55 to 65 percent of peripheral blood T cells. T_5 and T_8

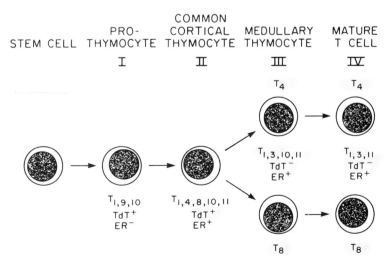

Figure 3–24 T cell differentiation stages. OK-T markers are represented. TdT = terminal deoxynucleotidyl transferase; ER = rosette formation with sheep erythrocytes. At stages III and IV, common markers are shown in the middle, and subset markers are indicated above and below the diagrammed cells.

positive cells are the suppressor/cytotoxic subset, accounting for about 20 to 30 percent of peripheral blood T cells.

The enzyme TdT is present in immature T cells but is lost during T cell development as the cells become ER+. Class-specific Fc receptors are found on some mature T cells. The Fc receptor for IgM heavy chain has been associated with helper/inducer cells, and that for IgG heavy chain has been asociated with the suppressor/cytotoxic subset, but these relationships are not absolute. Activation of mature T cells exposes not only T_9 and T_{10} but also class II antigens. However, the resting T cells have receptors that recognize their own class II antigens on other cell surfaces.

The antigen-recognition mechanism on the T cell surface consists of a T cell receptor joined to a receptor for the histocompatibility antigens. The receptor for class I antigens is found on suppressor/cytotoxic $T_8{}^+$ cells. The class II antigen receptor is associated with the T_4 marker on helper/inducer cells. Regulatory responses of $T_8{}^+$ cells require recognition both of the foreign antigen and of class I antigens on antigen presenting cells or target cells, whereas the responses of $T_4{}^+$ cells depend on interaction with foreign antigen and class II cellular antigens. The T cell receptor is associated with the T_3 membrane surface marker and contains constant- and variable-region gene products analogous to those of immunoglobulins (Reinherz et al., 1983). It is undoubtedly just as specific as the surface immunoglobulin that serves as the antigen receptor on B cells.

The Major Histocompatibility (MHC) Locus

The gene products of the MHC complex are proteins expressed on cell membranes (Dausset, 1981). They serve to identify self from nonself and thus are critical in the immune system's decision whether or not to reject foreign tissue. Accurate identification of these cell surface antigens is accordingly central to the successful transplantation of kidney, marrow, and other tissues from one individual to another. In addition, MHC gene products facilitate normal immune responses by specifying certain cellular interactions, as already discussed.

The genes of the MHC locus, designated HLA in the human, are located close to one another on the short arm of chromosome 6 (Fig. 3–25). The HLA-A, -B, and -C genes are clustered in a site closely linked with the D/DR genes as well as with those for several components of the complement system (Steinmetz and Hood, 1983). Also close by are the genes for the enzymes glycoxylase, phosphoglucomutase-3 and 21-hydroxylase. Both HLA alleles in any one individual are expressed.

The HLA-A, -B, and -C gene products are determined serologically, but the identification of HLA-D type demands the use of a mixed lymphocyte culture (MLC) test. When isolated lymphocytes from two individuals are mixed together, differences in this HLA sublocus are detected by observing the induction of cell proliferation as measured by the incorporation of tritiated thymidine. One can analyze the

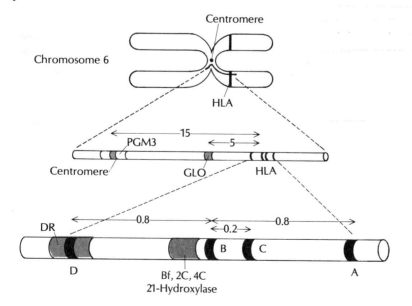

Figure 3–25 The genetic locus of the MHC complex (HLA) on the short arm of chromosome 6. Relative distances are shown in recombination units. GLO = glyoxylase; PGM3 = phosphoglucomutase-3. Bf, 2C, 4C are genes for complement factors. The HLA DR (D-related) region is very near the HLA D locus. (From Schaller, J. G., and Hansen, J. A.: Hosp. Pract., *16(5)*:42, 1981.)

Table 3–12 WORLD HEALTH ORGANIZATION HLA-SPECIFIC ANTIGENS AS OF 1980*

HLA-A	HLA-B	HLA-B	HLA-C	HLA-D	HLA-DR
A1	B5	Bw45 (12)	Cw1	Dw1	DR1
A2	B7	Bw46	Cw2	Dw2	DR2
A3	B8	Bw47	Cw3	Dw3	DR3
A9	B12	Bw48	Cw4	Dw4	DR4
A10	B13	Bw49 (w21)	Cw5	Dw5	DR5
A11	B14	Bw50 (w21)	Cw6	Dw6	DRw6
Aw19	B15	Bw51 (5)	Cw7	Dw7	DR7
Aw23 (9)	Bw16	Bw52 (5)	Cw8	Dw8	DRw8
Aw24 (9)	B17	Bw53		Dw9	DRw9
A25 (10)	B18	Bw54 (w22)		Dw10	DRw10
A26 (10)	Bw21	Bw55 (w22)		Dw11	
A28	Bw22	Bw56 (w22)		Dw12	
A29	B27	Bw57 (17)			
Aw30	Bw35	Bw58 (17)			
Aw31	B37	Bw59			
Aw32	Bw38 (w16)	Bw60 (40)			
Aw33	Bw39 (w16)	Bw61 (40)			
Aw34	B40	Bw62 (15)			
Aw36	Bw41	Bw63 (15)			
Aw43	Bw42				
	Bw44 (12)	Bw4			
		Bw6			

*The letter "w" stands for "workshop" and indicates the tentative nature of certain antigens not yet universally accepted as accurately identified. (From Dick, H. M. *In* Holborow, E. J., and Reeves, W. G. (Eds.): Immunology in Medicine. 2nd ed. New York, Grune & Stratton, 1983, p. 214.)

lymphocyte populations separately by blocking DNA synthesis in one of them through the addition of mitomycin. This lymphocyte population then becomes the *stimulators* and the nonblocked lymphocytes become the *responders*. A large number of different HLA alleles have been recognized in the population (Table 3–12). Thus, there is little likelihood that any two unrelated persons will by chance bear the same HLA antigens on their cell surfaces. However, since the MHC locus is stable and is inherited en bloc with relatively little chance for crossover, there is a one-in-four chance that two siblings will share identical HLA antigens, with one haplotype inherited from the mother and the other from the father (Fig. 3–26). Thus, siblings provide the

best chance for finding an optimal match for tissue transplantation. Such matches are graded from A (the best) to F (the worst) (Table 3–13).

The cell surface antigens of the MHC complex are classed according to differences in tissue distribution, biochemical structure, and immunologic function. Class I antigens in the human include the gene products of the HLA-A, -B, and -C gene subloci. They are found on all cell types except mature red blood cells. They have a common structure consisting of a heavy chain of 45,000 daltons, combined with a β_2-microglobulin of 12,000 daltons, the gene for which is located on chromosome 15. Class I antigens are important in the recognition of foreign antigens located on cell surfaces, in-

Figure 3–26 An example of the inheritance of histocompatibility antigens.

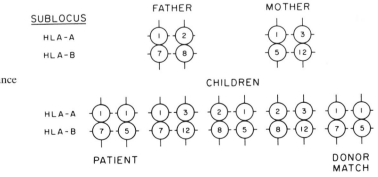

Table 3–13 MATCHING GRADES FOR HL-A SYSTEM

Grade	
A	Identical siblings
B	Identical unrelated or no antigen in donor not present in recipient
C	One incompatibility
D	Two incompatibilities
E	Three incompatibilities
F	Positive crossmatch or ABO incompatibility

ducing destruction of such cells by cytotoxic T lymphocytes.

Class II antigens in the human refer to the gene products of the HLA-D/HLA-DR system. They are often called Ia, or immune-associated antigens, although this designation originally referred only to the murine model. The HLA-D/HLA-DR genes play decisive roles in immunity. They are *immune-response-*genes, and their gene products are *immune-associated* because, for most immune responses to occur, the antigen-presenting cell and the regulatory helper/inducer T cells must share the same class II antigens on their cell surfaces. If this requirement is not met, the immune response does not occur (Benacerraf, 1981). Class II antigens are limited to only a few specialized cell types, including B lymphocytes, monocytes, macrophages and antigen-presenting cells, granulocytic and erythroid precursors, endothelial cells, and activated T cells. Class II antigens also have a structure in common, consisting of an α chain and a β chain that closely resemble each other and a smaller γ chain. Both class I and class II antigens have cytoplasmic, intramembranous, and cell surface components.

There are extensive phenotypic and genotypic similarities between immunoglobulins and the MHC antigens. This homology has suggested that class I and class II antigens, β_2-microglobulin, immunoglobulin, and T cell receptor genes may all share a common genetic origin (Cushley and Owen, 1983).

The HLA system of antigens bears a statistical correlation with the development of certain disease states (Schaller and Hansen, 1981). For example, ankylosing spondylitis is associated with B_{27}, hereditary hemochromatosis with A_3, and myasthenia gravis with B_8. For the most part, the mechanism of the association is obscure. In the case of hemochromatosis, it is one of gene linkage.

FUNCTION

The presentation of antigen to antigen-specific receptors on the surfaces of lympho-cytes—sIg on B cells and T cell receptor on T cells—triggers a selective clonal expansion of those B and T cell lines with receptors for the particular antigen, leaving the remaining clones with other specificities in the resting state. As a result of this antigen-specific clonal expansion, a multifaceted humoral and cellular effector response contains and destroys the particular antigen. Lymphocyte secretions called lymphokines facilitate activation, growth, and differentiation of immunocytes. They also have important functional effects on other cells engaged in the immune response.

Regulation of the Immune Response

Foreign soluble or particulate antigens are initially engulfed, degraded, and disposed of by phagocytes. If the degradation is complete, no immunologic reaction occurs. However, some phagocytes (especially dendritic macrophages in the lymph nodes) are less efficient, and antigenic fragments are fixed to their exterior surfaces. These antigens attract and activate a subset of T cells characterized by the presence of T_4^+ surface markers (Unanue, 1980; Reinherz and Schlossman, 1981). The attraction of these helper/inducer T cells is genetically restricted to T cells belonging to the same class of HLA-D as the antigen-presenting cell because of the presence of specific receptors, as already described (Fig. 3–27). The activated clone of helper/inducer cells is further stimulated by the release from the macrophages of a soluble factor, interleukin-1 (IL-1) (Müller, 1982). The activated helper/inducer cells in turn release factors that facilitate the activation of antigen-specific suppressor T cells and the development of clones of antigen-specific B lymphocytes and cytotoxic T lymphocytes. They also release a number of soluble factors that activate various effector cells involved in the elimination of the offending antigen. Thus, the helper/inducer T cells are the gatekeepers of immune reaction.

The suppressor T cells in turn require helper/inducer cells for induction of their suppressor activity. Once activated, they secrete suppressor factors, which (like helper factors) are antigen-specific (Ballieux and Heijnen, 1982; Kapp et al., 1984). Their suppressive effects ordinarily dampen only the specific immune response and not immune responsiveness in general. The suppressor cells complete the negative feedback loop by inhibiting the helper/inducer cells that activated them, quenching the immune response at its source. Most B cell responses to antigen are also

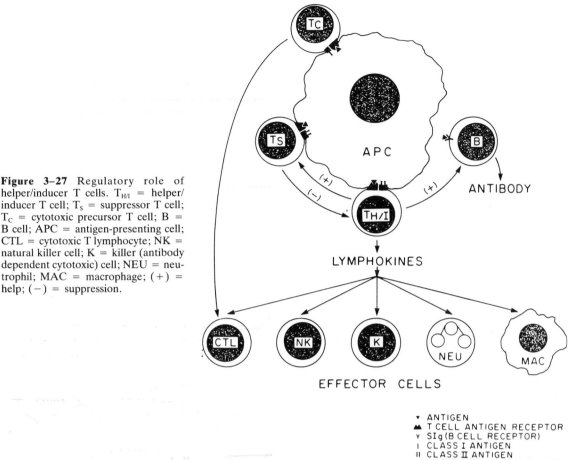

Figure 3–27 Regulatory role of helper/inducer T cells. $T_{H/I}$ = helper/inducer T cell; T_s = suppressor T cell; T_C = cytotoxic precursor T cell; B = B cell; APC = antigen-presenting cell; CTL = cytotoxic T lymphocyte; NK = natural killer cell; K = killer (antibody dependent cytotoxic) cell; NEU = neutrophil; MAC = macrophage; (+) = help; (−) = suppression.

▾ ANTIGEN
▲▲ T CELL ANTIGEN RECEPTOR
Y SIg(B CELL RECEPTOR)
I CLASS I ANTIGEN
II CLASS II ANTIGEN
▯ T CELL CLASS I RECEPTOR
▯ T CELL CLASS II RECEPTOR

dependent on helper/inducer cells, with one exception being their response to certain polysaccharide antigens. B cell interaction with antigen and with specific helper factor excites the cell and initiates IgM synthesis. The activated B cells expose a surface receptor for a lymphokine, B cell growth factor (BCGF), which binds to the cell and stimulates cell division in conjunction with interleukin-l. Then another lymphokine, B cell differentiation factor (BCDF), promotes B cell differentiation into plasma cells along with class-switching of immunoglobulin heavy chains (Fig. 3–28).

Cytotoxic T lymphocytes (CTL), like suppressor cells, are T_8^+ and are capable of lysing target cells by surface-to-surface contact independent of antibody. The target cells carry the same HLA-A, -B and -C antigens as the cytotoxic T cell but bear foreign antigens such as virus particles. The activation of a precursor of the CTL is initiated by an antigen on such cells and further stimulated by interleukin-2

Figure 3–28 B cell regulation. B = B cell; a-B = activated B cell; PC = plasma cell; Ab = antibody; HF = helper factor; BCGF = B cell growth factor; BCDF = B cell differentiation factor; IL-1 = interleukin-1. Symbols are as in Figure 3–27.

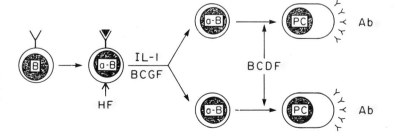

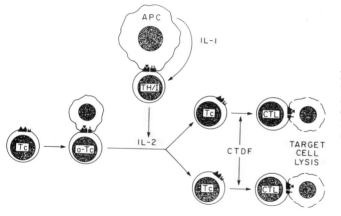

Figure 3–29 Cytotoxic T lymphocyte (CTL) regulation. T_C = cytotoxic T lymphocyte precursor; a-T_C = activated T_C; APC = antigen-presenting cell; $T_{H/I}$ = helper/inducer T cell; IL-2 = interleukin-2; CTDF = cytotoxic T lymphocyte differentiation factor. Symbols are as in Figure 3–27.

(IL-2), or T cell growth factor, a substance analogous to BCGF. The IL-2 is released by activated helper/inducer cells after antigenic exposure, as already described. Finally, the CTL precursors are acted on by CTL differentiation factor (CTDF), which renders the T cells actively cytotoxic against the target cells to which they were sensitized (Fig. 3–29).

Three classes of cytotoxic lymphocytes are recognized, fighting alongside mononuclear phagocytes and neutrophils (see Fig. 3–27). Cytotoxic T lymphocytes, already described, require prior activation in a class I MHC-restricted response. Natural killer (NK) cells and antibody-dependent cytotoxic cells (ADCC, or K for killer cells) are not MHC-restricted and do not require prior activation. NK cells attack certain target cells such as virus-transformed and tumor cells (Herberman, 1982). They are thought to play a role in immune surveillance. The surface determinants on the target cells against which they react are unknown. ADCC cells require antibody on the surface of the target cells for direction of their specificity. NK and ADCC cells appear to belong to null (i.e., typing as neither T nor B) and T lymphocyte subsets.

Effector Responses

The effector limb of the immune response mobilizes not only the various classes of cytotoxic lymphocytes but also the granulocytes and the cells of the mononuclear-macrophage complex in an inflammatory reaction that contains and then usually destroys the invading antigen. Many of these attack mechanisms are directed by the various classes of immunoglobulins acting in concert with complement (Feld-

bush et al., 1984). Whereas the variable regions of the immunoglobulins determine antigen specificity, the constant regions govern functional activity, most notably Fc receptor and complement-binding.

IgG is quantitatively the most important of the immunoglobulin classes, but IgM is the first to appear, and, because of its intravascular location and agglutinating ability, it is especially effective in clearing antigen from the blood stream. IgA protects mucosal surfaces from antigen intrusions, including those of food allergens. Because of its smaller size, IgG crosses the placenta and penetrates well into extravascular spaces. It is most effective in neutralizing toxins. The bulk of IgE is attached to Fc receptors on basophils and mast cells, mediating the release of histamine, slow-reacting substance, eosinophilic chemotactic factor, and other substances (Buisseret, 1982). Its protective role against parasitic diseases and its pathogenic role in allergic diseases are still not thoroughly understood. IgD functions as a membrane receptor and has no known effector function.

The immunoglobulin classes and subclasses vary in potency and specificity for Fc receptor and complement-binding (Table 3–14). The most effective complement binders are IgG_1, IgG_3, and IgM. IgG_2 has only weak activity. Complement activation destroys targets by direct cell lysis and also by attachment to C3b receptors on the surfaces of monocytes, macrophages, and neutrophils. Fc receptor binding is a function of both cell type and heavy chain class. IgG_1 and IgG_3 attach to mononuclear phagocytes; IgG_1, IgG_3, IgG_4, and IgA to neutrophils; all classes but IgD to subpopulations of lymphocytes; and, as noted, IgE to basophils and mast cells.

Certain lymphokines also directly participate

Table 3–14 IMMUNOGLOBULIN CLASS FUNCTIONS

	Complement Fixation	Cell-Binding			
		Mononuclear Phagocytes	Neutrophils	Mast Cells and Basophils	T and B Lymphocytes
IgG$_1$	+ +	+	+	−	+
IgG$_2$	+	−	−	−	+
IgG$_3$	+ + +	+	+	−	+
IgG$_4$	−	−	+	?	+
IgM	+ + +	−	−	−	+ *
IgA	−	−	+	−	+ *
IgD	−	−	−	−	−
IgE	−	?	−	+ + +	+ *

*Subpopulations only.

in the effector response by localizing and activating mononuclear and polymorphonuclear phagocytes. Interferon-γ stimulates NK cells, macrophages, and cytotoxic T cells. Lymphotoxin causes cytolysis of target cells. Colony-stimulating factor enhances the growth of macrophages and granulocytes. Lymphokines and their actions are summarized in Table 3–15.

Self-Tolerance and Autoimmunity

The repertoire of immunocompetent cells is comprehensive and encompasses complementary V region gene products for all possible antigenic configurations. However, cellular clones directed against intrinsic self-antigens are restrained from fratricidal missions against normal cohabitating cells. How such clones are prevented from producing autoimmune disease is still not well understood (Schoenfeld and Schwartz, 1984). Populations of suppressor cells may in some manner be specifically programmed to quench autoimmune responses (Miller and Schwartz, 1982). Disruption of this suppression would then lead to autoimmune disease. Immune tolerance might also come about through structural or functional deletion of those clones that are directed against self. Some sort of "clonal escape" might then lead to autoimmunity. Some self-antigens may be immunologically silent because they are located on a cell membrane that lacks the immunologically restrictive class II antigens.

The induction of some degree of tolerance is a requirement for successful tissue transplantation for all those donor-recipient pairs of less than syngeneic match. A variety of nonspecific measures are used in an effort to induce tolerance. These include radiation, antibodies against lymphocytes, and immunosuppressive agents, such as corticosteroids, methotrexate, azathioprine, and cyclosporin. The last is of particular interest because of its specificity for T cells (Cohen et al., 1984).

Table 3–15 LYMPHOKINES AND MONOKINES

Current Name	Target Cell	Function
Interleukin-1 (IL-1)	T cells	T cell activation
Interleukin-2 (IL-2)	CTL	Proliferation of activated CTL
Interferon-γ (IFNγ)	Many cells	Many (enhances CTL, macrophages, NK cells)
Colony-stimulating factor (CSF)	Granulocytes and mononuclear phagocytes	Growth of granulocytes and macrophages
B cell growth factor (BCGF)	B cells	B cell growth
B cell differentiation factor (BCDF)	B cells	B cell differentiation
CTL differentiation factor (CTDF)	CTL	CTL differentiation
Migration inhibition factor (MIF)	Macrophages	Immobilization of macrophages
Macrophage activation factor (MAF)	Macrophages	Activation of macrophages
Leukocyte inhibition factor (LIF)	Neutrophils	Immobilization of neutrophils
Chemotactic factor (CF)	Neutrophils	Attraction of neutrophils
Lymphotoxin (LT)	Target cells	Cytolysis
Osteoclast activity factor (OAF)	Osteoclasts	Bone resorption
Helper factors	T and B cells	Antigen-specific help
Suppressor factors	Helper T cells	Antigen-specific suppression

PATHOPHYSIOLOGY

Classification and General Considerations

The fixed and circulating immunocytes of the secondary lymphatic tissues are specialized to meet the challenge of invasion by any number of foreign antigens. Reactive changes are seen in response to challenges, such as local or systemic infections. The reaction may be one of lymph node enlargement, increase in spleen size, the presence of large lymphocytes or plasmacytoid cells in the circulation, or an elevation of absolute lymphocyte count. A generalized increase in the concentration of all immunoglobulin classes may also occur.

When immunocytes undergo neoplastic transformation, their proliferation is inappropriate and may be associated with either an increase or a decrease in the concentration of immunoglobulins. Impairment of cellular or humoral immunity causes susceptibility to infections. These "opportunistic" infections are quite different from those commonly seen in patients with intact immunity. Autoimmune disorders, such as hemolytic anemia and thrombocytopenia, also occur with increased frequency.

In clinical practice, the distinction of a neoplastic lymphoproliferative disorder from a reactive state is important because of the vast differences in treatment and prognosis.

A summarized classification of immunocyte disorders is given in Table 3–16.

Table 3–16 CLASSIFICATION OF IMMUNOCYTE DISORDERS

I. *Quantitative Disorders*
  A. Lymphocytopenia and hypogammaglobulinemia
    1. Primary
      (a) Congenital
      (b) Acquired
    2. Secondary
  B. Lymphocytosis and hypergammaglobulinemia
    1. Reactive
    2. Immunoproliferative

II. *Qualitative Disorders*

III. *Immunoproliferative Disorders*
  A. Leukemia
    1. Chronic lymphocytic
    2. Acute lymphoblastic
  B. Lymphoma
    1. Hodgkin's
    2. Non-Hodgkin's
  C. M-component disorders
    1. Plasma cell myeloma
    2. Macroglobulinemia
    3. Benign monoclonal gammopathy

Quantitative Disorders

Lymphocytopenia and Hypogammaglobulinemia. The normal concentration of lymphocytes in the blood is 2500 per mm^3 (range: 1500 to 4000). A reduction below 1500 per $mm.^3$ affects primarily T cells because they are the predominant lymphocytes in blood. The mechanism may be increased loss, decreased production, or a shift in distribution.

One can produce mechanical loss of lymphocytes by tapping the circulating stream at the thoracic duct and draining off the lymph. A similar mechanism may explain the lymphocytopenia of intestinal lymphangiectasia and other disorders associated with leakage of lymph into the gastrointestinal tract. Lymphocytes are extraordinarily radiosensitive, and a fall in the lymphocyte count of the peripheral blood precedes the decrease in either granulocytes or platelets caused by radiation. Lymphocytopenia is often present in patients during acute stress or therapy with corticoids. The studies of Fauci and Dale (1975) have demonstrated that glucocorticoids produce lymphocytopenia by shifting the distribution of lymphocytes from the intravascular to the extravascular space. The effect is transitory. In patients with certain lymphoproliferative disorders, however, glucocorticoids may produce the opposite effect and temporarily raise the blood lymphocyte count by means of altering the body distribution from extra- to intravascular sites. Adrenal steroids also cause cell lysis and inhibit cell proliferation, but these actions are limited to certain sensitive lymphocyte subpopulations (Claman, 1983).

The secondary lymphatic tissue is the immediate source of the circulating lymphocytes as described in the section on Lymphatic Tissue. Malignant replacement by advanced Hodgkin's disease or widespread metastatic carcinoma, or destruction by irradiation of the lymph node–bearing regions of the body, leads to an inability of these regions to return adequate numbers of lymphocytes into the blood through the lymphatics. Chemotherapeutic alkylating agents will also affect lymphocyte replacement by interfering with the proliferating and the short-lived small lymphocyte pools.

A relatively new disorder has appeared, primarily affecting male homosexuals. It has been termed *acquired immunodeficiency syndrome (AIDS)*. Characteristic features include lymphadenopathy, the development of opportunistic infections such as *Pneumocystis carinii* pneumonia, and a high incidence of disseminated Kaposi syndrome (Gottlieb et al., 1981). The outcome is usually fatal. There is a lack of helper/inducer T lymphocytes and the ratio of T^{4+} to T^{8+} lymphocytes is decreased below the normal value of 2 to levels as low as 0.1. Despite polyclonal hypergammaglobulinemia, specific humoral immune responsiveness is impaired. A minority of the patients have been recipients of blood products (e.g., hemophiliacs) (Curran et al., 1984). These cases have led to the supposition that the disorder is caused by a transmissible agent passed on to a susceptible host. AIDS has also occurred among immigrants from Haiti, suggesting an epidemiologic relationship. The deficiency in cellular immunity resembles that seen commonly in patients with lymphoma.

Reduced levels of serum immunoglobulin may be found secondary to increased losses in the urine in nephrotic syndrome or in the gastrointestinal tract in protein-losing enteropathy. More frequently, the reduction occurs secondary to immunoproliferative disease, most notably chronic lymphocytic leukemia, plasma cell myeloma, or lymphoma. The deficiency may be due to insufficient numbers of normal B cells or to defective B cell differentiation (Filipovich and Kersey, 1983).

In addition to the secondary disorders discussed, there is an array of primary immunodeficiency states, some congenital and some others acquired (Rosen et al., 1984). Despite quantum leaps in knowledge about immunologic control mechanisms, some of these disorders still defy adequate explanation (Table 3–17).

X-linked agammaglobulinemia (Bruton type) is a familial disorder affecting males with a developmental defect of B cells. The B cell zones of the secondary lymphatic tissues are depopulated, whereas T cell zones remain intact. Circulating lymphocytes are present in normal numbers, but plasma immunoglobulin concentrations are markedly depressed. Patients are afflicted with recurrent infections, often sinupulmonary, preventable by the therapeutic use of parenteral immunoglobulin fractions.

The physiological *hypogammaglobulinemia of infancy* must be distinguished from the familial disorder. Following the gradual disappearance of maternal IgG from the infant's circulation, endogenous synthesis raises IgG and IgM levels to about three fourths the adult level by 1 year of age. IgA levels increase more slowly, reaching adult levels by about age 2 years. Occasionally, some infants have more profound immunoglobulin deficiency associated with delayed onset of synthesis, and they experience recurrent infections. The hypogammaglobulinemia of infancy is transient, however, and spontaneously remits, usually by 2 years of age (Geha and Rosen, 1983).

Late onset common variable primary hypogammaglobulinemia usually presents during the third decade of life. It varies a great deal in severity and in the pattern of immunoglobulin deficiency. The defect appears to be one involving the terminal differentiation of B lymphocytes into plasma cells. Recurrent sinupulmonary infections and gastrointestinal malabsorption are common complications. There is also an increased incidence of autoimmune blood disorders. A small proportion of patients have increased numbers of suppressor T lymphocytes, but whether these play a primary role in pathogenesis or are a secondary phenomenon is still not clear.

Selective deficiency of certain immunoglobulin classes occurs occasionally in otherwise healthy individuals. One of the more prevalent is selective lack of IgA, a condition associated with anaphylactic reactions to the IgA present in infused plasma. These occur because of the development of anti-IgA antibodies. Individuals with deficiency of the subclass IgG2 are prone to recurrent respiratory infections and will go undetected unless the levels of the IgG subclasses are measured. Thymoma has also been associated with hypogammaglobulinemia, at times together with such autoimmune phenomena as myasthenia gravis and red cell aplasia.

Thymic aplasia (di George's syndrome) is a severe developmental defect of the third and fourth pharyngeal pouches causing a lack of

Table 3–17 PRIMARY IMMUNODEFICIENCY DISORDERS

Immunoglobulin deficiency
X-linked agammaglobulinemia (Bruton type)
Transient hypogammaglobulinemia of infancy
Late-onset hypogammaglobulinemia (common variable)
Selective immunoglobulin deficiency (IgA, IgG subclass, IgM)
Thymoma with hypogammaglobulinemia

T cell deficiency
Thymic aplasia (diGeorge's syndrome)
Purine nucleoside phosphorylase deficiency

Combined deficiency
Severe combined immunodeficiency (Swiss type)

Miscellaneous
Wiskott-Aldrich syndrome
Ataxia telangiectasia

thymus and parathyroid formation together with other structural defects. The T-dependent zones of the lymphatic system are depleted, and there is lymphocytopenia. Immunoglobulin levels are usually normal. Thymus transplantation is considered for the more severely affected infants. Deficiency of the enzyme purine nucleoside phosphorylase also causes a T cell deficiency syndrome. The pathogenesis apparently is related to the accumulation of the metabolite deoxyguanosine triphosphate, exerting a selective toxicity on T cells.

Severe combined immune deficiency (SCID) affects a common stem cell that leads to profound deficiency of both T and B cells. Most affected infants fail to thrive, and they succumb to recurrent infections by the age of 2 years. A number of cases have occurred in association with deficiency of the enzyme adenosine deaminase (ADA). Deoxyadenosine accumulates and is the probable lymphocyte toxin. Transfusions of red blood cells have been helpful because they contain ADA, which metabolizes circulating deoxyadenosine. Marrow transplantation may correct the defect in SCID by supplying the required stem cells.

Other miscellaneous deficiency states are even less well understood. *Wiskott-Aldrich syndrome* is a sex-linked familial disorder involving thrombocytopenia, eczema, and a susceptibility to the development of malignant lymphoma. Infections are common. Antibody production in response to polysaccharide antigens is poor. IgM levels and isohemagglutinin titers are low. IgG concentrations are normal. IgA and IgE levels may be increased. In *ataxia telangiectasia* there is selective IgA deficiency along with defects in cell-mediated immunity (Waldman et al., 1983). Malignant lymphoma is once again a common complication.

Lymphocytosis and Hypergammaglobulinemia. Lymphocytosis is defined as an increase in the absolute lymphocyte count above 4000 per mm.^{3} in adults, above 7000 mm.^{3} in young children, and above 9000 per mm.^{3} in infants. In "relative" lymphocytosis, the proportion of lymphocytes in the peripheral blood is increased because of concomitant granulocytopenia, but the absolute number is not above the normal range.

The leukocyte response evoked by a particular infection varies with the particular organism and also with the stage of the infection. Some infections, mostly viral but including some bacterial, are noted for their ability to evoke a lymphocytic response. *Pertussis* and

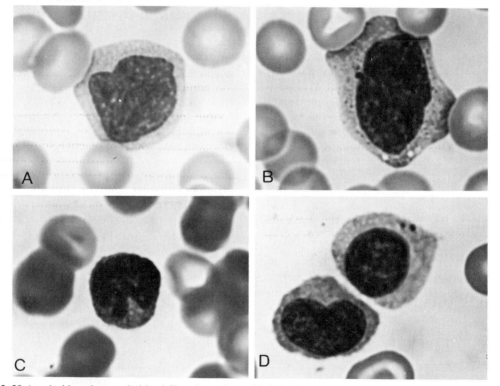

Figure 3–30 Atypical lymphocytes in blood film of a patient with infectious mononucleosis. *A* and *B*, Cytoplasm adherent to red cells. *C* and *D*, Notched and irregular nuclei with cytoplasmic vacuoles.

acute infectious lymphocytosis are two childhood illnesses with a particularly striking tendency to raise the blood lymphocyte count—predominantly small mature forms—to very high levels usually in the range of 15,000 to 50,000 per mm.^{3} but occasionally to as high as 100,000 per mm.^{3}

Infectious mononucleosis is associated with a more modest lymphocytosis, usually not in excess of 20,000 per mm.^{3}, but there is a greater proportion (usually about 20 percent) of young and "atypical" forms (Lai, 1977). These are as large as 15 to 25 μm in diameter, with a generous rim of cytoplasm, often deep blue, foamy, and containing vacuoles, with an irregular outline that tends to cling to adjacent red cells. The nucleus is also larger, its chromatin clumps are somewhat more widely spread, and its outline is often indented, irregular, or lobulated into "monocytoid" forms. One or two nucleoli per nucleus are occasionally seen (Fig. 3–30).

Infectious mononucleosis is caused by the Epstein-Barr virus (EBV). B lymphocytes become infected with EBV. T lymphocytes then undergo a reactive proliferative response, giving rise to the atypical lymphocytes in the peripheral blood. EBV antigen can be identified on B cell membranes but is absent from the T cells. The humoral response is of use in establishing the diagnosis by means of a significantly positive heterophile antibody titer.

During this period of T cell response in infectious mononucleosis, as in other viral infections, there is a temporary period of anergy associated with loss of the delayed hypersensitivity response. This occurs because the T cell response against the EBV-infected B cells is primarily an increase in cytotoxic/suppressor lymphocytes. This state of temporary immune deficiency lasts only for a few weeks (deWaele et al., 1981).

When EBV infection occurs in individuals with immunodeficiency disorders, the T cell response may be lacking, and the EBV-infected B cells cannot be restrained. They continue to proliferate and cause a malignant lymphoma, if not an earlier demise as a direct result of the infection (Purtilo et al., 1982).

The EBV also appears to be of importance in the African type of *Burkitt's lymphoma* and in *nasopharyngeal carcinoma* (Pearson et al., 1983). It is constantly associated with both these neoplasias (Henle et al., 1979). EBV is also commonly associated with Hodgkin's disease.

The heterophile antibody test is positive in the great majority of cases, distinguishing infectious mononucleosis from a large number of other infections that may give rise to a similar blood picture, although usually with fewer atypical lymphocytes (Horwitz et al., 1977). These infections include measles, mumps, adenovirus, viral hepatitis, cytomegalovirus, toxoplasmosis, brucellosis, typhoid fever, *Listeria monocytogenes,* and even tuberculosis. These infections sometimes cause only a relative lymphocytosis, with the most prominent change being a reduction in circulating granulocytes. Relative lymphocytosis is also a feature of the very early (usually preclinical) stages of bacterial infection, as granulocytes begin to leave the circulation to enter the infected tissues, or the very late stages of severe and overwhelming bacterial infection after exhaustion of granulocyte reserves. In the latter circumstance, the relative lymphocytosis is an ominous prognostic indicator. As one would predict from the effect of adrenal steroids on lymphocytes, adrenal insufficiency may cause a rise in the blood lymphocytes.

An inappropriate increase in the absolute lymphocyte count, not explainable on the basis of immunoreactive states, may be indicative of a lymphoproliferative disorder, usually lymphatic leukemia. Small mature lymphocytes predominate in chronic lymphocytic leukemia. The leukocytosis of acute lymphoblastic leukemia features immature lymphoblasts.

One of the most important problems in clinical hematologic diagnosis is the distinction between leukemia and "leukemoid" reactions. The clinical course, whether benign and self-limited or persistent and progressive, is one obvious point of difference. Another is the morphologic appearance of lymphocytes and lymphoblasts, which in reactive states is varied and atypical but in leukemias is clonal and almost identical. The association of anemia, thrombocytopenia, and/or granulocytopenia suggests leukemia, but these findings singly or in combination are sometimes seen in infections. Perhaps the most salient pathophysiologic point of distinction lies in the fact that replacement of the primary lymphatic organ, the marrow, is a prominent feature of leukemia. Reactive states cause proliferation mostly in the secondary lymphatic tissue; the reactive young and "atypical" lymphocytes that characterize infectious mononucleosis and other infections do not replace the normal marrow cells to any significant degree. Lymphocytes and plasma cells may increase in the marrow as a reactive change, but they usually are in the range of 5 to 15 percent of the total marrow cells, hardly ever above 30 percent, and never replace the marrow tissue as leukemic proliferation usually does.

An increase in plasma immunoglobulin concentration above the normal range is a common response not only in many infectious diseases but also in other conditions, such as liver cirrhosis, carcinoma, sarcoidosis, and lupus erythematosus, to name a few. Such responses are polyclonal and affect a variety of immunoglobulins. This is reflected in the serum electrophoretic pattern by a diffuse increase, or broad-band hypergammaglobulinemia. Immunoelectrophoretic analysis shows increases in all immunoglobulin families, IgG, IgA, and IgM. The finding in a serum electrophoretic pattern of hypergammaglobulinemia due to a narrow dense band in the broad region where the gamma globulins are normally found has a different significance. It is the secretory product of a monoclonal line of B cells producing only one type of immunoglobulin. This narrow band is often referred to as a *spike,* but the term *M-component*, for monoclonal component, is more appropriate (Fig. 3–31). The presence of an M-component in the serum or urine requires investigation of the patient for a malignant proliferative disorder of the B

cells, namely, myeloma or primary macroglobulinemia. However, the mere presence of such a component does not by itself establish such a diagnosis.

Qualitative Disorders

For immunocytes, it is difficult to separate qualitative from quantitative disorders. These cells are geared for clonal selection and proliferation under the influence of specific antigenic stimulation, and a qualitative disorder at one stage of cellular differentiation may be reflected by deficient cell numbers at a functionally more mature stage. It might be predicted, however, that functional defects will be discovered that affect one or another of the lymphocyte subsets at terminal stages of cellular differentiation after proliferation has been completed. Some of the hypogammaglobulinemic immunodeficiency disorders may indeed be defects of terminal B cell differentiation.

Immunoproliferative Disorders

The neoplastic alterations of the lymphoid tissue produce an array of conditions quite

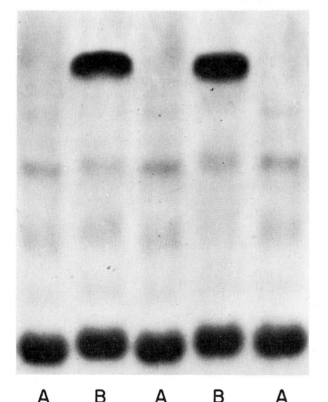

A   B   A   B   A

Figure 3–31 Electrophoretic separation of serum proteins on cellulose acetate. *A* is normal serum. *B* is abnormal serum containing an M-component located near the cathodal end of the strip in the gamma zone. (The cathodal end is at the top and the anodal at the bottom of the picture.)

Table 3–18 CLASSIFICATION OF IMMUNOPROLIFERATIVE DISORDERS ACCORDING TO STAGE OF DIFFERENTIATION (EXCLUDING HODGKIN'S DISEASE)

	T cell disorders
T precursor cell	? Some cases of acute lymphoblastic leukemia
Intermediate T cell	T cell acute lymphoblastic leukemia/lymphoma
Mature T cells	Sézary syndrome/mycosis fungoides T_4^+
	HTLV lymphoma/leukemia T_4^+
	T cell chronic lymphocytic leukemia T_8^+
	B cell disorders
B precursor cell and pre–B cell	CALLA$^+$ acute lymphoblastic leukemia
Differentiated B cell	Non-Hodgkin's lymphoma (most cases)
	B cell chronic lymphocytic leukemia
	B cell acute lymphoblastic leukemia/lymphoma (Burkitt's lymphoma)
Secretory B cell and plasma cell	Waldenström's macroglobulinemia
	Plasma cell myeloma

distinct from, but as rich in diversity as, the myeloproliferative group of hematologic syndromes. The rapid expansion of basic knowledge about lymphocytes has produced a flurry of concepts of lymphoproliferative disorders that rely on cell markers as well as traditional histopathology. The rapidly emerging concepts are forcing reappraisal of old ideas.

The lymphocytic leukemias primarily invade the marrow, with a prominent tendency to infiltrate the circulating bloodstream. The condition spreads to involve lymph nodes, spleen, and indeed many other tissues in the body. The lymphomas are a group of related conditions that affect the secondary lymphatic tissue first with tumor formation that subsequently spreads to the other tissues including the marrow, without much tendency in most cases to release significant numbers of malignant cells into the circulation. The entities in the third major group of immunoproliferative conditions, plasma cell myeloma and primary macroglobulinemia, cause extensive marrow replacement but show little tendency to infiltrate the blood. They do give rise to a high frequency of aberrations of immunoglobulin synthesis.

Lymphoproliferative disorders may be classified according to their origins from a T or B cell line and also with respect to the functional stage of cell differentiation from which the monoclonal neoplasia springs. Hodgkin's disease continues to elude a niche in this schema (Table 3–18).

B Cell Chronic Lymphocytic Leukemia (CLL). This disease increases in frequency with advancing age, whereas acute lymphoblastic leukemia is mostly a disease of childhood. The terms *chronic* and *acute* were originally descriptive of the clinical courses, but therapeutic advances in the management of the acute variety have narrowed the gap in life expectancy between the two. As a result, the terms are now more indicative of the morphology of the leukemic cell than of the prognosis. The small mature lymphocyte is the hallmark of chronic lymphocytic leukemia; the lymphoblast is the sign of the acute variety.

The disorder is a monoclonal expansion in the numbers of B cells. The cell proliferation rate is slow, and the excess is more one of gradual cell accumulation than of rapid cell division. The neoplastic cells express membrane sIg more weakly than normal B lymphocytes (Foon et al., 1982). When sIgM is coexpressed with sIgD, they share the same variable region and light chain structures, as expected from their monoclonal origin. The relatively weak expression of sIg has suggested that these cells are arrested at a relatively early stage of their maturation. However, about 5 percent of patients develop secretory capacity and produce a monoclonal IgM component demonstrable by serum protein electrophoresis. Hypogammaglobulinemia is probably most often due to arrested maturation of B cells, although increased numbers of suppressor T cells or decreased numbers of helper T cells have also been blamed. Signs of marrow failure have traditionally been attributed to encroachment by the expanding clone of neoplastic B cells, but anemia in some cases seems to have been the result of hemopoietic suppression caused by increased numbers of suppressor T lymphocytes. The explanation for expansion of T cell numbers in this B cell neoplasm is obscure (Fernandez et al., 1983).

The rarity of B cell CLL among individuals of Oriental extraction along with the significant occurrence of multiple cases within families has suggested that genetic factors are important in pathogenesis. Indeed, chromosomal abnormalities are present in the neoplastic cells of a large proportion of cases, most often trisomy 12.

CLL is rare in childhood but not uncommon in mature and older adults; two thirds of patients are over the age of 60 years (Skinnider et al., 1982). There is a 2:1 sex predominance in favor of males. The diagnosis is usually easily made by the observation that large numbers of small mature lymphocytes have accumulated in the blood and bone marrow. In comparison with the normal cells, these lymphocytes are often more friable, have deeper nuclear clefts, and sometimes have more cytoplasm. Immature lymphoid cells account for less than 5 percent of the total. The absolute lymphocyte count in the blood is usually elevated to 10,000 to 150,000 per mm.^{3} or even higher at the time of initial diagnosis, although a "subleukemic" (or "aleukemic") variety may be seen in which the cellular infiltration is confined to the marrow. Generalized lymphadenopathy and splenomegaly are common. Lymphocytic infiltration of the liver and other body tissues increases as the disease progresses.

Staging systems have been devised that allow categorization of patients into prognostic groups. The criteria for staging include lymphadenopathy, hepatosplenomegaly, anemia, and thrombocytopenia. Absence of these correlates well with a relatively benign clinical course that may not shorten life expectancy much, if at all. The median survival time for patients lacking these criteria is almost 20 years. At the other extreme, only about half the patients in the most unfavorable group survive 2 years. Thus, although the median survival time for all patients is approximately 5½ years, this figure has little meaning because it does not take into account disease stage.

Although years may pass without the occurrence of significant symptoms, some patients report anorexia, fatigue, weight loss, and sweats. Growth of lymphatic tumors may cause mechanical symptoms due to obstruction or compression. Massive splenic enlargement may add to the severity of the cytopenia by trapping and sequestering or destroying any one or a combination of the blood cells. About 5 to 10 percent of patients have an associated Coombs-positive autoimmune hemolytic anemia, with spherocytosis, reticulocytosis, and erythroid hyperplasia in an otherwise lymphocytic marrow, along with the other usual signs of hemolysis. Susceptibility to infection may stem either from severe neutropenia or from the impediment to the production of circulating antibody. The loss of humoral immunity makes the patient susceptible to recurrent bacterial infections such as pneumococcal pneumonia. More profound immunocompromise may break down defenses against infections by opportunistic invaders that usually do not cause significant infections in healthy people. These are a frequent cause of mortality in the severely immunodeficient patient.

The goals of therapy are to relieve symptoms and to improve anemia, thrombocytopenia, and granulocytopenia by reducing the size of the lymphocyte mass. Because rapid cell proliferation is not a prominent feature, chemotherapeutic agents that depend on the DNA synthetic or mitotic phases of cycling cells are usually not useful. Chemotherapeutic destruction of the lymphocyte mass by alkylating agents (chlorambucil or cyclophosphamide) and adrenal glucocorticoids used singly or in combination are the mainstay of treatment. Radiation therapy is effective for localized symptoms.

Therapy has no doubt decreased morbidity and improved quality of life in CLL, but it seems likely that it has not dramatically increased life expectancy. Although peripheral blood counts improve, hypogammaglobulinemia is often not affected by treatment. The goal is to achieve "control" of the disease rather than "complete remission," since there is no evidence that added clinical benefit would accrue from the additional therapy that would be necessary. If properly managed, many patients may live out their normal life span with this disease. It rarely changes character, and the danger lies almost entirely in the immunodeficiency and in marrow and organ impairment from lymphocyte encroachment.

CLL Variants. Fewer than 5 percent of cases in the United States are *T cell CLL*, although in Japan this variety is seen more often than *B cell CLL*. In T cell CLL, hepatosplenomegaly and cutaneous involvement are more frequent, and the patients tend to be younger. In many cases, the disease follows a more relentless course, although this is not invariably so. The proliferation appears to involve well-differentiated T cells that are ER^+ and Tdt^-. $Fc\gamma$ receptors or T_8 markers may be demonstrable on the cell membranes, and some cell populations show cytotoxic or suppressor activity. A number of cases have been reported in association with red cell aplasia or neutropenia, suggesting that the expanded population of T cells suppresses hemopoiesis. In some of

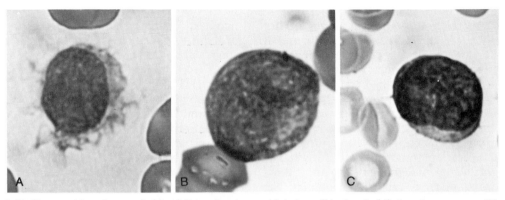

Figure 3–32 Abnormal lymphocytes in blood films of patients with hairy cell leukemia (*A*), lymphosarcoma cell leukemia (*B*), and prolymphocytic leukemia (*C*).

these cases, the neoplastic nature of the disorder has not been firmly established.

Hairy cell leukemia was originally called *leukemic reticuloendotheliosis* because the proliferating cells were thought to be derived from the mononuclear phagocyte complex, then known as reticuloendothelial cells. However, it is now apparent that most cases exhibit B cell surface characteristics (Catovsky, 1977). The abnormal cells resemble small lymphocytes, but the cytoplasm has a hairy fringed border that earns the disorder its name (Fig. 3–32). Nuclear chromatin is less compact than that in the small lymphocyte. The cytoplasm stains positively for tartrate-resistant acid phosphatase. The neoplastic cells show a predilection for invasion of the marrow and spleen. Lymph node enlargement is not impressive. Leukocytosis may occur, although pancytopenia is common. The latter may be caused by hypersplenism, and splenectomy is often helpful in relieving the situation (Jansen and Hermans, 1981). The clinical course is usually slow. Resistance to chemotherapy has been reported, but some cases do respond well when such treatment is indicated.

Lymphosarcoma cell leukemia refers to lymphocytic lymphoma that has transformed to a leukemic phase with diffuse invasion of the marrow, peripheral blood, and of many other tissues (Mintzer and Hauptman, 1983). The clinical course is usually more aggressive than that in B cell CLL. The proliferating cells are of B cell origin but are morphologically distinct from those of CLL. They show more cytoplasm, nuclear cleavage and lobulation, less compact nuclear chromatin, and distinct nucleoli (Fig. 3–32). In contrast to B cell CLL, this variant is characterized by strong expression of sIg.

Prolymphocytic leukemia is a disorder of

older males characterized by marked splenomegaly without significant lymph node enlargement. Marked leukocytosis is the rule. The neoplastic cell line is usually of B cell origin and shows strongly expressed sIg, and the cells are relatively large and are intermediate between lymphoblasts and small lymphocytes in their morphologic features. Nucleoli are prominent (Fig. 3–32). The clinical course is subacute and relatively resistant to treatment (Taylor et al., 1982).

Sézary syndrome is also considered a CLL variant, but it will be discussed later under cutaneous T cell lymphoma.

Acute Lymphoblastic Leukemia (ALL). Primarily a disease of childhood with peak incidence at the age of 4 years, ALL affects 20- to 30-year-old adults with a frequency about equal to that of acute granulocytic leukemia (Chessells, 1982). Above that age, 90 percent or more of the acute leukemias are granulocytic. It is the most common malignancy of childhood. The onset is relatively sudden, with symptoms of anemia, bleeding, or fever. Preleukemic manifestations are absent. Bone pain is not uncommon. The white blood cell count is usually increased, occasionally to values of 100,000 per mm.[3] or higher, with infiltration of the blood with lymphoblasts, but about one third of the patients present with a normal or low white cell count. Anemia and thrombocytopenia are the rule, but immunodeficiency is uncommon, except that it may come later as a result of the immunosuppressive effects of therapy. Intracranial hemorrhage is a life-threatening event, the likelihood of which is increased if severe thrombocytopenia occurs together with extreme elevations of the white cell count. Serum uric acid concentrations often are high, and precautions are necessary to avoid urate nephropathy. Neurologic manifestations due to infiltration of the central nervous system or of peripheral nerves are not uncommon. A slight to moderate degree of lymphadenopathy and hepatosplenomegaly is often present. Many other body tissues also become infiltrated with leukemic cells. Slow but unrestrained proliferation of the lymphoblasts crowds out normal blood precursor cells and produces death within a few months from hemorrhage or infection if the condition is not treated. Successful treatment eradicates all visible evidence of malignant tissue and allows the normal marrow cells to repopulate the marrow and to restore peripheral blood counts to normal, a state called *complete remission.*

Several subclasses of ALL have been defined by means of membrane surface markers (Table 3–19). The most common of these does not show the surface features of either B or T cells but has the "common ALL antigen" (CALLA) on the blast cell membranes. This antigen is leukemia-associated rather than leukemia-specific. It is present on the surfaces of a small percentage of normal marrow cells. A small proportion of children and a larger proportion of adults with non-T non-B cell ALL lack CALLA, and their disease is classified as null cell ALL. Actually, most cases of non-T non-B cell ALL appear to involve B precursor or pre–B cells, since their lymphoblasts show immunoglobulin gene rearrangements and sometimes cytoplasmic μ chains (Arnold et al., 1983).

T cell ALL is characterized by a high frequency of mediastinal tumor, skin and central nervous system involvement, a high initial white cell count, and a relatively poor prognosis. The disorder affects males more commonly than females and has a predilection for older children and young adults. The syndrome may present as a lymphoma, usually mediastinal, without leukemia at onset. However, the tendency to leukemic conversion is marked, and the term *T cell lymphoblastic lymphoma/leukemia* is often used as a synonym for *T cell ALL* (Nathwani et al., 1981). The neoplastic cells are of an intermediate degree of maturity. They are ER + but have not lost their TdT. T cell ALL should be considered apart from human T cell leukemia/lymphoma virus (HTLV)-associated malignancy, which has distinguishing clinical and phenotypic features and will be discussed later.

The rarest subclass is B cell ALL, also a poor prognosis group, diagnosed by the presence of sIg on the lymphoblasts. This type probably represents Burkitt's lymphoma in the leukemic phase.

Terminal deoxyribonucleotidyl transferase (TdT) is a useful cellular marker that helps one distinguish ALL from acute myelogenous leukemia (AML). This enzyme is a DNA polymerase that adds deoxyribonucleoside monophosphates to preformed DNA without the need for a template. It appears to be a sign of lymphoid cell immaturity and is normally restricted in tissue distribution to cortical thymocytes and a small subpopulation of marrow lymphocytes. It is found in 95 percent of ALL cases.

Chromosomal abnormalities are commonly present in ALL clones, and of these aneuploidy (usually hyperploidy) is the most frequent. About 20 to 30 percent of cases of blast crisis of chronic myelogenous leukemia (CML) are TdT positive and are of lymphoid origin. Their blast cells are Philadelphia chromosome (Ph[1]) positive. In fact, about 5 percent of children and 25 percent of adults with de novo ALL are Ph[1] positive without having passed through a previous clinically recognized phase of CML. The presence of the Ph[1] chromosome in ALL is an indication of poor prognosis. B cell ALL blasts may show the translocation characteristic of Burkitt's lymphoma, as discussed subsequently.

The FAB (French-American-British) morphologic classification of ALL includes three categories. In L1 the cells are microlymphoblasts, small relatively uniform cells with skimpy rims of cytoplasm. In L2 the lymphoblasts are larger and more varied in size and shape, with more prominent nucleoli. Most cases of CALLA positive ALL are of L1 morphology, but the correlation beween morphology and surface antigens is not good. Most cases of L3 morphology are B cell (Burkitt's) ALL. The blasts are large and round and show numerous small cytoplasmic vacuoles. If the blast nucleus has a convoluted cerebriform appearance, it suggests T cell origin, but this sign is an unreliable indicator of cell lineage.

Table 3–19 SUBCLASSES OF ACUTE LYMPHOBLASTIC LEUKEMIA

Subclass	Children (<15 yrs.)	Adults
CALLA	76%	50%
T-ALL	12%	10%
B-ALL	1%	2%
Null-ALL	11%	38%

(From Greaves, M. F., and Lister, T. A.: New Engl. J. Med., *304*:119, 1981.)

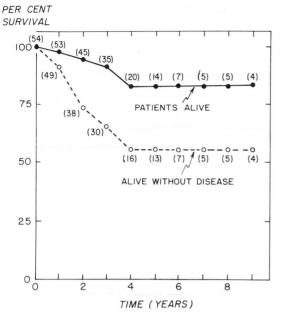

PER CENT SURVIVAL

TIME (YEARS)

Figure 3–38 Survival in patients with localized Hodgkin's disease treated with radical radiation therapy. Most of the deaths and recurrences occurred within 3 years. A similar group of patients not treated radically had a 5-year survival of 35 percent, but no survivor was free of disease. (Redrawn from Prosnitz, L. R., et al.: Am. J. Roentgenol., *105*:618, 1969. Courtesy of Charles C Thomas, Publisher.)

are sometimes used, for example, if tumor masses are very large. The proper role of combined modality management is still under investigation. Although localized palliation is sometimes necessary, the major goal of radiotherapy is the cure of the patient. For many years, chemotherapy had been assigned a purely palliative role, but the development of combination chemotherapy has dramatically changed the outlook for many patients with advanced disease. Treatment with multiple agents is carried out for a number of months to induce complete remission, which can be accomplished in about 80 percent of patients, the majority of whom do not relapse. Treatment regimens are based on the alkylating agents (nitrogen mustard, cyclophosphamide), the vinca alkaloids, the nitrosoureas, the anthracyclines, procarbazine, dacarbazine, bleomycin, and the adrenal glucocorticoids.

Without treatment, very few patients with Hodgkin's disease survive 10 years, according to old data. This bleak picture has been radically changed with modern treatment methods. Now, about 85 per cent of patients with asymptomatic localized disease are cured. For those with advanced disease, the cure rate appears to be in the range of 50 percent. Survival differences among the various histopathologic

types have practically disappeared, although disease stage, age, and the presence or absence of symptoms are still significant determinants of survival. (See Proceedings of the Symposium on Contemporary Issues in Hodgkin's Disease, 1982).

Non-Hodgkin's Lymphomas. These heterogeneous disorders are clonal proliferations of lymphocytes that have undergone malignant transformation at an arrested stage of their differentiation. They are mostly neoplasms of B cell lines and occur predominantly in middle and older age. They are more likely to present at an advanced stage than Hodgkin's disease, yet in many instances this may not necessarily indicate a poor prognosis. Although staging is necessary in the evaluation of non-Hodgkin's lymphoma patients, surgical laparotomy is rarely, if ever, done because the results will not influence therapy. In many cases, the neoplastic lymphocytes retain their functional and migratory properties.

For several decades, the histopathologic classification of the non-Hodgkin's lymphomas has been a pathologist's nightmare because of frequent discordance in pathologic diagnosis from one observer to the next. Rapid advances in immunologic research uncovered scientific inaccuracies in nomenclature. These same advances have helped in the design of new systems, but a number of controversial issues are still not resolved.

The system of Rappaport has been, and continues to be, in widespread clinical use because of its relative simplicity and clinical utility. The Kiel system devised in Europe and its American counterpart, the Lukes-Collins system, attempted to overcome errors and shortcomings of the earlier nomenclature of Rappaport. Both Kiel and Lukes-Collins recognized that the "poorly differentiated lymphocyte" was really a follicular center cell ("cleaved cell" according to Lukes-Collins and "centrocyte" according to Kiel). The "histiocyte" was really a large lymphoid cell in a more active state of proliferation. "Undifferentiated" cells were lymphoblasts. In order to reconcile these and other new classification systems, a *Working Formulation* was devised with international cooperation in the hope that a uniform nomenclature would be acceptable to all. (See The Non-Hodgkin's Lymphoma Pathologic Classification Project, 1982.) It is based primarily on clinical behavior and on conventional histopathologic appearance without the assistance of immunologic techniques (Table 3–21). In the discussion to follow, the Working Formulation designations will be

Table 3–21 WORKING FORMULATION CLASSIFICATION OF NON-HODGKIN'S LYMPHOMA*

Low-grade
Follicular, small cleaved cell (nodular poorly differentiated)
Follicular, mixed small cleaved and large cell (nodular mixed lymphocytic-histiocytic)
Diffuse, small cell (diffuse, well-differentiated lymphocytic)

Intermediate-grade
Follicular, large cell (nodular histiocytic)
Diffuse, small cleaved cell (diffuse, poorly differentiated lymphocytic)
Diffuse, mixed small and large cell (diffuse, mixed lymphocytic-histiocytic)
Diffuse, large cell (diffuse, histiocytic)

High-grade
Lymphoblastic (lymphoblastic)
Small noncleaved (undifferentiated Burkitt's and non-Burkitt's)
Immunoblastic large cell (diffuse histiocytic lymphoma)

Other variants
Cutaneous T cell lymphoma—mycosis fungoides/Sézary type
Cutaneous T cell lymphoma—HTLV associated variant
Extramedullary plasmacytoma
Histiocytic lymphoma

*Rappaport nomenclature given in parentheses.

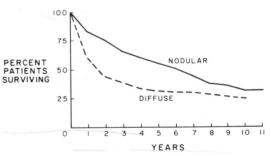

Figure 3–39 Survival of patients with nodular (favorable) and diffuse (unfavorable) non-Hodgkin's lymphoma. (Adapted from Horwich, A., and Peckham, M.: Semin. Hematol., *20*:36, 1983.)

used, with the Rappaport equivalents cited in parentheses.

The architecture of the lymph node, whether follicular or diffuse, and the size and character of the predominating cells, whether small and slowly proliferating or large and rapidly proliferating, determine prognosis. A follicular pattern and small cell size correlate with a relatively indolent clinical course, with median survival time of about 8 years and some patients alive and well, although not free of disease, even after 20 years (Portlock, 1983). Diffuse obliteration of the nodal architecture and a large cell size go together with a more aggressive clinical course that may shorten life expectancy to less than a year. The survival curve for the more aggressive lymphomas falls off rapidly but then plateaus after 2 to 4 years. For lymphomas associated with a more favorable prognosis, the curve follows a more gradual downward slope. The two meet at about 12 years, at which point the survival statistics are about the same for the two groups, about 35 percent (Fig. 3–39).

About half the non-Hodgkin's lymphomas are *follicular,* a pattern that indicates that the follicular center cells have retained their natural behavior for "homing" in germinal centers. Large numbers of nonmalignant T cells are associated with the neoplastic follicular center cells in a reactive or interactive relationship. The *small cleaved cell type* (nodular poorly differentiated) is the most common of the *follicular lymphomas.* It is classified as low-grade, despite the fact that 90 percent of the patients are Stage III or IV at initial presentation. The marrow is involved in about 60 per cent of cases. Lymph node involvement is usually widely disseminated. Mesenteric nodal enlargement is more common (Fig. 3–40) and massive mediastinal tumor formation much less common than in Hodgkin's disease. Patients with the condition are often asymptomatic, and symptoms, when they do occur, are often related to a local tumor enlargement that is causing obstruction or compression. This may affect the kidney, the gastrointestinal tract, the spinal cord or other aspects of the nervous system, the orbit, or the sinuses, among other areas. After some years, the condition may convert to a more aggressive histologic pattern, with a predominance of large cells in a nodular or diffuse pattern. Although small numbers of circulating neoplastic cells can be demonstrated by cytofluorometry in earlier phases of the disease (Smith et al., 1984), gross leukemic conversion occurs only occasionally after heavy cellular infiltration of the marrow. Survival at that point is usually measured in weeks or months (Hubbard et al., 1982).

The term *follicular lymphoma, mixed small cleaved cell and large cell* (nodular mixed lymphocytic-histiocytic) is used when there is no predominant cell type. However, if the dominant cell type is the *large cell* in a *follicular* pattern (nodular histiocytic), the clinical behavior is more aggressive and the lymphoma is classified as *intermediate grade.*

Virtually all the follicular lymphomas are B cell neoplasms. The cells express sIg strongly and have class II MHC antigens and B cell

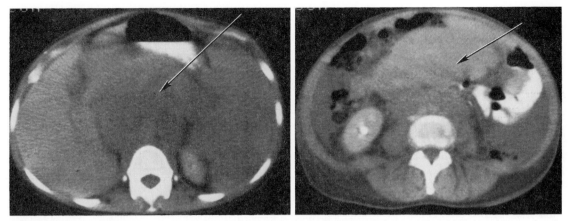

Figure 3–40 Computerized tomography of the abdomen of a patient with nodular non-Hodgkin's lymphoma, showing massive mesenteric and retroperitoneal lymph node enlargement (arrow). The liver is to the left, and the enlarged spleen to the right, of the enlarged nodes.

lineage markers on their membranes. Some are also CALLA positive.

The management of the low-grade lymphomas is conservative. Often, no treatment at all is possible when there are no symptoms and the clinical course is nonprogressive (Horning and Rosenberg, 1984). Local radiotherapy may be used for Stage I or II disease and for palliation of symptoms due to local tumor growth. However, the neoplastic proliferation is also sensitive to chemotherapy. Conservative chemotherapy regimens may be used. Although aggressive regimens bring about complete remission more quickly, there is no convincing evidence that they significantly prolong survival time.

Among the *diffuse* lymphomas, one type stands out among the others for its relatively good prognosis and for its low-grade classification, namely *small cell lymphocytic lymphoma* (well-differentiated diffuse). It is the same disorder as B cell CLL, a widely disseminated, relatively indolent proliferation of monoclonal, weakly sIg positive B lymphocytes of medullary cord origin. However, the peripheral blood is not grossly invaded as it is in B cell CLL, and the infiltration is limited to the tissues, usually including the marrow. Hypogammaglobulinemia and autoimmune blood dyscrasias may occur as in B cell CLL.

The remainder of the diffuse lymphomas are of intermediate- or high-grade clinical severity. *Diffuse lymphoma, small cleaved cell type* (diffuse poorly differentiated) is a neoplasia of small follicular center cells, but the cells no longer follow their follicular instincts and instead assemble in sheets. The clinical course is more aggressive and invasive. In *diffuse large*

cell lymphoma (diffuse histiocytic), the clinical nature is even more aggressive, but in about 20 to 30 percent of cases the process is localized in a lymph node or extralymphatic site, such as the skin, bone, gastrointestinal tract, central nervous system, or some other tissue. Marrow involvement is less common in comparison with that seen in the low-grade lymphomas. There is a greater tendency for presentation as a large abdominal or mediastinal mass. The presence of systemic symptoms, bulky tumors, more advanced stages of the disease, and marked elevation of the serum lactic dehydrogenase are all predictors of a worse prognosis. About half the cases are of B cell origin, one fourth are of T cell origin, and the remainder are neither T nor B cells ("null"). When the predominating cell type is neither small nor large, the histologic classification is *diffuse, mixed small and large cell* (diffuse mixed lymphocytic-histiocytic).

Treatment is indicated for all the intermediate- and high-grade lymphomas with intent to cure. Aggressive combination chemotherapy is used with a high rate of complete remission. Radiation therapy may be used for localized disease, but survival statistics are less satisfactory than those achieved by combination chemotherapy with or without radiation. Radiation may also be used in conjunction with chemotherapy for the treatment of bulk disease. With these modern techniques, prolonged survivals are attained in about 90 percent of patients with localized disease and in 35 to 50 percent of those with more advanced stages. In those who fail treatment, there is progressive visceral invasion associated with weight loss, fever, anemia, and paralysis of the immune system, inviting infection by opportunistic organisms.

The more infrequent *high-grade malignancies* are all diffuse and have the most rapid cell proliferation rates. These lymphomas are more likely to give rise to such metabolic complications as extreme hyperuricemia, hyperkalemia, and lactic acidosis. They tend to convert to a leukemic phase rather rapidly. *Lymphoblastic lymphoma* is usually of T cell origin and commonly presents in late childhood or early adult life as a mediastinal tumor. As previously discussed, this tumor appears to be essentially a tissue phase of acute lymphoblastic leukemia.

Burkitt's lymphoma (undifferentiated) and a cytologically and clinically similar variant called *non-Burkitt lymphoma* are *small non–cleaved cell diffuse lymphomas* with extremely rapid cell proliferation rates. In the endemic African variety, extralymphatic presentation is the rule in younger children, particularly in the jaw or abdomen. In the nonendemic cases, lymph node presentation is more common in older children, adolescents, and young adults, usually in the abdomen or neck (Ziegler, 1981). The neoplastic B cells are of follicular center origin.

Immunoblastic lymphoma (diffuse histiocytic lymphoma) is a type of diffuse large cell lymphoma that occurs in a setting of chronic immune stimulation, anemia, polyclonal hypergammaglobulinemia, systemic symptoms, poor response to treatment, and short survival.

With aggressive treatment programs that follow the general principles outlined for the management of acute lymphoblastic leukemia (including prophylactic treatment of the central nervous system), a significant number of patients with high-grade lymphoma may be cured of an otherwise rapidly fatal disorder (Weinstein et al., 1979).

Other Lymphoma Variants. The cutaneous T cell lymphomas are neoplasms of mature cells of helper/inducer phenotype (T_4^+, ER^+ TdT^-) with a homing instinct for the skin (Haynes et al., 1981). *Mycosis fungoides* follows a chronic but slowly progressive course, and is associated with a median survival time of about 9 years. Skin involvement progresses, lymph nodes enlarge, and the disease finally spreads to viscera. The *Sézary variant* is a stage of the disease characterized by diffuse erythrodermia and infiltration of the blood with monocytoid T lymphocytes that have convoluted nuclei and PAS positive cytoplasmic vacuoles (Lamberg et al., 1984). The marrow is spared until late in the disease. Intraepider-

mal nests of the abnormal cells (Pautrier's abscesses) are seen in skin biopsy specimens.

A variety of T cell lymphoma has been recognized with certain distinctive features, including adult onset, disseminated skin lesions, lytic bone disease, hypercalcemia, aggressive clinical course, and resistance to treatment (Bunn et al., 1983). Most of the cases have been reported in southwest Japan, with smaller numbers found in the Caribbean region and the southeastern United States (Blayney et al., 1983). The malignant cells bear the helper/inducer phenotype but, paradoxically, have suppressor activity. The disorder is associated with the human T cell leukemia/lymphoma virus (HTLV).

The true histiocytic lymphomas are rare neoplasms of the monocyte/macrophage complex, described in the discussion of phagocytes.

Pathogenesis. For most cases of non-Hodgkin's lymphoma, a cause is not evident. However, the immunocompromised state, whether due to inborn factors or to immunosuppressive therapy (e.g., for transplant recipients), markedly increases the incidence. The interaction of chronic immune stimulation with deficient immune responses appears to be particularly provocative. Given these observations together with the known concurrence of lymphoma with autoimmune disorders, the genesis of the neoplasia appears to be closely associated with a defect in immune regulation.

The viral etiology theory has been given substantial support by the discovery of the two virus-associated entities, Burkitt's lymphoma and HTLV leukemia/lymphoma. EBV is a DNA virus of the herpes family with a strong affinity for B cells. In cell culture, this virus propagates B cell growth. In humans, EBV infection is almost ubiquitous, but the B cell proliferation is usually restrained by cytotoxic T cells. When this response is deficient, unrestrained B cell growth can result in lymphoma. EBV is found in the cellular genome of almost all patients with African Burkitt's lymphoma but only in the minority of those with the nonendemic variety, suggesting that EBV infection may be only an adjunctive or secondary phenomenon.

The HTLV is a RNA retrovirus, so called because it is transcribed into cellular DNA through the auspices of an enzyme, reverse transcriptase. This virus has a tropism for T cells. It has been identified in cell lines of patients with HTLV leukemia/lymphoma, and almost all these patients have high antibody titers against the virus. About 1 to 2 per cent of normal individuals from nonendemic areas and higher proportions of family members and of apparently normal people from endemic areas also have elevated titers. Several varieties of HTLV have been identified, revealing an intriguing relationship between HTLV leukemia/lymphoma and AIDS. One type (HTLV-I) promotes T_4^+ cell growth and causes malignancy. Another (HTLV-III) produces T_4^+ cell lysis and helper cell deficiency and is presumably the cause of AIDS.

Chromosome abnormalities are present in most cases of non-Hodgkin's lymphoma, and of these the most common is an exchange of genetic material between the long arm of chromosome 14, where the genes for Ig heavy chains are located, and chromosome 8, 11, or 18 (Yunis et al., 1982). Most cases of Burkitt's lymphoma are marked by a translocation between the long arms of chromosomes 8 and 14 ($8q^-$, $14q^+$). In a smaller number, the translocation is between chromosome 8 and a chromosome that carries the loci for light chain immunoglobulin genes, either 2 or 22 (Fig. 3–41). The tip of chromosome 8 that is translocated bears a proto-oncogene called *c-myc*. Proto-oncogenes are normal constituents of cellular DNA that, when activated, become oncogenes that have the capacity to bring about malignant transformation. So far, about 24 proto-oncogenes have been described, of which c-myc is only one. They are highly conserved segments of DNA found in many diverse species and also in retroviruses that have the capacity to steal them from their native cellular habitats. In Burkitt's lymphoma, the c-myc gene segment is spliced into the midst of immunoglobulin gene regions. Presumably, this changed location brings the segment under the control of new regulatory effects that stimulate it, causing activation and growth of a B cell line.

M-Component Disorders. An "M-component" is the secretory product of a single monoclonal line of immunoglobulin-producing immunocytes. The abnormal protein is recognized as a narrow homogeneous band, or "spike," in the electrophoretic pattern of serum or concentrated urine (see Fig. 3–31). It is the product of a cellular clone that has undergone an unusual degree of proliferation, often of a neoplastic character. The absolute production rate of the M-component can be used as a measure of the mass of the abnormal cell line, assuming that each cell produces a fixed quantity of immunoglobulin per unit time. The production rate can be estimated from measurement of its concentration and a knowledge of its turnover rate. An imbalance in the production rates of the subunits that combine to make up the immunoglobulin molecule causes overproduction of one of the subunits, usually L chains, which spill out readily into the urine because of their low molecular weight. The L chains, called *Bence Jones protein* in the premolecular era, are either κ or λ in type, but not both, a further demonstration of the monoclonal character of the cell of origin. Excesses of H chains in the serum and urine occur more rarely.

These abnormal proteins often are discovered accidentally because of the frequency with which serum electrophoresis is done. The heat

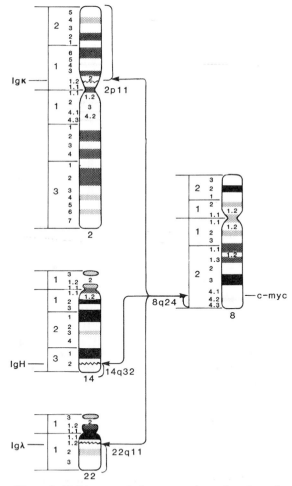

Figure 3–41 Diagram of chromosomal translocations observed in Burkitt's lymphoma. The arrows designate the break points at which translocations occur between the distal segment of chromosome 8, which bears the c-myc gene, and the immunoglobulin gene regions of chromosomes 2, 14, or 22. Most of the translocations are between chromosomes 8 and 14. (From Leder, P., Battey, J., Lenoir, G., et al.: Science, 222:767, 1983.)

test for Bence Jones protein in the urine is unreliable. Detection of urinary L chains should be by electrophoresis of sufficiently concentrated urine. Paper dip techniques in common use for the routine detection of albuminuria are not sensitive to the presence in the urine of other proteins, such as L chains. This is a persuasive argument for using sulfosalicylic acid for the detection of proteinuria. L chains may be detected in the serum, but since they are so rapidly excreted by the kidney, their concentration is very low unless there is renal insufficiency. The concentration of the serum M-component varies from the range of 1 gm. per 100 ml. to more than 10 gm per 100 ml. The daily urinary excretion of L chains may vary from less than 1 gm. per day to 15 to 20 gm. per day. Immunoelectrophoretic techniques are now in common use to classify the M-components of the serum and urine. Quantitation of immunoglobulins shows depressed serum concentrations of the uninvolved types. The ability to produce specific antibody is often impaired. Recurrent bacterial pneumonia and other infectious complications then appear.

M-components in the serum sometimes confer strange properties upon it that may be of pathophysiologic significance. If the M-component is a cryoglobulin, reversible precipitation or gelation at reduced temperatures may cause circulatory embarrassment in exposed body parts. Red cells readily aggregate into "rouleaux," and the erythrocyte sedimentation rate is often rapid, but significant hemolysis usually does not occur. Bleeding may stem from antagonistic effects on plasma coagulation factors, fibrin polymerization, and platelet function. The M-component, especially if it is an IgM type, may increase plasma viscosity by eight- to tenfold. The "hyperviscosity syndrome" causes visual disturbances, retinal venous congestion and a sausage-like periodicity of the vein walls ("boxcar effect"), mental confusion, stupor, and even coma (Bloch and Maki, 1973). Symptoms are quickly ameliorated by plasmapheresis. The excretion in the urine of large amounts of L chains is significantly related to the development of renal insufficiency, presumably through tissue deposition of L chains as amyloid or by a direct toxic effect of this small protein on the renal tubule epithelial cells. Hypercalcemia and hyperuricemia also contribute to the multifactorial renal disease that complicates plasma cell myeloma.

Plasma cell myeloma is a malignant prolif-eration of plasma cells, usually in the marrow, somtimes forming solitary or multiple tumors, but almost always going on to widespread dissemination as diffuse "myelomatosis" (Bloch and Franklin, 1982). Destructive bone disease is the major pathologic consequence, possibly because of the local secretion of an osteoclast-stimulating factor. Localized osteolytic punched-out lesions affecting the skull, ribs, pelvis, or proximal portions of the long bones, as well as diffuse osteoporosis of the whole skeletal system, are common (Durie and Salmon, 1975). Extramedullary myelomas may rarely form almost anywhere. Lymphatic involvement is not a feature of the disease, and hepatosplenomegaly is generally not detected. Localized bone pain and pathologic fractures are the most fearsome consequences. Symptomatic hypercalcemia, apparently related to bone dissolution, is common and may require emergency treatment.

Amyloidosis associated with plasma cell myeloma usually assumes the clinical features of the primary rather than the secondary form. Fragments of the L chains are invariably found in the tissue deposits (Solomon et al., 1982). Musculoskeletal involvement is impressive and causes symptoms of arthritis, carpal tunnel syndrome, myocardial weakness, and macroglossia.

A moderate normocytic and normochromic anemia is common, and about one third of patients have pancytopenia related to replacement of the marrow by the neoplastic plasma cells. Morphologic confirmation of the diagnosis is always necessary, either by biopsy of a plasma cell tumor or by random aspiration of marrow. If sheets of immature plasma cells replace the normal marrow cellular elements, the morphologic picture is diagnostic, but if the plasma cells are fewer, great care must be exercised in morphologic interpretation. Reactive plasmacytosis may increase the marrow plasma cells to 25 to 30 percent of the total, although usually a reactive plasmacytosis is not in excess of 10 to 15 percent. *Benign monoclonal gammopathy* and *primary amyloidosis* must also be distinguished from plasma cell myeloma. Increasing degrees of plasma cell immaturity along with frequent polyploid forms favor the latter diagnosis.

Depressed concentrations of the normal serum immunoglobulins are a constant feature of plasma cell myeloma. For quite some time, this has been explained mechanistically as a "crowding out" of normal plasma cells by the neoplastic clone. Other possible explanations include deficiencies of B cell surface receptors for antigen causing a block in B cell differentiation; excessive negative feedback from the high level of monoclonal protein or plasma cell mass or both; and depression of humoral immunity by a population of suppressor cells.

Three fourths of plasma cell myeloma patients have either an IgG or an IgA M-component in the serum, with IgG occurring twice as commonly as IgA. Almost all of the remaining patients who lack such a serum component will have an M-component in the urine, with decreased serum immunoglobulin concentrations. In all, about one half to two thirds have demonstrable L chains in the urine. Rare cases of IgD and IgE myeloma have been reported. A few plasma cells are commonly seen in the peripheral blood in myeloma, but overt plasma cell leukemia is a rare and rapidly fatal variant.

Primary macroglobulinemia of Waldenström typically affects older people in their eighties. The clinical picture overlaps that of chronic lymphocytic leukemia and lymphocytic lymphoma, in which about 5 percent of patients have an M-component, usually IgM. The typical presentation of primary macroglobulinemia is one of a dense infiltration of the marrow with small mature lymphoid cells, many of which have plasmacytoid features. A number of typical plasma cells may also be seen. There is no leukemic infiltration of the blood; generalized lymphadenopathy and splenomegaly are present but are not marked. The diagnosis is confirmed by demonstrating the presence in the serum of an IgM M-component in excess of 2 gm. per 100 ml. L chains may be found in the urine. Anemia is common and may be severe, although in part it is dilutional owing to increased plasma volume. Pancytopenia is not uncommon. Osteolytic bone lesions are exceptionally rare.

Finding an M-component in the serum or urine alone cannot be considered diagnostic of either of the aforementioned immunoproliferative conditions without the assistance of supporting information (Kyle, 1978). The term *benign monoclonal gammopathy* has been applied to those patients with an M-component in the serum, usually less than 2 gm. per 100 ml., without decreases in the other serum immunoglobulins, significant abnormalities in blood counts, bone disease, or more than a minority of mostly mature plasma cells in the marrow. In some instances, the M-component spontaneously disappears, suggesting that it may have been evoked as a physiologic but monoclonal response to some undetermined but highly specific antigen. A low concentration of monoclonal IgM occurs with cold agglutinin hemolytic anemia. *Amyloidosis* is thought to bear some relationship to an underlying process of plasma cell proliferation either of a secondary reactive nature, as in chronic infections, Hodgkin's lymphoma, or rheumatoid arthritis, or of a primary nature. Indeed, one school of thought contends that primary amyloidosis is an expression of plasma cell myeloma, even in the absence of osteolytic bone disease and other diagnostic criteria of myeloma. M-components and marrow plasmacytosis are common findings in primary amyloidosis, the diagnosis of which is most readily confirmed by biopsy of the gum or rectal mucosa. In the absence of these associated conditions, patients with benign monoclonal gammopathy commonly remain stable and asymptomatic for many years and require no treatment, but in some instances the condition exists as the asymptomatic preclinical stage of plasma cell myeloma.

Heavy chain diseases are rare, having been first described by Franklin and associates (1964), who observed γ type H chains in the serum and urine of a patient with a lymphoma-like illness. Another variant of H chain disease is the α type, which presents as a lymphoma of the small intestine in association with the signs and symptoms of sprue. The relationship is particularly intriguing because of the known abundance of IgA-secreting plasma cells in the normal gastrointestinal tract.

Therapy of the symptomatic M-component disorders is often successful and may arrest progression of the disease for years. The chemotherapeutic agents of greatest utility have been aklylating agents (melphalan and cyclophosphamide) and adrenal glucocorticoids. Palliative radiation therapy is helpful for local bone pain and for such dreaded complications as spinal cord compression, for which surgical decompression may also be necessary.

Pseudolymphoma. Some patients present clinical syndromes that lie in a twilight zone between lymphoma and chronic inflammatory states. These may be of a chronic autoimmune nature with an occasional subsequent lymphomatous transformation (e.g., *Sjögren's syndrome*). Others are idiopathic or drug-induced hypersensitivity states. Both clinicians and pathologists are faced with confusion and consternation in trying to arrive at a definite decision that only time will resolve. The term *pseudolymphoma* conveys the uncertainty.

Lukes and Tindle (1975) have described the syndrome of *immunoblastic lymphadenopathy,* with lymph node enlargement, fever, sweats, an increase in polyclonal immunoglobulin, and a characteristic histopathologic picture. They postulate that it is a hypersensitivity state that may become transformed into an immunoblastic lymphoma (Pangalis et al., 1983). Chronic pulmonary lymphocytic infilrates also fall in this general category *(lymphomatoid granulomatosis, lymphoid interstitial pneumonitis)* (Israel et al., 1977). Similarly, lymphocytic infiltrations in the stomach, parotid, thyroid, or orbit may cause confusion when one is attempting to distinguish correctly between a chronic inflammatory state and a lymphocytic lymphoma. Special studies of tissue sections conducted to determine whether the lymphocyte population is monoclonal or polyclonal may help one differentiate the neoplastic conditions from those that are reactive.

References

Arnold, A., Cossman, J., Bakhshi, A., et al.: Immunoglobulin-gene rearrangements as unique clonal markers in human lymphoid neoplasms. New Engl. J. Med., *309*:1593, 1983.

Ballieux, R. E., and Heijnen, C. J.: Antigen-specific helper and suppressor T cell factors in man. Clin. Haematol., *11*:711, 1982.

Benacerraf, B.: Role of MHC gene products in immune regulation. Science, *212*:1229, 1981.

Blayney, D. W., Blattner, W. A., Robert-Guroff, M., et al.: The human T cell leukemia-lymphoma virus in Southeastern United States. J.A.M.A., *250*:1048, 1983.

Bloch, K. J., and Franklin, E.: Plasma cell dyscrasias and cryoglobulins. J.A.M.A., *248*:2670, 1982.

Bloch, K. J., and Maki, D. G.: Hyperviscosity syndromes associated with immunoglobulin abnormalities. Semin. Hematol., *10*:113, 1973.

Buisseret, P. D : Allergy. Sci. Am., *247*(2):86, 1982.

Bunn, P. A., Jr., Schechter, G. P., Jaffe, E., et al.: Clinical course of retrovirus associated adult T cell lymphoma in the United States. New Engl. J. Med., *309*:257, 1983.

Calvert, J. E., Maruyama, S., Tedder, T. F., et al.: Cellular events in the differentiation of antibody secreting cells. Semin. Hematol., *21*:226, 1984.

Catovsky, D.: Hairy cell leukemia and prolymphocytic leukemia. Clin. Haematol., *6*:245, 1977.

Chessells, J. M.: Acute lymphoblastic leukemia. Semin. Hematol., *19*:155, 1982.

Claman, H. N.: Glucocorticosteroids. I. Anti-inflammatory mechanisms. Hosp. Pract., *18*(7):123, 1983.

Cohen, D. J., Loertscher, R., Rubin, M. F., et al.: Cyclosporine: a new immunosuppressive agent for organ transplantation. Ann. Int. Med., *101*:667, 1984.

Curran, J. W., Lawrence, D. N., Jaffe, H., et al.: Acquired immunodeficiency syndrome (AIDS) associated with transfusions. New Engl. J. Med., *310*:69, 1984.

Cushley, W., and Owen, M. J.: Structural and genetic similarities between immunoglobulins and class-1 histocompatibility antigens. Immun. Today, *4*:88, 1983.

Dausset, J.: The major histocompatibility complex in man. Science, *213*:1469, 1981.

deWaele, M., Thielemans, C., and van Camp, B. K. G.: Characterization of immunoregulatory T cells in EBV induced infectious mononucleosis by monoclonal antibodies. New Engl. J. Med., *304*:460, 1981.

Durie, B., and Salmon, S. E.: A clinical staging system for multiple myeloma. Cancer, *36*:842, 1975.

Fauci, A. S., and Dale, D. C.: The effect of hydrocortisone on the kinetics of normal human lymphocytes. Blood, *46*:235, 1975.

Feldbush, T. L., Hobbs, M. V., Severson, C. D., Ballas, Z. K., and Weiler, J. M.: Role of complement in the immune response. Fed. Proc., *43*:2548, 1984.

Fernandez, L. A., Jr., MacSween, J. M., and Langley, G. R.: Immunoglobulin secretory function of B cells from untreated patients with chronic lymphocytic leukemia and hypogammaglobulinemia: role of T cells. Blood, *62*:767, 1983.

Filipovich, A. H., and Kersey, J. H.: B lymphocyte function in immunodeficiency disease. Immun. Today, *4*:50, 1983.

Foon, K. A., Schroff, R. W., and Gale, R. P.: Surface markers on leukemia and lyphoma cells: recent advances. Blood, *60*:1, 1982.

Franklin, E. C., Lowenstein, J., Bigelow, B., et al.: Heavy chain disease, a new disorder of serum gamma-globulins. Report of the first case. Am. J. Med., *37*:332, 1964.

Geha, R. S., and Rosen, F. S.: Immunoregulatory T cell defects. Immun. Today, *4*:233, 1983.

Gottlieb, M. S., Schroff, R., Schanker, H. M., et al.: *Pneumocystis carinii* pneumonia and mucosal candidiasis in previously healthy homosexual men: evidence of a new acquired cellular immunodeficiency. New Engl. J. Med., *305*:1425, 1981.

Haynes, B. F., Metzgar, R. S., Minna, J. D., and Bunn, P. A.: Phenotypic characterization of cutaneous T cell lymphoma. New Engl. J. Med., *304*:1319, 1981.

Henle, W., Henle, G., and Lennette, E. T.: The Epstein-Barr virus. Sci. Am., *241*(1):48, 1979.

Herberman, R. B.: Natural killer cells. Hosp. Pract., *17*(4):93, 1982.

Horning, S. J., and Rosenberg, S. A.: The natural history of initially untreated low grade non-Hodgkin's lymphomas. New Engl. J. Med., *311*:1471, 1984.

Horwich, A., and Peckham, M.: "Bad risk" non-Hodgkin's lymphomas. Semin. Hematol., *20*:35, 1983.

Horwitz, C. A., Henle, W., Henle, G., et al.: Heterophile negative infectious mononucleosis and mononucleosis-like illnesses: laboratory confirmation of 43 cases. Am. J. Med., *63*:947, 1977.

Hubbard, S. M., Chebner, B. A., DeVita, V. T., Jr., et al.: Histologic progression in non-Hodgkin's lymphoma. Blood, *59*:258, 1982.

Israel, H. L., Patchevsky, A. S., and Saldana, M. J.: Wegener's granulomatosis, lymphoid granulomatosis, and benign lymphocytic angiitis and granulomatosis of lung. Ann. Int. Med., *87*:691, 1977.

Jacobs, A. D., and Gale, R. P.: Recent advances in the biology and treatment of acute lymphoblastic leukemia in adults. New Engl. J. Med., *31*:1219, 1984.

Jansen, J., and Hermans, J.: Splenectomy in hairy cell leukemia: retrospective multicenter analysis. Cancer, *47*:2066, 1981.

Kapp, J. A., Pierce, C. W., and Sorensen, C. M.: Antigen specific suppressor T-cell factors. Hosp. Pract., *19*(8):85, 1984.

Kyle, R. A.: Monoclonal gammopathy of undetermined significance. Natural history of 241 cases. Am. J. Med., *64*:814, 1978.

Lai, P. K.: Infectious mononucleosis: recognition and management. Hosp. Pract., *12*(8):47, 1977.

Lamberg, S. I., Green, S. B., Byar, D. P., et al.: Clinical staging for cutaneous T cell lymphoma. Ann. Int. Med., *100*:187, 1984.

Leder, P.: Genetic control of immunoglobulin production. Hosp. Pract., *18*(2):73, 1983.

Lukes, R. J., and Tindle, B. H.: Immunoblastic lymphadenopathy. A hyperimmune entity resembling Hodgkin's disease. New Engl. J. Med., *292*:1, 1975.

Mauer, A. M., Saunders, E. F., and Lampkin, B. C.: Possible significance of non-proliferating leukemic cells. *In* Perry, S. (ed.): Human Tumor Cell Kinetics. Natl. Cancer Inst. Monogr., *30*:63, 1969.

Miller, K. B., and Schwartz, R. S.: Autoimmunity and suppressor T lymphocytes. Adv. Int. Med., *27*:281, 1982.

Mintzer, D. M., and Hauptman, S. P.: Lymphosarcoma cell leukemia and other non-Hodgkin's lymphomas in leukemic phase. Am. J. Med., *75*:110, 1983.

Müller, G. (Ed.): Interleukins and lymphocyte activation. Immun. Rev., *63*:1, 1982.

Nathwani, B. N., Diamond, L. W., Winberg, C. D., et al.: Lymphoblastic lymphoma. A clinicopathologic study of 95 patients. Cancer, *48*:2347, 1981.

Pangalis, G. A., Moran, E. M., Nathwani, B. N., et al.: Angioimmunoblastic lymphadenopathy. Long term follow up study. Cancer, *52*:318, 1983.

Pearson, G. R., Weiland, L. H., Neel, H. B., et al.: Application of Epstein-Barr virus (EBV) serology to the diagnosis of North American nasopharyngeal carcinoma. Cancer, *51*:260, 1983.

Portlock, C. S.: "Good risk" non-Hodgkin's lymphomas. Approaches to management. Semin. Hematol., *20*:25, 1983.

Proceedings of the Symposium on Contemporary Issues in Hodgkin's Disease: Biology, Staging, and Treatment. Cancer Treat. Rep., *66*:601, 1982.

Purtilo, D. T., Sakamoto, K., Barnabei, V., et al.: Epstein-Barr virus–induced diseases in boys with the X-linked lymphoproliferative syndrome (XLP). Am. J. Med., *73*:49, 1982.

Reinherz, E. L., Meuer, S. C., and Schlossman, S. F.: The delineation of antigen receptors on human T lymphocytes. Immun. Today, *4*:5, 1983.

Reinherz, E. L., and Schlossman, S. F.: The characterization and function of human immunoregulatory T lymphocyte subsets. Immun. Today, *2*:69, 1981.

Rosen, F. S., Cooper, M. D., and Wedgewood, R. J. P.: The primary immunodeficiencies. New Engl. J. Med., *311*:235, 1984.

Schaller, J. G., and Hansen, J. A.: HLA relationship to disease. Hosp. Pract., *16*(5):41, 1981.

Schoenfeld, Y., and Schwartz, R. S.: Immunologic and genetic factors in autoimmune diseases. New Engl. J. Med., *311*:1019, 1984.

Skinnider, L. F., Tan, L., Schmidt, J., and Armitage, G.: Chronic lymphocytic leukemia. A review of 745 cases and assessment of clinical staging. Cancer, *50*:2951, 1982.

Smith, B. R., Weinberg, D. S., Robert, N. J., et al.: Circulating monoclonal B lymphocytes in non-Hodgkin's lymphoma. New Engl. J. Med., *311*:1476, 1984.

Solomon, A., Frangione, B., and Franklin, E. C.: Bence Jones proteins and light chains of immunoglobulins. Preferential association of the VλVI subgroup of human light chains with amyloidosis AL(λ). J. Clin. Invest., *70*:453, 1982.

Steinmetz, M., and Hood, L.: Genes of the major histocompatibility complex in mouse and man. Science, *222*:727, 1983.

Taylor, H. G., Butler, W. M., Rhoads, J., et al.: Prolymphocytic leukemia: Treatment with combination chemotherapy to include doxorubicin. Cancer, *49*:1524, 1982.

The Non-Hodgkin's Lymphoma Pathologic Classification Project. National Cancer Institute sponsored study of classifications of non-Hodgkin's lymphomas. Cancer, *49*:2112, 1982.

Turner, M. W.: Immunoglobulins. *In* Holborow, E. J., and Reeves, W. G. (Eds.): Immunology in Medicine. New York, Grune and Stratton, 1983, p. 35.

Unanue, E. R.: Cooperation between mononuclear phagocytes and lymphocytes in immunity. New Engl. J. Med., *303*:977, 1980.

Vogler, L. B.: Bone marrow B cell development. Clin. Haematol., *11*:509, 1982.

Waldman, T. A., Broder, S., Goldman, C. K., et al.: Disorders of B cells and helper T cells in the pathogenesis of the immunoglobulin deficiency of patients with ataxia telangiectasia. J. Clin. Invest., *71*:282, 1983.

Weinstein, H. J., Vance, Z. B., Jaffe, N., et al.: Improved prognosis for patients with mediastinal lymphoblastic lymphoma. Blood, *53*:687, 1979.

Yunis, J. J., Oken, M. M., Kaplan, M. E., et al.: Distinctive chromosomal abnormalities in histologic subtypes of non-Hodgkin's lymphoma. New Engl. J. Med., *307*:1231, 1982.

Ziegler, J. L. Burkitt's lymphoma. New Engl. J. Med., *305*:735, 1981.

4

Hemostasis and Thrombosis

Thrombocytes

STRUCTURE

In 1906, Wright first proposed that the megakaryocyte, a well-known but mysterious bone marrow giant cell, produced blood platelets. Numerous subsequent morphologic and kinetic studies have supported this proposal and shown that this cell plays a key role in hemostasis. The average megakaryocyte measures about 5000 μ^3 in volume (see Fig. 1–10), but cells almost twice that size and with diameters of more than 100 μ are often seen. Like other differentiated precursor cells, the megakaryocyte descends from a committed progenitor cell (CFU-Meg) programmed to undergo blast transformation to a megakaryoblast. This blast cell is morphologically similar to other blast cells, but the nucleus is engaged in rapid DNA synthesis without cell cleavage, so-called endomitosis. Within a few days, the blast cell has grown considerably in size, and the single dense nucleus may contain 2, 4, 8, or even 16 times the normal diploid content of DNA. At any one of these stages, further DNA synthesis and nuclear endomitosis may cease, and cellular maturation commences. The nucleus becomes lobulated, and the cytoplasm increases in volume, with both processes occurring in rough proportionality to the ploidy of the cell. Specific cytoplasmic organelles appear, and the cytoplasm takes on a pale granular appearance. At this stage, the cytoplasm becomes burrowed out by invaginated surface membrane that transforms the cytoplasm into a honeycomb of granulated fragments. These are then peeled off in long ribbons into the bone marrow sinusoids, where they finally break up into individual platelets. After the lobulated megakaryocytic nucleus has become depleted of cytoplasm, it is rapidly disposed of by macrophages.

It has been generally accepted that young platelets, like young red cells, are larger than the more mature forms. However, careful sizing of platelets by Levin and Bessman suggests that platelets in thrombocytopenic patients are always larger than platelets in normals, regardless of the age of platelets. Nevertheless, at a given platelet count it appears that the young platelets seen in patients with peripheral platelet destruction are larger than those seen in patients with decreased platelet production.

The mature platelets are disk-shaped, measure about 2 to 3 μ in diameter, and on a Wright's stained smear are pale blue with a granular core. On electron microscopy (Fig. 4–1), the core is found to consist of fields of glycogen particles, mitochondria, vacuoles, and a variety of granules. The glycogen and mitochondria provide energy essential to viability and function. The vacuoles appear to be part of a spongelike canalicular system covered by interiorized phospholipid-containing surface membrane. This system facilitates the absorption of and interaction with various coagulation factors and also serves as a conduit for substances released from the granules. These granules can be divided into three classes: (1) the lysosomes containing hydrolytic enzymes; (2) the α-granules containing contact-promoting proteins such as fibrinogen, von Willebrand's factor, fibronectin, and throm-

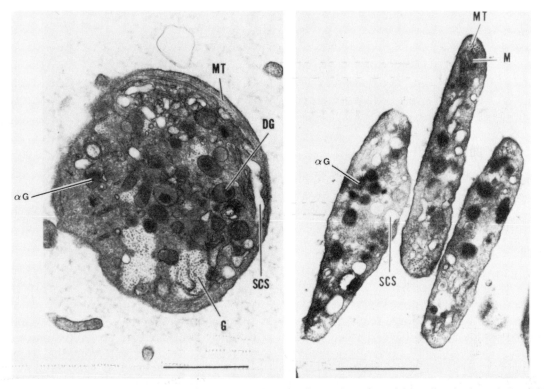

Figure 4–1 Electron microscopic picture of normal platelets showing a circumferential bundle of microtubules (MT), dense granules (DG), α granules (αG), glycogen (G), mitochondrias (M), and the cannicular surface connected system (SCS). (From Murphy, S., and Gardner, F. H.: Platelet physiology. *In* Nathan, D. G., and Oski, F. A. [Eds.]: Hematology of Infancy and Childhood. Philadelphia, W. B. Saunders Co., 1974, p. 626.)

bospondin as well as other proteins such as Factor V, platelet factor 4, and platelet-derived growth factor; and (3) the dense granules containing nonproteins such as serotonin, calcium, and adenine nucleotides, especially ADP. The cytoplasm contains large amounts of actin monomers in dynamic equilibrium with filamentous actin polymers. The monomers are added slowly to the leading end of the polymer and dissociated from its tail end. This "treadmilling" of monomers maintains a random distribution of short actin filaments throughout the cytoplasm. As is the case for most other cells, the actin polymers are attached to the membrane by various proteins such as ankyrins and spectrins and contribute to its discoid shape. However, a more definitive shape-controlling factor is the ring of microtubules situated under the equator of the platelet. The membrane, with its canalicular extensions, consists of the usual lipid bilayer with suspended lipoprotein and glycoprotein particles. Membrane components of special importance for subsequent platelet activation are phospholipase A_2, which can generate free arachidonic acid for prostaglandin synthesis, and the gly-

coprotein complexes Ib and IIb IIIa, which act as receptors for von Willebrand's factor and fibrinogen. Because these coagulation proteins are present in plasma, it is believed that the receptors are concealed in "resting" platelets and made accessible only after molecular reorientation in the activated platelet membrane.

FUNCTION

Platelets constitute our first and foremost line of defense against accidental blood loss. They accumulate almost instantaneously at the site of a vascular injury and attempt first to provide a temporary seal by plugging the vascular leak and then to promote the formation of a permanent seal by facilitating the local conversion of fibrinogen to fibrin. The rapid aggregation of nonsticky, circulating platelets into a firm platelet plug is a remarkable feat triggered by contact of the platelets with exposed subendothelial tissue. This in turn causes adhesion of platelets to the injured tissue, disk-to-sphere transformation of the attached platelets, release of their granular contents to the

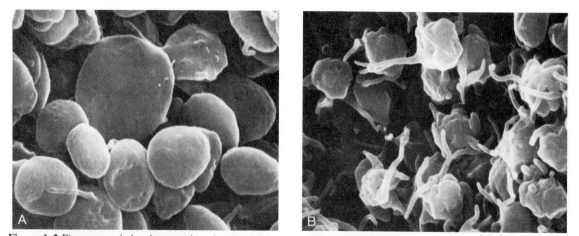

Figure 4–2 Pictures made by the scanning electron microscope of free disk-shaped platelets *(A)* and aggregates of spiny transformed platelets *(B)*.

immediate environment, aggregation of platelets to each other, and finally formation and consolidation of a thrombus (see reviews by Zucker, 1980 and by George et al., 1984).

Observations in vitro have clarified certain aspects of these events. They have demonstrated that some agents such as ADP, thrombin, and collagen will cause a change in the light transmission through a platelet-rich suspension by transforming smooth disk-shaped platelets into aggregates of spiny, sticky degranulated spheres (Fig. 4–2). The addition of ADP and thrombin will induce immediate aggregation of platelets in vitro, followed shortly afterwards by a second wave of aggregation that reflects release of endogenous ADP from the dense granules. Conversely, the effect of collagen is not immediate but is delayed until endogenous ADP has been released (Fig. 4–3). These observations, however, have been made in a completely artifactual in vitro milieu, and conclusions based on their biochemical and ultramicroscopic dissection have had to be modified by in vivo observations of thrombus formation in normal individuals and in patients with genetically abnormal platelets.

Currently, it is believed that endothelial damage exposes subendothelial tissue containing collagen and contact-promoting proteins such as fibronectin and von Willebrand's factor (Fig. 4–4). These elements will "activate" platelets and expose concealed glycoprotein Ib, which will bind to subendothelial von Willebrand's factor and cause adhesion of platelets to exposed tissue. This adhesion will in turn initiate cytoplasmic ionization of calcium and stimulate ATP production by glycogenolysis and oxidative phosphorylation. Calcium ions and ATP will increase the growth of actin fibrils, actin-binding proteins such as the calcium-dependent gelsolin will organize the fibrils into bundles, and the small amount of myosin present in the platelets will be phosphorylated and become attached to actin filaments. The production of both contractile actin bundles and actomyosin fibrils makes directed

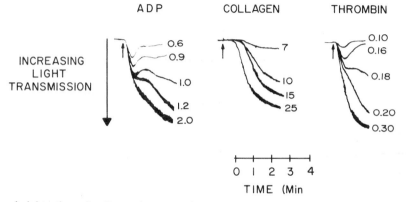

Figure 4–3 Aggregation of human platelets in citrated platelet-rich plasma at 37° C. ADP, collagen suspension, or thrombin was added (arrow) to give the fluid concentrations shown (μ moles/L., μ L./ml., or units/ml., respectively). Photometric recordings indicate the increase in light transmission as the platelets aggregate over a period of about 3 minutes. At low concentrations, ADP or thrombin administration is followed by disaggregation. At intermediate concentrations this disaggregation is prevented by release of endogenous ADP. The

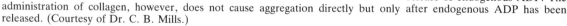

administration of collagen, however, does not cause aggregation directly but only after endogenous ADP has been released. (Courtesy of Dr. C. B. Mills.)

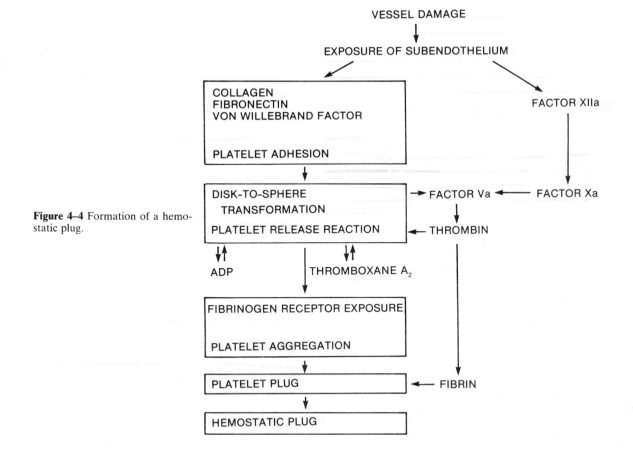

VESSEL DAMAGE

EXPOSURE OF SUBENDOTHELIUM

COLLAGEN
FIBRONECTIN
VON WILLEBRAND FACTOR

PLATELET ADHESION

FACTOR XIIa

DISK-TO-SPHERE
TRANSFORMATION
PLATELET RELEASE REACTION

FACTOR Va ← FACTOR Xa

THROMBIN

ADP   THROMBOXANE A_2

FIBRINOGEN RECEPTOR EXPOSURE

PLATELET AGGREGATION

PLATELET PLUG ← FIBRIN

HEMOSTATIC PLUG

Figure 4–4 Formation of a hemostatic plug.

shape changes possible and causes a centripetal movement of the microtubular ring until it has corralled all the granules in the center of the platelets and squeezed their contents into the canaliculi and out of the cell. Contact-promoting proteins and ADP in the squeezed-out material will promote further adhesion as well as shape change and granule release in adjoining platelets. Concomitantly, membrane receptors for fibrinogen (glycoprotein complex IIa–IIIb) will be unmasked, and the ever-present fibrinogen will cause aggregation of degranulated platelets and the formation of a platelet plug.

Although released ADP plays a major role in in vitro aggregation, it seems to be of less importance in vivo, where thromboxane A_2 and thrombin are primarily responsible for secondary aggregation. Thromboxane A_2 is a prostaglandin derived from arachidonic acid, an unsaturated 20-carbon fatty acid present in 20 percent of all membrane phospholipids. This fatty acid is released from phospholipid by phospholipase A_2, transformed to cyclic endoperoxides by a cyclo-oxygenase, and finally changed into the potent but short-lived aggregating agent, thromboxane A_2, by a

thromboxane synthetase (Fig. 4–5). It is believed that one effect of collagen or von Willebrand's factor is to unmask and activate membrane-bound phospholipase A_2. Thrombin, formed on the platelet membrane by released Factor V, will in minute amounts act as an additional aggregation agent.

The growth of the aggregate is eventually stopped by flowing blood, which will wash away aggregating factors, and by adjoining intact vessel walls, which produce a platelet-aggregation inhibitor, prostacyclin (PGI_2). The final platelet aggregate is consolidated into a plug by further contraction of shape-changed platelets, and their fused lipoprotein membranes will form a matrix on which secreted and circulating coagulation factors can interact to form fibrin and provide a firm seal.

In addition to sealing vascular breaks, platelets appear to play an almost continuous role in maintaining normal vascular integrity. Patients with thrombocytopenia have a decreased capillary resistance, and petechiae appear following the slightest trauma or change in blood pressure. It seems probable that these petechiae are caused by superficial endothelial desquamations that under normal conditions are

↑ capillary fragility

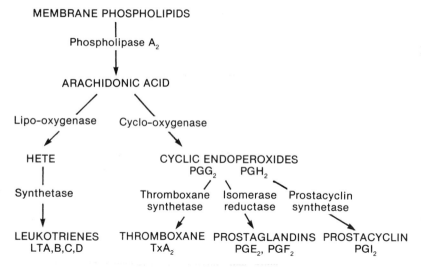

MEMBRANE PHOSPHOLIPIDS

|
Phospholipase A$_2$

↓

ARACHIDONIC ACID

Lipo-oxygenase   Cyclo-oxygenase

↓   ↓

HETE   CYCLIC ENDOPEROXIDES
                      PGG$_2$ PGH$_2$

Synthetase   Thromboxane Isomerase Prostacyclin
                 synthetase   reductase synthetase

↓

LEUKOTRIENES   THROMBOXANE PROSTAGLANDINS PROSTACYCLIN
LTA,B,C,D   TxA$_2$ PGE$_2$, PGF$_2$ PGI$_2$

Figure 4–5 Arachidonic acid metabolism in blood cells. Phospholipids in cellular membranes will, when exposed to phospholipase A$_2$, release arachidonic acid, which in turn will form cyclic endoperoxides or hydroxyeicosatetraenoic acid (HETE). In platelets, the endoperoxides will form thromboxane A$_2$ or prostaglandins; in endothelial cells and smooth muscle cells, the endoperoxides will form prostacyclin; and in granulocytes, the HETE will form leukotrienes.

sealed immediately by platelets but in patients with thrombocytopenia remain open and permit the escape of a small amount of blood. Platelets, through their release of prostaglandins, serotonin and lysosomal enzymes, may in part also be responsible for the inflammatory reaction that occurs around a newly formed thrombus (i.e., thrombophlebitis).

KINETICS

Until recently, kinetic studies of megakaryocytes and thrombocytes have appeared quite forbidding because of difficulties in quantitating the rate of production of platelets, the size of the circulating platelet mass, and the life span of individual platelets. However, careful planimetric measurements of megakaryocytes in bone marrow sections, the introduction of phase contrast microscopic measurements, automatic particle counting, and the use of random and cohort labeling with various isotopes have provided valuable and reproducible kinetic data. These data indicate that platelet production, like red cell production, is controlled by feedback systems that regulate the transformation of a committed but undifferentiated progenitor cell to a differentiated blast cell.

As previously emphasized, our current concept of the bone marrow stem cell pool is that it is made up of a multipotential compartment and several unipotential compartments, one of them committed to the megakaryocytic cell line (Fig. 1–7). The interrelationship between these compartments is not clear, but it appears that the multipotential stem cells are predom-

inantly dormant (G$_O$) and are called into supportive action only if the committed progenitor cell compartments become depleted. Because increased erythropoiesis after blood loss or hemolysis is often associated with increased thrombopoiesis and under certain conditions with decreased granulocytopoiesis, questions have been raised, but not answered, about specific cooperation or competition among the committed progenitor compartments. In response to demands for platelets, the progenitor cells committed to megakaryocytes undergo blast transformation and differentiate to megakaryoblasts. During the next 2 to 3 days and before visible cytoplasmic maturation, the nucleus divides two to four times, resulting in the formation of a large blast cell. After the endomitotic division has ceased, the nucleus becomes lobulated, the cytoplasm matures, granulated material segregates, and platelets are finally peeled off 2 to 3 days later. It has been estimated (Table 1–1) that the normal human marrow contains about 15×10^6 megakaryocytes per kg. body weight, with each megakaryocyte producing about 2000 to 7000 platelets. Since the average megakaryocytic volume is about 5000 μ^3, the total megakaryocytic mass is about 75×10^9 μ^3 per kg. body weight, about one fifth the total mass of nucleated red cell precursors ($5 \times 10^9 \times 90$ μ^3). However, the daily production of platelets, about 2.5×10^9 per kg. body weight, is close to that of erythrocytes, about 3.1×10^9 per kg. body weight.

After the release from the bone marrow, the platelets will circulate for about 8 to 10 days before they are removed and destroyed by the macrophages, primarily in liver and spleen. During their circulating life span, the platelets are distributed between the spleen and the bloodstream. Aster has pointed out that, at any one time, about one third of the circulating platelets are present in the spleen, probably in a slow transit through the tortuous splenic cords rather than as trapped and starved cells. A transit time of merely 8 minutes would explain such a segregation of the total platelet mass between spleen and blood. Certainly, the sequestration of platelets in the spleen does not appear to last long enough to produce cellular injury, and splenic contraction induced by epinephrine will expel perfectly normal platelets into the circulation. The physiologic significance, if any, of the splenic pooling of platelets is not known, but its existence does explain that the platelet count almost invariably is higher in splenectomized than in normal individuals. In patients with splenomegaly, a significant proportion of the circulating platelets is slowly meandering through the large spleen, and although total platelet mass may be normal, the platelet count can be quite low. This splenomegalic thrombocytopenia is rarely as severe as thrombocytopenia caused by hypersplenic destruction of platelets. However, hemostasis depends on the number of circulating platelets, and if a large spleen cannot mobilize its content of platelets in time, the effect is the same as if the platelets had been permanently destroyed.

Since platelets are consumed during their function as hemostatic agents, it could have been anticipated that their destruction would be random rather than age-dependent. In other words, survival curves should be exponential rather than linear with time. Somewhat surprisingly, however, most studies of platelet life span utilizing random labels such as ^{51}chromium or cohort labels such as ^{32}phosphorus have indicated an age-dependent linear life span (Fig. 4–6). Furthermore, studies by Abrahamsen of individuals receiving anticoagulants have failed to show a change in the slope of the survival curve or a prolongation of the platelet life span. This would tend to rule out the existence of major continuous intravascular coagulation with random platelet utilization. However, the spread of the survival curve is wide enough to conceal the presence of some minor random utilization in addition to the major age-dependent destruction.

Under physiologic conditions, the platelet count and especially the platelet mass are kept constant, indicating the existence of a feedback system adjusting platelet production to platelet destruction. This feedback has a built-in delay

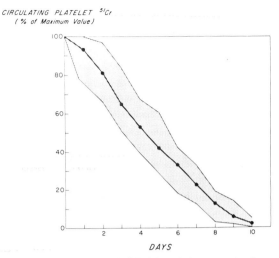

CIRCULATING PLATELET ^{51}Cr (% of Maximum Value)

Figure 4–6 Survival of ^{51}Cr-labeled human platelets. Shaded area from 30 normal subjects. (From Aster, R. H.: J. Clin. Invest., *45*:645, 1966.)

that causes a considerable rebound thrombocytosis after induced thrombocytopenia and rebound thrombocytopenia after induced thrombocytosis (Fig. 4–7). Delayed feedback may, under certain conditions, result in oscillating platelet counts (Fig. 3–9), causing seemingly capricious variations in platelet counts obtained intermittently in patients with hematologic disorders.

The feedback stimulus could act either on

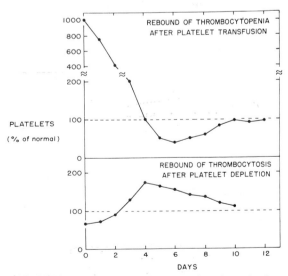

Figure 4–7 Rebound thrombocytopenia after platelet transfusion and rebound thrombocytosis after platelet depletion in normal rats. (Adapted from Odell, T. T., Jr., et al.: Acta Haematol., *38*:34, 1967, and Odell, T. T., Jr., et al.: Acta Haematol., *27*:171, 1962.)

the megakaryoblasts, causing them to undergo additional endomitotic divisions, thereby increasing their volume and producing more platelets, or on committed progenitor cells, causing the production of an increased number of megakaryoblasts. Because the megakaryocytes of patients with thrombocytopenia due to increased platelet destruction are both larger and more numerous than normal, Harker concluded that the stimulus does both. It has also been suggested that the stimulus shortens maturation time, a suggestion more difficult to accept because the introduction of additional endomitotic divisions should lengthen the total maturation time, unless of course the generation time is cut way down.

Numerous investigators have suggested that the responsible stimulus is transmitted by a specific humoral factor, a so-called thrombopoietin. Evatt and Levin were the first, however, to provide convincing but still indirect experimental data in support of this suggestion. Utilizing [75]selenium methionine to label megakaryocytic cytoplasm, they showed that injection into normal animals of serum from donors with thrombocytopenia will cause a greater isotope incorporation into new platelets than injections of serum from normal donors. The difference becomes more pronounced if endogenous thrombopoiesis of the recipient is suppressed by platelet transfusions (Fig. 4–8). Although the technique is similar to that which has been used successfully in the study of erythropoietin, the logistic problems of maintaining a preparatory thrombocytosis

are so large that it has yielded little additional information. In vitro studies of the effect of thrombopoietin on megakaryocyte progenitors (CFU-Meg) have been confusing. Thrombopoietin raised in animals rendered thrombocytopenic by means of a platelet antibody has been found to stimulate not only CFU-Meg but also CFU-GM and BFU-E. Thrombopoietin generated by nonimmunologic means, however, does not appear to stimulate any progenitor cells, and currently it is believed that the action of thrombopoietin is directed solely at the rate of nuclear endoduplication of megakaryocytes, which in turn controls their size and platelet output (see review by Levin, 1983). In order to expand the megakaryocyte population and support a sustained increased platelet production, the megakaryocyte progenitors need to be stimulated as well, but this stimulus is believed to be mediated by cell-to-cell interactions in the marrow. It may involve macrophages and lymphocytes and be similar to the stimulation envisioned for BFU-E after erythropoietin-induced depletion of CFU-E. Hoffman and coworkers have identified a factor in serum of patients with depleted numbers of marrow megakaryocytes, suggesting somewhat surprisingly a long-range effect of a supposedly short-range cell-to-cell signal.

If a thrombopoietin influences the production of platelets, what controls the production of thrombopoietin? Obviously, platelets are needed for the maintenance of vascular integrity, and it would seem likely that impaired hemostasis causes the release of a thrombopoietin in the same way that impaired oxygenation of the kidney causes the release of erythropoietin. However, as shown by the age-dependent life span of platelets, most platelets do not get involved in hemostatic activities. Furthermore, hemostatic function remains normal until the platelet count is reduced far below the level at which a compensatory increase in platelet production is initiated. Finally, the patients with congestive splenomegaly in whom up to 80 percent of the total platelet mass is in the spleen fail to show a compensatory increase in platelet production despite low circulating platelet count and impaired hemostatic function. These observations suggest that it is the platelet mass rather than the platelet count that triggers the release of thrombopoietin. However, it is very difficult to envision a sensor that can perceive the size of the platelet mass, distributed as it is between the spleen and the circulating blood. Furthermore, it seems possible that rather than being

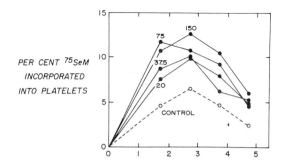

PER CENT [75]SeM INCORPORATED INTO PLATELETS

DAYS AFTER ADMINISTRATION OF [75]SeM

Figure 4–8 Effect of plasma from thrombocytopenic donor rabbits upon incorporation of selenomethionine-75 ([75]SeM) into the platelets of rabbits previously transfused with platelet concentrates. The plasma, in volume from 20 ml. to 150 ml., was administered in three divided doses, and [75]SeM was given 6 hours after the last infusion (solid lines). The broken line is the mean [75]SeM utilization in six platelet-transfused control rabbits. (From Shreiner, D. P., and Levin, J.: J. Clin. Invest., *49*:1709, 1970.)

BONE MARROW

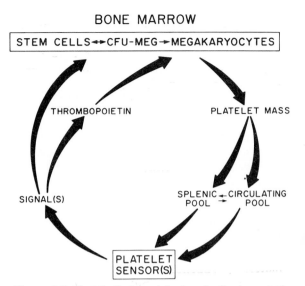

Figure 4-9 Hypothetical model of a feedback control system for platelets.

the number or mass, it is the surface area that is involved in sensing and adjusting the concentration of thrombopoietin. The platelet surface is well known to act as a sponge and absorb a variety of plasma factors. Actually, deGabriele and Penington have shown that thrombopoietic activity of plasma could be removed by preincubation with normal platelets. Consequently, platelet function, mass, and surface in addition to the mass and number of megakaryocytes must be incorporated into a still very hypothetical model of the feedback circuit controlling platelet production (Fig. 4-9).

PATHOPHYSIOLOGY

Classification and General Considerations

The thrombocytic disorders are usually classified according to number and function of platelets into "quantitative abnormalities," "qualitative abnormalities," and "myeloproliferative disorders" (Table 4-1).

In general, patients with platelets in inadequate numbers or with inadequate functional competence will have petechiae, hemorrhages, prolonged bleeding time, and impaired clot retraction. Because platelets are primarily responsible for hemostasis in small superficial vessels, petechiae are the hallmark of platelet deficiency disorders. Local pressure from tissue tension will tend to diminish blood loss

from deep vessels, and the presence of many petechiae and hemorrhages on the skin or visible mucous membrane does not necessarily mean that similar bleedings are present throughout the body. Actually, deep bleedings into tissues or joint spaces are much more characteristic of a deficiency in coagulation proteins than of a deficiency in platelets. The minimal number of platelets needed for normal hemostasis is usually considered to be about 50,000 per mm³. However, spontaneous hemorrhages are rare until the platelet count is reduced to less than 20,000 per mm³. Observations by Karpatkin and others indicate that the hemostatic competence of young platelets is greater than that of old platelets, explaining that hemorrhagic problems tend to be less at a given platelet level for individuals with thrombocytopenia due to peripheral destruction than for those with thrombocytopenia due to decreased production.

Elevated platelet counts are usually tolerated well but may cause either thrombosis or bleeding. The thrombotic tendency is probably related to an excessive hemostatic response to minor vascular injury, but the reason for the bleeding tendency in the face of an increased number of functional platelets is still unknown.

Quantitative Abnormalities

Thrombocytopenia. *Decreased platelet production* occurs in a bewildering array of congenital and acquired disorders. In some the pathogenesis has been unraveled, but in most the responsible dysfunction of the megakaryocytes awaits identification.

Table 4-1 CLASSIFICATION OF THROMBOCYTIC DISORDERS

I. *Quantitative Abnormalities*
  A. Thrombocytopenia
    1. Decreased production
      (a) Congenital
      (b) Acquired
        (1) Megakaryocytic disorders
        (2) Bone marrow replacement
    2. Increased destruction
      (a) Immune
      (b) Consumptive
    3. Uneven distribution
      (a) Hypersplenism
  B. Thrombocytosis
    1. Reactive
    2. Myeloproliferative disorders
II. *Qualitative Abnormalities*
  A. Congenital
  B. Acquired

Of special interest among the many descriptions of individual cases is a report by Shulman and coworkers about a child with severe congenital thrombocytopenia who was found to respond to infusions of normal plasma with brief increases in platelet count and who for many years has been kept alive and functioning on regularly spaced plasma infusions. The responsible plasma factor was named *thrombopoietin* and was believed to cause maturation of existing megakaryocytes. Re-evaluation of this case, however, has suggested a link to thrombotic thrombocytopenic purpura and to the responsiveness of this disease to plasma.

Acquired abnormalities of megakaryocytes causing moderately severe thrombocytopenia are usually found in patients with megaloblastic anemia due to folic acid or B_{12} deficiency, and specific treatment causes a prompt return of platelet count to normal. Patients with chronic alcoholism also may have maturation problems of both nucleated red cells and megakaryocytes, but the cause is difficult to pinpoint, since such patients usually suffer from a multitude of nutritional deficiencies and hepatic abnormalities. Nevertheless, metabolic studies by Post and Des Forges have demonstrated that one cause may be alcohol itself, which apparently impairs megakaryocytic function directly. Although iron deficiency has been associated with thrombocytopenia, thrombocytosis is observed far more commonly. If decreased platelet production is found in iron-deficient patients, complicating deficiency of folic acid or B_{12} should be excluded.

Viral infections and exposures to certain drugs are often associated with megakaryocytic dysfunction and thrombocytopenia. During pregnancy, such infections and exposures may lead to neonatal thrombocytopenia, usually of short duration. However, if the bone marrow insult occurs during the first trimester, a specific syndrome characterized by *amegakaryocytic thrombocytopenia,* malfunction of the heart, and absence of the radius may occur. Since the megakaryocytes, heart, and radius all appear at about the sixth to eighth week of gestation, an infectious or toxic insult at that time may explain the development of this seemingly unrelated triad. In both children and adults, viral infections frequently cause thrombocytopenia. For example, inoculation with live measles vaccine will, as Oski and Naiman have shown, regularly cause a temporary decrease in platelet production. As a general principle, a self-limited viral infection should always be suspected as the etiology in every patient with unexplained thrombocytopenia. Despite this frequent association, drugs are actually the most common cause of defective platelet production. The many myelosuppressive agents used in the treatment of neoplastic and autoimmune disorders make up the majority of drugs causing thrombocytopenia. The anticipated response to such drugs is a general bone marrow suppression, but certain drugs such as cytosine arabinoside and busulfan have a reputation for causing particularly marked suppression of platelet production. More capricious and still unexplained is the mild megakaryocytic suppression that may follow the use of thiazide diuretics. It has been suggested that they may bring about a process of immunologic "rejection" of megakaryocytes akin to the "rejection" of nucleated red cells observed in patients with pure red cell aplasia. However, drug-induced immunologic injury of megakaryocytes is a far less common cause of thrombocytopenias than drug-induced, immunologic destruction of circulating platelets.

2) *Increased platelet destruction* is mediated primarily by antibodies. Immunologic destruction of platelets can cause thrombocytopenia at any age. In the newborn, the pathogenetic mechanism is similar to that causing erythroblastosis fetalis in that an antibody produced in the mother crosses the placenta and causes destruction of the infant's platelets. During pregnancy and at the time of delivery, platelets from the fetus pass into the circulatory system of the mother, and if they contain antigens different from hers, they will evoke an antibody response. The subsequent transfer of the antibody across the placenta results in platelet destruction and thrombocytopenia in the infant. Maternal platelets are safe from antibody-induced destruction and may be used to arrest hemorrhages in the infant. Such isoimmune thrombocytopenia does not depend on ABO or Rh incompatibility but on incompatibility in the platelet specific antigen (Pl^{A1}) or the more general HL-A tissue antigen system. Because tests for antigens and antibodies in this system are time-consuming and difficult, the diagnosis is usually made by exclusion. First, thrombocytopenia due to infections must be ruled out immediately. Maternal viremia, such as cytomegalic inclusion disease and rubella, can cause changes in the fetal production and destruction of platelets, and bacteremia in the newborn may be associated with disseminated intravascular coagulation and thrombocytopenia. Other infectious etiologies to be

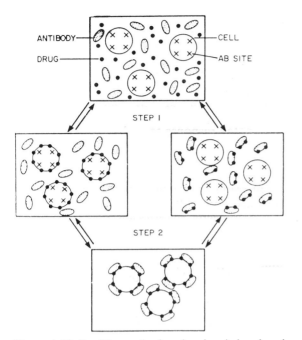

Figure 4–10 Possible mechanism for drug-induced and other immunologic thrombocytopenias. *Left,* the platelets are directly involved by initially being coated by antigen. *Right,* the platelets act as "innocent bystanders." (From Shulman, N. R.: Ann. Intern. Med., *60*:506, 1964.)

excluded are congenital syphilis and toxoplasmosis. Second, the possibility that the mother has idiopathic thrombocytopenic purpura with an antiplatelet autoantibody crossing the placenta and nonspecifically attacking the infant's platelets must be excluded by obtaining a thorough history and a platelet count on the mother. Finally, maternal drug ingestion must be looked into as a possible cause.

In children and adults, the cause for immunologic destruction of platelets is usually idiopathic, but the possibility that it is drug-related should always be considered. Quinidine is the most widely recognized offender, and its mechanism of action is slowly being unraveled. When attached to a protein the drug acts as a hapten, causing the production of antibodies in sensitized individuals. It was first assumed that the hapten attached itself to a platelet protein and that this hapten-platelet complex elicited and responded to antibody. However, subsequent data suggest that the hapten is bound to a plasma protein carrier and that it is this complex that elicits and combines with antibody. The eventual binding of the antigen-antibody complex to platelet membrane is due to a chance affinity between the immune complex and the membrane, and the platelet is

actually an "innocent bystander" in the immunologic reaction (Fig. 4–10). Unfortunately for the platelets, the coating with antigen-antibody complexes causes agglutination, complement fixation, and destruction. A great number of drugs have been implicated in immunologic platelet destruction, but only in a few instances have in vivo and in vitro testing convincingly shown a drug to be causative (Miescher, 1973). In addition to quinidine, quinine, stibophen, digitoxin, methyldopa, sulfonamides, sedormid, and gold have been so identified. The association of aspirin and birth control pills with thrombocytopenia has been of interest, but the possibility of a mere coincidence rather than a cause-effect relationship has not been ruled out. It has been recognized that heparin may be a major offender. Since heparin-induced thrombocytopenia rarely is associated with demonstrable antibodies and commonly with thromboembolic phenomena, it appears that heparin may cause thrombocytopenia both by being an antigen and by inducing platelet aggregation, leading to local or disseminated coagulation (King and Kelton, 1984). In order to establish a diagnosis of drug-induced thrombocytopenia several in vitro tests have been developed. These are based on detection of impaired platelet function after the addition of the drug to the patient's plasma. Inhibition of normal clot retraction is the easiest test (Fig. 4–11), but it is less sensitive than tests depending on agglutination, lysis, complement fixation, or direct demonstration of IgG on the platelet surface.

Idiopathic thrombocytopenic purpura (ITP) is a disorder characterized by increased platelet destruction in an otherwise healthy individual. In childhood, ITP is usually acute and time-limited, and many studies have related it immunologically to a preceding viral infection. In adults, ITP is usually chronic, and, although also believed to be immunologically determined, its etiology is still truly idiopathic.

Acute thrombocytopenia may follow well-established viral infections such as rubella, rubeola, and chickenpox, but in most cases the preceding illness consists merely of a mild respiratory or gastrointestinal upset, so frequently experienced in childhood that it is often overlooked. The thrombocytopenia is usually first noticed after the "viral symptoms" have subsided, suggesting that the platelet injury is caused by antibodies rather than by the virus itself. It has been proposed that platelet antibodies are elicited by platelet membranes that have been antigenetically altered by the

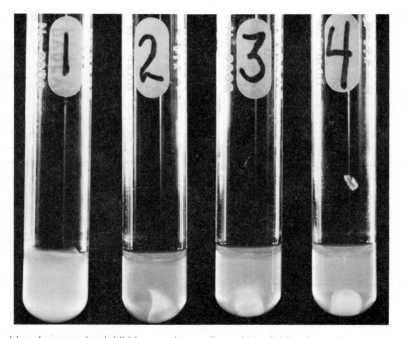

Figure 4–11 A positive clot retraction inhibition test in a patient with quinidine-induced purpura. The four test tubes were prepared as follows:

Serum	Quinidine	Normal Platelet-Rich Plasma
(1) Patient	+	+
(2) Patient	–	+
(3) Control	+	+
(4) Control	–	+

After 1 hour of incubation, $CaCl_2$ was added, and the degree of clot retraction inhibition was observed 1 hour later. Inhibition of clot retraction is seen in tube 1.

attachment of viral particles. However, as in drug-induced thrombocytopenia, the platelets may merely be "innocent bystanders" with a fatal affinity for viral antigen-antibody complexes. In either case, the antibody production and action would depend on the presence of a circulating viral antigen, and the disease would be of limited duration. Complete recovery can be expected if the patient is carried though the dangerous thrombocytopenic period by the judicious use of careful observation, protection against trauma, platelet transfusions, and corticosteroids. Splenectomy, although undoubtedly effective, need rarely be contemplated in the acute time-limited ITP of childhood.

The chronic variety of ITP is a disease of adults, although children who fail to recover from acute ITP must be included. Like acute ITP, it is believed to be immunologically induced and it is often found associated with immune illnesses such as disseminated lupus erythematosus and lymphoproliferative disorders.

The immunologic nature of this disorder was first suspected when Harrington and coworkers found that plasma or its gamma globulin fraction from patients with chronic ITP caused thrombocytopenia when infused into normal subjects. Supportive evidence for the existence of an autoimmune mechanism was provided by the fact that infants of mothers with chronic ITP often have transient thrombocytopenia at birth and that in vitro immunologic tests indicate the presence of an antiplatelet antibody in plasma from a large number of patients with chronic ITP. Recently IgG coating has been demonstrated directly with the use of a monoclonal IgG antibody (see review by Murphy, 1983). So far the antibody has reacted with all platelets, regardless of antigenic composition, and it appears that it is directed against a common platelet component rather than a type-specific antigen. In a few cases, this component has been identified as the membrane glycoprotein complex IIa-IIIb. The agent responsible for the production of autoantibodies is unknown, but the life-long presence of certain viral antigens in tissue cells makes a viral etiology an attractive hypothesis.

The severity of chronic ITP and its response to splenectomy seems to depend on the amount of antibody coating the platelets. Heavy coating will cause agglutination with easy recognition, sequestration, and destruction by all macrophages, and splenectomy by removing merely a fraction of these will be of only moderate therapeutic benefit. Light coating, however, will not cause significant agglutination of circulating platelets, and only the spleen with its slow percolation of blood through vessels densely lined with macrophages will recognize, sequester, and destroy coated platelets. In this condition, splenectomy will be of definite benefit, and the life span and function of lightly coated platelets will be almost normal after surgery. In a few cases, the titer of antiplatelet antibodies has decreased after splenectomy, suggesting that the spleen preferentially produces these antibodies and that splenectomy not only removes a filter but also eliminates a major site of antiplatelet antibody production (McMillan et al., 1974).

One of the most controversial findings in chronic ITP has been the presence of megakaryocytes of unusual morphologic appearance. Not only are they increased in number (Fig. 4–12), as would be expected as a compensation for increased destruction of mature platelets, but many are immature, are devoid of intracytoplasmic demarcations, and show no evidence of active platelet production. It has been suggested that the antibody to circulating platelets also reacts with megakaryocytes and prevents platelet formation. However, platelet turnover studies suggest an increased rate of platelet production, and it seems more likely that accelerated thrombopoietic activity causes an early release of platelets from still immature cells and a shift to the left in the megakaryocytic series. The presence of unusually large platelets in the blood of patients with chronic ITP also suggests a hurried production, with the release of unfinished pieces of megakaryocytic cytoplasm.

The clinical manifestations of chronic ITP are determined entirely by the number of available platelets, and the treatment is directed toward maintaining the number at an asymptomatic level. As expected, platelet transfusions are of very brief effect because transfused platelets are destroyed as fast as endogenous platelets. Adrenocorticosteroids are usually quite effective in increasing the platelet count in patients with chronic ITP. They may act by suppressing phagocytic activity, but the exact reason for their beneficial

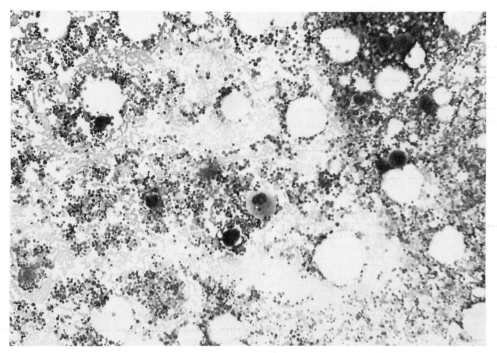

Figure 4–12 Megakaryocytic hyperplasia in patient with chronic ITP.

effect still has not been established (Handin and Stossel, 1978). In patients who do not respond to steroids with an increase in platelet count, the bleeding manifestations are nevertheless reduced, as if the steroids in some way enhance capillary stability. In the treatment of chronic ITP, steroids usually are administered for a few months in the hope that the disease will remit spontaneously. If the thrombocytopenia recurs immediately after discontinuation of the drug or if the patient is only partly responsive, splenectomy is the treatment of choice. Splenectomy will result in a sustained improvement in 70 to 90 percent of patients. In almost all, the operation will be followed by a brief thrombocytosis that reaches its peak at about the tenth day and then slowly decreases over the next few months (Fig. 4–13). This sequence corresponds well to the fact that in the absence of the spleen the platelets produced by the increased number of megakaryocytes live a normal 10-day life span, and it suggests that it must take some time to adjust the number of megakaryocytes in the bone marrow to the actual need for platelets in the circulation. Postsplenectomy thrombocytosis may be of concern in patients in whom postoperative complications force them to rest immobile in bed, and in such patients the use of preventive anticoagulants or platelet antiaggregating agents may be indicated. It is assumed that platelets of patients who do not derive lasting benefit from splenectomy are so heavily coated with antibody that they are removed by the total mononuclear phagocyte system, not merely by the spleen. In such patients, immunosuppression has been attempted, using drugs developed for the treatment of neoplastic disorders. In some patients, gratifying remissions have been obtained, especially after the use of vincristine and vinblastine. These two agents may be delivered directly to the phagocyting macrophages by use of normal platelets, "soaked" or "loaded" with vinca alkaloids, as vehicles (see comments by Rosse, 1984). The decision to use these potentially dangerous agents certainly must be made with great reluctance and only if other methods of treatment fail.

Post-transfusion purpura is an unusual syndrome consisting of a temporary period of thrombocytopenia with onset about a week after blood transfusion. The disorder occurs only in individuals lacking the platelet-specific antigen (Pl^{A1}), a circumstance found in only 1 to 2 percent of the population. The presence of this antigen in platelet material present in the transfused blood evokes the production of an antibody in the recipient. Immune complexes adhere to the patient's own platelets ("innocent bystanders"), bringing about their destruction as in quinidine purpura. Spontaneous remission occurs when the immune complexes are cleared from the circulation.

Nonimmunologic destruction of circulating platelets in bacterial or viral infections is often difficult to separate from immunologic destruction because these infections may be associated with both. However, nonimmunologic destruction usually occurs at the height of the infectious illness and is accompanied by decreased levels of several coagulation proteins such as fibrinogen and Factors V and VIII. The pathogenesis is believed to be increased platelet consumption due to *disseminated intravascular coagulation* (DIC) (Colman et al., 1979). Despite the presence of purpura and increased bleeding tendency, heparin may be the treatment of choice whenever laboratory studies indicate an increased rate of consumption of platelets and coagulation proteins. The thrombocytopenia characterizing *thrombotic thrombocytopenia purpura* and the *hemolytic uremic syndrome* is probably caused by excessive intravascular deposition of platelets in cerebral and renal vessels. However, there is little evidence of excessive consumption of coagulation proteins, and it appears that these diseases are caused by a vascular wall dysfunction, possibly due to immunologic damage to endothelial cells (Machin, 1984). The therapeutic use of exchange transfusions and of plasma infusions appears most promising in these otherwise highly fatal diseases (Bukowski et al., 1981). Surgery accompanied by major blood loss that is replaced by transfusions of stored, platelet-poor blood is often associated with a washout, dilutional thrombocytopenia. Platelet transfusions may be life-saving.

Thrombocytopenia is observed regularly in

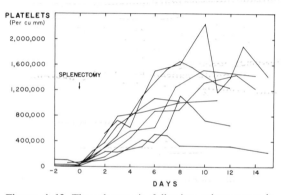

Figure 4–13 Thrombocytosis following splenectomy in patients with ITP.

patients with splenomegaly, and in the past many explanations were given for the development of this *hypersplenic thrombocytopenia.* The most obvious explanation for the thrombocytopenia would appear to be increased platelet destruction by the large spleen, but this explanation was made untenable some years ago when Cohen and coworkers found that the platelet life span in patients with hypersplenic thrombocytopenia was normal. The alternate explanation, that platelet production was decreased owing to the effect of megakaryocytic inhibitors released by the large spleen, was also found to be untenable because platelet turnover studies did not suggest a decreased rate of platelet production. Studies by Aster of platelet kinetics have provided a third and much more likely explanation.

As described earlier, the spleen, because of its tortuous vascular channels, always contains a considerable number of platelets in slow transit. In patients with splenomegaly, the transit time becomes longer, and instead of containing about 30 percent of all circulating platelets, a large spleen may contain up to 80 percent of the platelets. Since platelet production appears to be aimed at maintaining a constant total platelet mass, the uneven distribution of platelets between spleen and circulating blood is not being compensated for by an increased rate of platelet production, and the splenomegalic patient will stay thrombo-

cytopenic. This explanation is supported by the observation that the infusion of platelets to patients with hypersplenic thrombocytopenia results in lower peripheral recovery than normal (Fig. 4–14) and that one can mobilize large numbers of viable platelets from an intact spleen by giving epinephrine and from an excised spleen by flushing its vascular system with saline. Supporting evidence is also provided by the fact that hypersplenic thrombocytopenia is not always proportional to the size of the spleen but is more closely related to its vascularity. For example, congestive splenomegaly secondary to liver cirrhosis is usually associated with lower platelet counts than "meaty" splenomegaly secondary to lymphomas. The potential availability of splenic platelets and the distributional limits to the number of platelets that can be present in the spleen make this thrombocytopenia rather mild and rarely in need of treatment per se.

Thrombocytosis. Thrombocytosis occurs as an obscure reactive response to a number of illnesses and as a manifestation of the myeloproliferative syndrome. As a general rule, "reactive" platelets are small and uniform in size, while large even giant platelets are present in "neoplastic" thrombocytosin. A high platelet count is a useful diagnostic clue in patients with anemia, since iron deficiency regularly causes an increase in platelet production, and counts in excess of one million per mm.^{3} may be found in children with nutritional iron-deficiency anemia. Other conditions in which a high platelet count may be of diagnostic help are Hodgkin's disease, disseminated malignant diseases, and chronic inflammatory disorders (Schloesser et al., 1965; Tranum and Haut, 1974; and Marchasin et al., 1964). Pronounced thrombocytosis with levels of several million platelets per mm.^{3} is usually seen only after splenectomy or in myeloproliferative disorders, such as polycythemia vera, myelofibrosis, chronic myelogenous leukemia, and essential thrombocytosis. The clinical manifestations of very high platelet counts consist of a capricious combination of thrombotic episodes and increased bleeding tendency. The thromboses are probably caused by platelet aggregation and coagulation factor activation, but the bleeding tendency is more difficult to explain. Cardamone and coworkers have found a platelet dysfunction in patients with the myeloproliferative syndrome, whereas in most cases of reactive thrombocytosis the only abnormality found has been an increase in the number of circulating platelets.

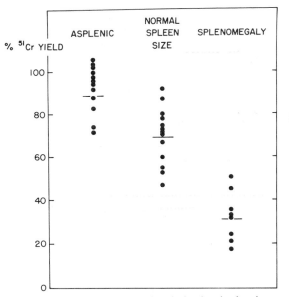

Figure 4–14 Recovery of transfused platelets in the circulating blood of asplenic patients, normal patients, and patients with congestive splenomegaly. (Gardner, F.: Clin. Haematol., *1*:307, 1972.)

Qualitative Abnormalities

Qualitative abnormalities of platelet function have been found in a number of rare hereditary disorders and more commonly in uremia and after ingestion of certain drugs such as aspirin, antihistamines, and anti-inflammatory agents (George et al., 1984). The inherited disorder most often found is *von Willebrand's disease*, described in the next chapter. *Glanzmann's thrombasthenia* is seen more rarely and is characterized by a prolonged bleeding time, impaired clot retraction, and absent ADP-induced aggregation. The number and morphology of platelets and megakaryocytes are normal, but the patients suffer from a mild life-long increased bleeding tendency. Studies of the glycoprotein composition of the platelet membrane have disclosed a decrease or absence of the fibrinogen receptor complex IIb–IIIa, possibly explaining impaired fibrinogen-mediated platelet aggregation. *Storage pool disease* is another congenital disorder of platelet structure. The platelets respond to exogenous ADP with a normal first-phase aggregation but fail to release endogenous ADP in response to collagen (second-phase aggregation). The number of ADP-containing dense particles is diminished, suggesting that the basic abnormality is a defect in the production, packaging, or storing of ADP. The clinical consequences are mild and consist primarily of increased bruising and excessive bleeding after trauma or surgery. Another rare disorder of platelet function is the so-called *Bernard-Soulier syndrome*, characterized by the presence of poorly functioning giant platelets. The membranes of these platelets lack glycoprotein Ib, the receptor for von Willebrand's factor. Consequently, they do not aggregate in vitro in response to von Willebrand's factor or ristocetin and they fail to adhere strongly in vivo to the subendothelium, a process primarily mediated by von Willebrand's factor.

Of the acquired disorders of platelet function, the clinically most important is the disorder found associated with chronic renal failure. Purpura and increased bleeding tendency are important manifestations of uremia and occur regularly despite normal platelet counts. Various changes in in vitro platelet function have been described, including decreased aggregation in response to ADP. Intensive dialysis rectifies this response and also normalizes the bleeding time, and it seems most likely that a retention product of small molecular size is responsible for the platelet defect.

Horowitz has proposed that this chemical is guanidinosuccinic acid, a metabolite of urea, but definite proof is still lacking.

The effect of aspirin on in vitro platelet function is quite remarkable. The ingestion of only one to two aspirin tablets will cause a week-long impairment in the release of platelet ADP in response to collagen or other aggregating agents such as epinephrine. Studies by Roth and Majerus suggest that this impaired ADP release is caused by irreversible aspirin-induced acetylation of platelet cyclo-oxygenase, necessary for the transformation of arachidonic acid to prostaglandin endoperoxides and in turn to the potent aggregating agent, thromboxane A_2 (see Fig. 4–5). Although aspirin clinically has been associated with an increased bleeding tendency, it must be conceded that bleeding problems, despite the striking in vitro changes, are rare among the millions who daily consume aspirin preparations.

References

Abrahamsen, A. F.: Platelet survival studies in man—with special reference to thrombosis and atherosclerosis. Scand. J. Haematol., Suppl. 3, 1968, p. 7.

Aster, R. H.: Pooling of platelets in the spleen: Role in the pathogenesis of "hypersplenic" thrombocytopenia. J. Clin. Invest., *45*:645, 1966.

Bukowski, R. M., et al.: Therapy of thrombotic-thrombocytopenic purpura. An overview. Semin. Thromb. Hemost., 7:1, 1981.

Cardamone, J. M., Edison, J. R., McArthur, J. R., and Jacob, H. S.: Abnormalities of platelet function in the myeloproliferative disorders. J.A.M.A., *221*:270, 1972.

Cohen, P., Gardner, F. H., and Barnett, G. O.: Reclassification of the thrombocytopenias by the ^{51}-Cr-labeling method for measuring platelet lifespan. N. Engl. J. Med., *264*:1294, 1961.

Colman, R. W., Robboy, S. J., and Minna, J. D.: Disseminated intravascular coagulation: A reappraisal. Ann. Rev. Med., *30*:359, 1979.

deGabriele, G., and Penington, D. G.: Regulation of platelet production. "Thrombopoietin." Br. J. Haematol., *13*:210, 1967.

Deykin, D.: Emerging concepts of platelet function. N. Engl. J. Med., *290*:144, 1974.

Evatt, B. L., and Levin, J.: Measurements of thrombopoiesis in rabbits using ^{75}selenomethionine. J. Clin. Invest., *48*:1615, 1969.

Fox, J. E. B., and Phillips, D. R.: Polymerization and organization of actin filaments within platelets. Semin. Hematol., *20*:243, 1983.

Gardner, F. H.: Platelet kinetics and lifespan. Clin. Haematol., *1*:307, 1972.

George, J. N., Nurden, A. T., and Phillips, D. R.: Molecular defects in interaction of platelets with the vessel wall. N. Engl. J. Med., *311*:1084, 1984.

Gerrard, J. M., et al.: Biochemical studies of two patients with the gray platelet syndrome. J. Clin. Invest., *66*:102, 1980.

Gewitz, A. M., et al.: In vitro studies of megakaryocytopoiesis in thrombocytotic disorders of man. Blood, *61*:384, 1983.

Handin, R. J., and Stossel, T. P.: Effect of corticosteroid therapy on the phagocytosis of antibody-coated platelets by human leukocytes. Blood, *51*:771, 1978.

Harker, L. A., and Finch, C. A.: Thrombokinetics in man. J. Clin. Invest., *48*:963, 1969.

Harrington, W. J., Minnich, V., Hollingsworth, J. W., and Moore, C. V.: Demonstration of a thrombocytopenic factor in the blood of patients with thrombocytopenic purpura. J. Lab. Clin. Med., *38*:1, 1951.

Hoffman, R., et al.: Assay of an activity in the serum of patients with disorders of thrombopoiesis that stimulates formation of megakaryocytic colonies. N. Engl. J. Med., *305*:533, 1981.

Horowitz, H. J.: Uremic toxins and platelet function. Arch. Intern. Med., *126*:823, 1970.

Karpatkin, S.: Heterogeneity of human platelets. II. J. Clin. Invest., *48*:1083, 1969.

King, D. J., and Kelton, J. G.: Heparin-associated thrombocytopenia. Ann. Intern. Med., *100*:535, 1984.

Legrand, Y. J., et al.: The molecular interaction between platelet and vascular wall. Blood Cells, *9*:263, 1983.

Levin, J.: Murine megakaryocytopoiesis in vitro: An analysis of culture systems used for the study of megakaryocyte colony-forming cells and the characteristics of megakaryocyte colonies. Blood, *61*:617, 1983.

Levin, J., and Bessman, J. D.: The inverse relation between platelet volume and platelet number. J. Lab. Clin. Med., *101*:295, 1983.

Machin, S. J.: Thrombotic thrombocytopenic purpura. Br. J. Haematol., *56*:191, 1984.

McMillan, R.: Chronic idiopathic thrombocytopenic purpura. N. Engl. J. Med., *304*:1135, 1981.

McMillan, R., Longmire, R. L., Yelenosky, R., et al.: Quantitation of platelet-binding IgG produced in vitro by spleens from patients with idiopathic thrombocytopenic purpura. N. Engl. J. Med., *291*:812, 1974.

Marchasin, S., Wallerstein, R. D., and Aggeler, P. M.: Variation of the platelet count in disease. Calif. Med., *101*:95, 1964.

Miescher, P. A.: Drug-induced thrombocytopenia. Semin. Hematol., *10*:311, 1973.

Moncada, S., Gryglewski, S., Bunting, S., and Vane, J. R.: An enzyme isolated from arteries transforms prostaglandin endoperoxides to an unstable substance that inhibits platelet aggregation. Nature, *263*:663, 1976.

Murphy, S.: In search of a platelet Coombs' test. N. Engl. J. Med., *309*:490, 1983.

Odell, T. T., Jr., Jackson, C. W., and Reiter, R. S.: Depression of the megakaryocyte platelet system in rats by transfusion of platelets. Acta Haematol., *38*:34, 1967.

Odell, T. T., Jr., McDonald, T. P., and Asano, M.: Response of rat megakaryocytes to bleeding. Acta Haematol., *27*:171, 1962.

Oski, F. A., and Naiman, J. L.: Effect of live measles vaccine on the platelet count. N. Engl. J. Med., *275*:352, 1966.

Peerschke, E. J., et al.: Correlation between fibrinogen binding to human platelets and platelet aggregability. Blood, *55*:841, 1980.

Post, R. M., and Des Forges, J. F.: Thrombocytopenia and alcoholism. Ann. Intern. Med., *68*:1230, 1968.

Rosse, W. F.: Whatever happened to vinca-loaded platelets? N. Engl. J. Med., *310*:1051, 1984.

Roth, G., and Majerus, P.: The mechanism of the effect of aspirin on human platelets. I. Acetylation of a particulate fraction protein. J. Clin. Invest., *56*:624, 1975.

Schloesser, L. L., Kipp, M. A., and Wenzel, F. J.: Thrombocytosis in iron-deficiency anemia. J. Lab. Clin. Med., *66*:107, 1965.

Shreiner, D. P., and Levin, J.: Detection of thrombopoietic activity in plasma by stimulation of suppressed thrombopoiesis. J. Clin. Invest., *49*:1709, 1970.

Shulman, L., Pierce, M., Lukens, A., and Currimbhoy, Z.: Studies on thrombopoiesis. I. A factor in normal human plasma required for platelet production; chronic thrombocytopenia due to its deficiency. Blood, *16*:943, 1960.

Shulman, N. R.: A mechanism of cell destruction in individuals sensitized to foreign antigens and its implications in autoimmunity. Ann. Intern. Med., *60*:506, 1964.

Smith, J. B., and Silver, M. J.: Prostaglandin synthesis by platelets and its biologic significance. *In* Gordon, J. L. (Ed.): Platelets in Biology and Pathology. Amsterdam, Elsevier, 1976, p. 331.

Smith, J. B., and Willis, A. L.: Aspirin selectivity inhibits prostaglandin production in human platelets. Nature, *231*:235, 1971.

Tranum, B. L., and Haut, A.: Thrombocytosis: platelet kinetics in neoplasia. J. Lab. Clin. Med., *84*:615, 1974.

Wright, J. H.: The histogenesis of the blood platelets. J. Morphol., *21*:263, 1910.

Zucker, M. B.: The functioning of blood platelets. Sci. Am., *242*:86, 1980.

Plasma Coagulation Factors

NORMAL STRUCTURE AND FUNCTION

The vascular system is self-healing because of the dynamic interaction of platelets and plasma coagulation factors with injured vessel walls. Within seconds of injury platelets will adhere to the site of endothelial damage, aggegate, and release vasoactive factors, leading to the formation of a "plug," or "white thrombus," and to local vasoconstriction. Thrombin is generated, causing fibrinogen activation and further platelet aggregation. These activities continue until platelets and red cells become entangled by fibrin polymers into a stable "red thrombus." Thrombin and fibrin activate clot-dissolution mechanisms, limiting and localizing the clot to the site of endothelial damage and reestablishing vascular patency. In wounds, fibrin clots establish the groundwork for fibrous organization and scar formation.

Breakdown in the hemostatic mechanism may provoke bleeding episodes ranging in severity from minor pinpoint petechiae to major life-threatening hemorrhages. Pathologic formation of clots within the circulatory system is an equal or even more serious problem, as evidenced by the high morbidity and mortality associated with stroke, myocardial infarction, and pulmonary embolism.

Although platelets, plasma coagulation factors, and vascular factors are discussed in separate sections, they in fact cooperate in closely integrated reactions. This section will concentrate on plasma coagulation factors, with emphasis placed on their interaction with platelets and the vascular wall. Most of these factors circulate as inactive precursor zymogens until they undergo sequential activation by cleavage at the site of vascular injury. Some are activated by conformational change. The activated clotting factors, designated by the letter "a," are usually serine proteases (i.e., they have serine at their active centers). Exceptions are Factors V, VIII, XIII and fibrinogen. The serine proteases have a high degree of substrate specificity, with reactions occurring on phospholipid surfaces such as the platelet and vascular lining cells. Some of the factors, notably V and VIII, are cofactors designed to bring reactants together to accelerate reaction rates. The entire sequence of activation of one factor leading to activation of the next has been compared to a waterfall, or cascade. Such a system has the advantages of rapid amplification as well as multiple points at which the reactions may be controlled.

The nomenclature of the plasma coagulation factors and some of their properties are given in Table 4–2. Factors V and VII through XIII are designated by their numbers. Factors I and II are most often called *fibrinogen* and *prothrombin*, respectively. Factor III is tissue factor and Factor IV is calcium. There is no Factor VI.

The discussion to follow will begin at the end of the clotting process, the conversion of fibrinogen to fibrin polymer and its subsequent dissolution by plasmin. The earlier reaction steps will then be considered. The structure of several of the clotting factors and their activation products will be illustrated as examples. Finally, the control mechanisms for limiting coagulation reactions will be discussed.

Fibrinogen

Fibrinogen, the raw material for the production of the clot, is a major constituent of the plasma, with a normal concentration of 150 to 400 mg. per 100 ml. The other plasma coagulation factors are present in much lower concentration. Most of the body pool of fibrinogen circulates in the plasma with a catabolic half-life of 4 days. The plasma concentration readily increases secondary to a large number of stimuli, including pregnancy, acute or chronic inflammatory states, and injury or surgical operation. The increase is entirely accounted for by increased synthesis, which takes place in the liver.

Fibrinogen spends an uneasy existence in

212

Table 4-2 PLASMA COAGULATION FACTORS

Factor	Synonyms	Half-Life*	Molecular Weight (Daltons)*	Normal Plasma Concentration (µg./ml.)†
I	Fibrinogen	3.7 days	340,000	1500–4000
II	Prothrombin	2.8 days	72,500	150
III	Tissue factor	—	—	—
IV	Calcium	—	—	—
V	Proaccelerin	15–24 hours	330,000	10
VII	Proconvertin, SPCA	1.2–6 hours	48,000	< 1
VIII:C	Antihemophilic factor	5–12 hours	>1,000,000	< .05
VIII:R	von Willebrand factor	24–40 hours		16
IX	Christmas factor, plasma thromboplastin component (PTC)	20–24 hours	57,000	5
X	Stuart-Prower factor	32–48 hours	59,000	8
XI	Plasma thromboplastin antecedent (PTA)	40–84 hours	160,000	5
XII	Hageman factor	48–52 hours	76,000	35
XIII	Fibrin stabilizing factor	5–12 days	320,000	20
Plasminogen		2.2 days	90,000	150
Prekallikrein	Fletcher factor	—	85,000	30
HMW Kininogen‡	Fitzgerald, Flaujeac, Williams factors	—	150,000	80

*Data from Martinez, J., and Palascak, J. E. *In* Zakim, D., and Boyer, T. D. (Eds.): Hepatology. A Textbook of Liver Disease. Philadelphia, W. B. Saunders Co., 1982, p. 557.

†Data from McKee, P. *In* Stanbury, J. B., et al. (Eds.): The Metabolic Basis of Inherited Disease. New York, McGraw-Hill Book Co., 1983, p. 1534.

‡HMW = high molecular weight.

the plasma, circulating between the forces of clot promotion, represented by thrombin, and those of clot dissolution, represented by plasmin. Its molecular weight of 340,000 daltons is equally divided between two identical subunits centrally bound together to give the molecule a symmetric mirror-image structure (Fig. 4–15). Each of the subunits consists of an Aα, a Bβ, and a γ polypeptide chain, the N-terminal ends of which are centrally bound together into a "disulfide knot." Three nodular domains can be identified, two identical D regions at either carboxyterminal end and a central E domain containing the N-terminal disulfide knot along with fibrinopeptides A and B. The E and D domains are connected by a coiled stretch of intertwined α, β, and γ chains, in the middle of which is a relatively unstructured region susceptible to enzymatic attack.

The carboxyterminal regions of the α chains are polar and free-floating.

Thrombin acts enzymatically on fibrinogen at arginine-glycine bonds by splitting off fibrinopeptides A and B from the N-terminal ends of the Aα and Bβ chains. These constitute approximately 3 per cent of the molecule, but their removal leads to a dramatic change in the functional state of the remaining fibrin monomer. The amino terminal peptides in the E domain exposed by thrombin cleavage react noncovalently with D regions of adjacent molecules to set in motion a process of polymerization with fibrin monomer molecules staggered bricklike in side-to-side association (Fig. 4–16). The electrostatic and hydrophobic bonds are easily disrupted by denaturing agents such as urea.

The polymer is then stabilized by the estab-

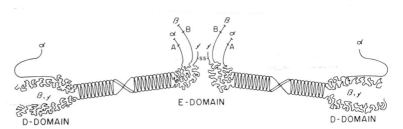

Figure 4–15 Diagram of fibrinogen structure. The molecule consists of three pairs of polypeptide chains, designated Aα, Bβ, and γ, joined into a mirror-image arrangement by disulfide bonds. Fibrinopeptides A and B are attached at the N-terminal regions of the α and β chains in the central region called the E domain. Nodular regions at the opposing carboxyl termini are on the D domains. The E and D domains are separated by a site where the molecule is susceptible to plasmin cleavage. (Adapted from Doolittle, R. F.: Sci. Am., *245(12)*:132, 1981.)

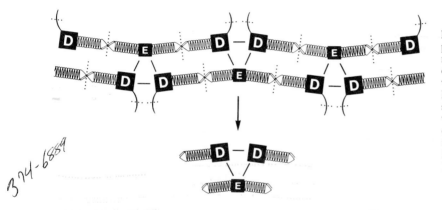

Figure 4–16 Demonstration of fibrin polymer formation showing the intermolecular arrangements of D and E domains of adjacent molecules. Covalent cross links are shown by straight heavy lines, and plasmin cleavage sites are indicated by dotted lines. A variety of fragments may be produced. In this example, a D2E fragment is illustrated. (Adapted from Doolittle, R. F.: Sci. Am., *245(12)*: 135, 1981.)

374-684

lishment of covalent linkages between lysine and glutamine residues of adjacent molecules in a transamidination reaction catalyzed by Factor XIIIa. End-to-end linkages are the first to form between the γ chains in adjacent D regions, followed by side-to-side connections between adjacent α chains, strengthening lateral growth (Fig. 4–16). The cross-linked fibrin clot is insoluble in 5M urea and is more resistant to plasmin degradation than the non–cross-linked clot. Factor XIII is activated by thrombin with the release of a small activation peptide followed by calcium-dependent subunit dissociation.

Certain snake venoms resemble thrombin in their action on fibrinogen (Russell, 1980). Reptilase hydrolyzes only the Aα polypeptide chains, releasing fibrinopeptide A. The parent molecule, like fibrin monomer, polymerizes into a clot. However, the clot is weak and is readily dissolved through the action of plasmin.

In contrast to the limited action of thrombin, plasmin attacks fibrinogen and fibrin more aggressively at a variety of arginine-lysine bonds. In this respect, plasmin resembles trypsin. Like trypsin, it attacks other proteins. The circulating plasma proteins are not physiologically exposed to its broadly destructive propensity because plasmin circulates as an inactive precursor, plasminogen, which is activated locally at the site of clot deposition. Plasmin attacks fibrinogen and fibrin with equal fervor. The degradation products of the two are referred to as *fibrinogen-fibrin degradation products,* or *split products.*

During the initial degradation of fibrinogen by plasmin, its molecular weight is reduced from 340,000 to about 250,000 daltons, with the release of low molecular weight fragments from the polar free-floating carboxyterminal appendages of the Aα chains. The macromo-

lecular structure that remains, called *fragment X,* retains the property of engaging in clot formation after exposure to thrombin. However, compared with fibrin monomer, fragment X clots slowly, and its presence weakens the clot structure. Fragment X undergoes additional asymmetric cleavage by plasmin, with further reduction of molecular weight to derivatives designated *fragment Y* (150,000 daltons) and *fragment D* (100,000 daltons). Both these fragments are nonclottable, but they interfere with fibrin strand formation and are potent anticoagulants. As degradation goes on to

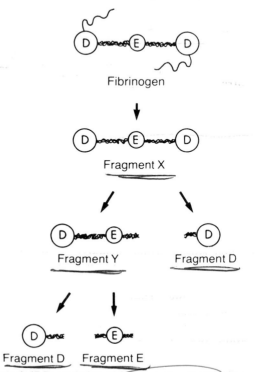

Figure 4–17 Degradation of fibrinogen by plasmin. (From Marder, V. J., Francis, C. W., and Doolittle, R. F. *In* Colman, R. W., et al. [Eds.]: Hemostasis and Thrombosis. Philadelphia, J. B. Lippincott Co., 1982, p. 149.)

completion fragment Y is further reduced to fragments D and E. The 50,000-dalton E fragment contains the N-terminal disulfide knot and is relatively less active as an anticoagulant (Fig. 4–17).

Plasmin attacks fibrin polymer at the same sites as it does fibrinogen, but the degradation products differ because of the presence of plasmin-resistant cross-links in the polymer (Fig. 4–16). The smallest complex released from fibrin polymer is D₂E, but larger complexes are also formed because of incomplete degradation.

One can best detect excessive action of plasmin in vivo by identifying elevated levels of fibrinogen-fibrin degradation products in serum from which all clottable material has been completely removed in the presence of a fibrinolytic inhibitor. Although excess plasmin activity most commonly occurs secondary to abnormal clotting, a high level of "split products" does not distinguish primary from secondary fibrinolysis. The presence of soluble complexes of fibrin monomer polymerized with fibrinogen-fibrin degradation products into higher molecular weight derivatives is demonstrated in plasma by tests for "paracoagulation." These include precipitation after addition of protamine sulfate, reversible insolubility in the cold (hence the term *cryofibrinogen*), and gelation after addition of ethanol. Excessive action of thrombin on fibrinogen in vivo might also be detected by assay of the plasma for fibrinopeptide A concentration.

Plasminogen Activation

Plasminogen is present in plasma at a concentration of 10 to 20 mg. per 100 ml. The structure of the zymogen is shown in Figure 4–18. The molecule is activated by cleavage at arginine 560–valine 561, changing the single-chain structure into a two-chain entity. There are five spirals called *kringles* on the heavy chain. These are lysine-binding sites that account for the binding affinity of the molecule for fibrin clots. They are also the sites of binding of ε-aminocaproic acid, a potent inhibitor of plasminogen activation. The light chain contains the active serine protease site responsible for plasmin activity.

There are several mechanisms for activating plasminogen. The most important of these is the release of tissue activator from endothelial cells at the site of clot formation (Fig. 4–19).

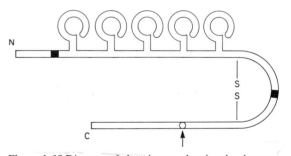

Figure 4–18 Diagram of plasminogen showing the cleavage sites (shaded areas) exposed by plasminogen activators. The N-terminal region of the molecule is susceptible to plasmin degradation, from which several derivatives arise. The heavy chain of plasmin contains the lysine binding sites as shown by the five "kringles," and the light chain has the active serine protease, as shown by the arrow. The two chains are held together by disulfide bonds. (Adapted from Francis, C. W., and Marder, V. J. *In* Williams, W. J., et al. [Eds.]: Hematology. New York, McGraw-Hill Book Co., 1983, p. 1267.)

Like plasminogen, tissue activator has an affinity for the fibrin clot. It is a fortunate occurrence that these two substances share such a similar attraction, keeping clot dissolution a local and not a systemic process. Because the ratio of endothelium to cross-sectional area is greater in the microcirculation than in large vessels, it is in this vascular site that plasminogen activation and fibrinolysis are the most active. Other safeguards help prevent plasmin from gaining access to the general circulation. These include the plasmin inhibitors, α-₂-antiplasmin and α-₂-macroglobulin, to be discussed later. Once activated, plasmin is very rapidly cleared from circulation.

Other plasminogen activators are of less

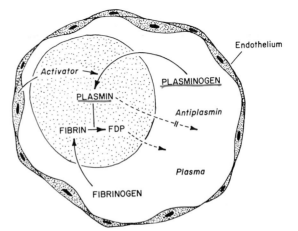

Figure 4–19 The local activation of plasminogen at the site of fibrin clot within a small blood vessel. (FDP = fibrin degradation products.)

physiologic importance. Lysosomes from white cells and other tissues contain large quantities of a tissue activator, but this is in a form not easily released. Surface activation of plasma coagulation factors causes plasmin to form. Plasmin in turn activates Factor XII, further amplifying the process. However, deficiencies of the surface-active factors do not lead to clinically apparent deficiencies of fibrinolysis. Urokinase is a plasminogen activator found in the urinary tract. It has the function of keeping this system free of clots and the potential harm they might cause as a result of obstruction. Streptokinase is a bacterial product that activates plasminogen by binding with it in a 1:1 molar ratio, forming a complex in which the active serine site apparently becomes exposed.

Streptokinase and, to a lesser extent, urokinase are used therapeutically for dissolving clots (Duckert, 1984). They can be given systemically with intent to establish a generalized state of fibrinolysis, or they can be perfused locally at the site of an obstructing pathologic clot (Laffel and Braunwald, 1984). These agents do not exhibit a particular affinity for localizing at the site of clot formation. Cultured cells have been used as a source of tissue activator, which can be given therapeutically with the advantage of clot localization without the need for establishing systemic fibrinolysis. Streptokinase-plasminogen complex also has an affinity for clot localization. It has been tested therapeutically with the same intent.

A variety of influences other than fibrin deposition also bring about the release of plasminogen activators from the endothelium. These include exercise, acute stress of almost any kind, and pharmacologic and other kinds of vasoreactive stimuli. The increase in plasma fibrinolytic activity, however, is transient and mild, since the plasminogen activators are rapidly cleared from the plasma by the liver with a half-life of only 13 minutes. The impairment of this clearing mechanism will lead to somewhat less transient and less mild degrees of systemic fibrinolysis, a situation that arises in shock or in the presence of liver disease.

Contact Activation

Endothelial disruption not only triggers the formation of a platelet plug but also initiates the contact activation of a group of plasma factors, beginning with Factor XII (Saito, 1980). The other participating principals are prekallikrein, Factor XI, and plasminogen. High molecular weight kininogen is an important cofactor in this series of reactions that link fibrin clot formation with its ultimate lysis and with the inflammatory response and complement activation (Colman, 1984) (Fig. 4–20).

Factor XII undergoes conformational change to expose its active serine center upon contact with a negatively charged surface. In the body, this surface is most often the subendothelium. In the laboratory, it is the surface of the test tube along with certain additives, such as kaolin, celite, and ellagic acid. Factor XIIa in turn activates prekallikrein and Factor XI, both of them requiring high molecular weight kininogen as cofactor with which they are in equimolar complex. This complex serves to attract them to the vascular surface site of bound Factor XIIa. Molecular cleavage converts the reactants to kallikrein and to Factor

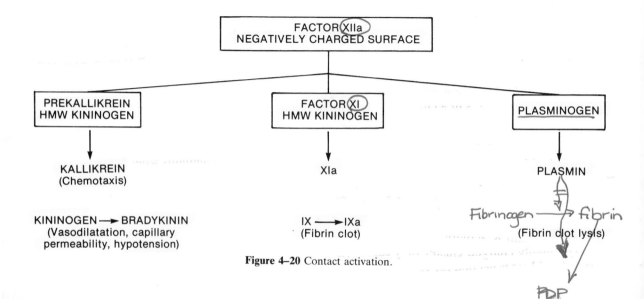

Figure 4–20 Contact activation.

XIa. Kallikrein converts kininogen to brady-kinin with vasoreactive and chemotactic consequences. Factor XIa activates Factor IX in the presence of calcium, and successive reactions occur so on through the remainder of the intrinsic and common pathways of coagulation. During the process of these reactions, plasminogen activation to plasmin occurs, but this is not as biologically important as the tissue activator pathway of plasminogen activation. The products of all three Factor XIIa-initiated reactions are autocatalytic. In a positive feedback relationship they activate Factor XII.

It is a curious fact, still not well understood, that although the contact system stands astride such a variety of biologically important reactions, deficiencies of Factor XII, of prekallikrein, and of high molecular weight kininogen do not give rise to clinically significant consequences, including bleeding, despite the fact that increased whole-blood clotting times and partial thromboplastin times are found in laboratory testing. Factor XI lack may be accompanied by a mild bleeding tendency.

Vitamin K–Dependent Factors

The biologic activities of Factors II, VII, IX, and X depend on an adequate supply of vitamin K, which comes mostly from the diet, with a smaller proportion from bacterial synthesis in the gastrointestinal tract. These four factors share similar amino acids in certain areas of their structure, and this homology has suggested a common genetic locus of origin early on in evolution, even though Factor IX is X-linked whereas the other three factors are autosomal. Vitamin K is not involved in the assembly of the amino acid backbones of these factors, but rather plays a key role in their postsynthetic transformation in the hepatocytes. This modification converts the factors from inert proteins to the biologically active forms present in normal plasma. The modification is a carboxylation of about 10 to 14 glutamic acid residues in a cluster located near the amino terminal end of the protein. The carboxylation occurs at the γ position, yielding γ-carboxyglutamyl derivatives. The reaction is coupled with the oxidation of reduced vitamin K to vitamin K epoxide (Fig. 4–21). After degradation of the protein, the γ-carboxyglutamyl derivatives are excreted in the urine. Their measurement can be used as an index of in vivo vitamin K activity.

The highly charged cluster of γ-carboxyglutamyl residues is needed for calcium- and phos-

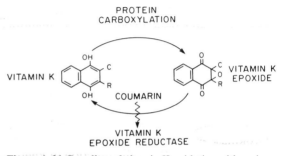

Figure 4–21 Coupling of vitamin K oxidation with carboxylation of protein γ-glutamyl residues. Coumarin anticoagulants interfere with the vitamin K cycle by preventing reduction of vitamin K epoxide. (Adapted from Walsh, P. N.: Hosp. Pract., *18(1)*:104, 1983.)

pholipid-binding. In the absence of this modification, the vitamin K–dependent factors are deficient when measured by functional tests of coagulation. However, they are present in adequate plasma concentrations if assayed by immunochemical methods that do not depend on the γ-carboxyglutamyl modification.

In addition to the procoagulant plasma proteins already mentioned, other body proteins are carboxylated in an analogous vitamin K–dependent fashion. These include the plasma anticoagulants, protein C, and protein S, to be discussed later, and osteocalcin, a protein of some importance in bone formation.

Certain adsorbents, such as barium sulfate, selectively remove the vitamin K–dependent factors from plasma. This process, like calcium-binding, is dependent on carboxylation. Adsorption is useful in preparing test plasma deficient in the vitamin K–dependent factors for use in laboratory diagnosis. Elution from the adsorbent yields factor concentrates therapeutically useful in the management of patients with hemophilia B as well as in certain other hemorrhagic circumstances.

The coumarin anticoagulants interfere with the action of vitamin K by inhibiting its reduction from the epoxide form (Fig. 4–21). They are of proven therapeutic value in the prevention of thromboembolic disorders (Gurevich, 1976). Correction of their anticoagulant effect follows within 6 hours of the administration of vitamin K and is complete soon after. In contrast to heparin, coumarin compounds are inactive as anticoagulants when added to plasma in vitro.

Factor VIII

The structure of Factor VIII has remained elusive for a long time, but the mystery has begun to unravel, giving rise to a picture of a most unorthodox molecule—or complex of molecules. Its instability and minute plasma concentration have been among the hindrances to its investigation.

The complex has an overall molecular weight in excess of one million daltons. It consists of subunits, each weighing about 200,000 daltons, arranged into a multimer. Two structurally distinct biologic activities are associated with the Factor VIII molecule. The first of these, designated VIII:C, contains the procoagulant activity deficient in the plasma of patients with hemophilia A. The second, designated VIII:R, for Factor VIII–related activity (or VIII:vWF for von Willebrand factor), contains the activity deficient in patients with von Willebrand's disease. Factor VIII:C and VIII:R are noncovalently bound and are separable under certain circumstances (Fig. 4–22).

Factor VIII:C is a sex-linked gene product that acts as a cofactor in the activation of Factor X by Factor IXa, accelerating the reaction rate by 500- to 1000-fold. It is activated by thrombin and inactivated by protein C. It is a relatively small piece of the Factor VIII molecule.

Factor VIII:R is an autosomal gene product that constitutes the bulk of the multimeric molecule. It supports the adhesion of platelets to vessel walls. This important platelet-related effect depends both on the carbohydrate portion of the molecule and on the multimeric configuration. When multimer formation is im-

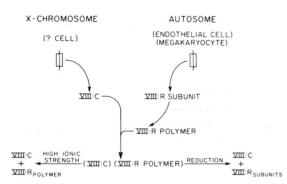

Figure 4–22 A summary of the properties of the Factor VIII complex. The small Factor VIII coagulant protein (VIII:C) interacts with the polymer form of the Factor VIII–related protein (VIII:R) in a noncovalent complex. Von Willebrand factor activity is a property of polymeric VIII:R. This activity is lost when VIII:R is dissociated into subunits by reduction. When dissociated by exposure to high ionic strength, the two components separate but retain their activities. The genetic control and sites of synthesis are indicated. (Adapted from Hoyer, L. W. *In* Colman, R. W., et al. [Eds.]: Hemostasis and Thrombosis. Philadelphia, J.B. Lippincott Co., 1982, p. 4.)

paired, activity is lost. Platelet aggregation induced by ristocetin in vitro depends on the interaction of VIII:R with its platelet receptor, glycoprotein-1. Measurement of ristocetin-induced platelet aggregation in vitro *(ristocetin cofactor activity)* is used as an index of VIII:R activity in plasma, since VIII:R activity cannot be measured directly. Factor VIII:R also appears to bind to platelet receptor glycoproteins IIb and IIIa in stimulated platelets.

Antibodies have been prepared that are specific for antigenic sites on either aspect of the molecule. The antigenic sites that can be detected immunochemically on the VIII:C portion of the molecule are designated VIII:CAg. Those that are detected immunochemically on the VIII:R portion of the molecule are called VIII:RAg.

Whether Factor VIII should be considered a complex molecule or a multimolecular complex is still uncertain. Under certain in vivo experimental conditions to be discussed later, VIII:C and VIII:R follow different metabolic patterns.

Intrinsic, Extrinsic, and Common Pathways

The terms *intrinsic* and *extrinsic* refer to clotting inside and outside the vascular system. This separation is useful conceptually, but in fact the two systems function together when coagulation is triggered by vascular damage. The intrinsic system is slow and the extrinsic system faster owing to the action of tissue factor. The end product of either system is Factor Xa. The conversion of prothrombin to thrombin by Factor Xa followed by the formation of a fibrin clot is the common pathway (Fig. 4–23). All three systems involve calcium-dependent complex formation with phospholipid. Calcium bridges and platelet receptors localize clot formation at phospholipid surfaces in the site of vascular damage.

The intrinsic system is initiated by contact activation of Factor XII, as already described. Factor XIa is formed and triggers coagulation by converting Factor IX to IXa, a potent coagulant that converts Factor X to Xa. The activity of Factor IXa is greatly enhanced by complex formation with Factor VIII:C, calcium, and phospholipid. Factor VIII:C is activated by the presence of small quantities of thrombin.

The extrinsic system is initiated through activation of Factor VII by tissue factor, a gly-

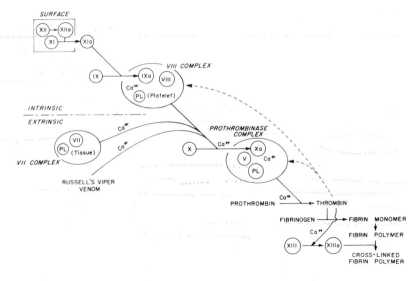

Figure 4–23 The sequence of reactions of the plasma coagulation factors. Details of the contact activation of Factor XII are shown in Figure 4–20. The intrinsic and extrinsic systems are separate pathways for the activation of Factor X. The common pathway refers to the conversion of prothrombin to thrombin by Factor Xa followed by the polymerization of fibrin. (PL = phospholipid.)

coprotein-phospholipid cofactor found in most cell membranes (Nemerson and Bach, 1982). Lung, brain, placenta, and the subintimal layer of blood vessels are particularly rich sources. Factor X is activated at the site of the tissue factor, phospholipid, calcium, Factor VIIa complex. The extrinsic system short-circuits the intrinsic pathway by bypassing contact activation and Factor IX activation (Fig. 4–23).

In the final common pathway, Factor Xa is capable of directly converting prothrombin to thrombin, but its activity is accelerated several thousand–fold by complex formation with Factor V as cofactor together with calcium and phospholipid.

Calcium, as noted, is required for many coagulation reactions. Citrate is an anticoagulant because it forms complexes with calcium. It is commonly used in the collection of plasma samples for coagulation testing. Its effect is readily reversed by addition of excess calcium. Hypocalcemia, however, is virtually never of sufficient clinical magnitude to cause abnormal bleeding.

Under the auspices of their vitamin K–dependent γ-carboxyglutamyl–rich regions, Factors IXa and VIIa are bound at phospholipid sites by calcium bridges. These sites in turn determine the local activation of Factor X and of prothrombin. In addition, specific platelet receptors play an important role in clot localization. For example, platelet membrane Factor Va acts as receptor for Factor Xa and for prothrombin.

Examples of activation mechanisms are given in Figures 4–24 and 4–25. A small peptide segment is spliced out of the Factor IX molecule during the course of its activation, leaving behind two polypeptide chains connected by a disulfide bridge. One chain contains the active serine center and the other the

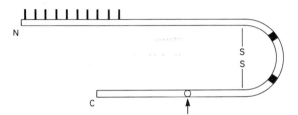

Figure 4–24 Activation of Factor IX. Two cleavage sites are indicated (shaded areas). The active serine center (arrow) remains connected by disulfide bonds to the γ-carboxyglutamyl–rich region (series of perpendicular lines) on the other chain of the active enzyme. (Adapted from Rosenberg, R. D. *In* Beck, W. S. [Ed.]: Hematology. 3rd ed. Cambridge, MA, M.I.T. Press, 1981, p. 378.)

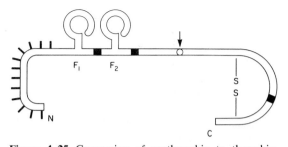

Figure 4–25 Conversion of prothrombin to thrombin. Three main cleavage sites are shown (shaded areas). The active serine (arrow) is present on one of the two chains of the thrombin molecule. Two kringles are illustrated. The F_1 region contains the γ-carboxyglutamyl–rich region (series of perpendicular lines). F_2 contains a binding site for platelet factor Va. (Adapted from Rosenberg, R. D. *In* Beck, W. S. [Ed.]: Hematology. 3rd ed. Cambridge, MA, M.I.T. Press, 1981, p. 383.)

γ-carboxyglutamyl–binding site. In the case of prothrombin, cleavage separates the active enzyme thrombin from both the phospholipid- and the platelet-binding sites, allowing the enzyme to diffuse some distance away from its activation site. Factor VII is activated both by conformational change and by cleavage. The cofactors V and VIII:C appear to activated by thrombin-mediated molecular cleavage.

Thrombin is the most versatile member of the coagulant team. It converts fibrinogen to fibrin monomer, activates Factor XIII, induces platelet aggregation, and exposes platelet-binding sites. It generates positive feedback by activating Factors V and VIII:C. It also triggers control reactions by activating protein C, as explained in the next discussion.

As noted, the intrinsic and extrinsic pathways operate in an interdependent relationship. The extrinsic system may activate the intrinsic system and vice versa. The crossovers involve activation reactions between Factors VIIa and IX, and between XIIa and VII.

Platelet Coagulation Factors

The activation of platelets and formation of a platelet plug consititute an essential part of in vivo hemostasis (see first section of Chapter 4). The activated platelets release fibrinogen, factor V, and factor VIII:R from their α-granules and unmask glycoprotein receptors for thrombin, fibrinogen, and Factors Xa and VIII:R (Walsh, 1981). These coagulation factors then interact on the fused phospholipid surface and form complexes (Fig. 4–23) leading to fibrin and thrombus formation. Thus, platelet and coagulation factors are dynamically linked and interdependent.

The Control of Coagulation Reactions: Heparin Cofactor

In addition to the localization of coagulants at phospholipid surfaces brought about by calcium bridges and specific receptors, a number of other factors collaborate to keep thrombus formation a local process (Rosenberg and Rosenberg, 1984). Rapid blood flow washes away local concentrations of activated factors. If perfusion is adequate, the liver rapidly clears the activated factors from the circulation, allowing them a half-life of only a few minutes. There they are quickly degraded. There are also present in normal plasma several inhibitors that neutralize activated coagulation fac-

tors (Table 4–3). These inhibitors interact with constituents of the intact endothelium to limit the thrombus to the site of damaged endothelium. The role of endothelial cell prostacyclin as an inhibitor of platelet thrombus formation has already been discussed in the preceding section.

The most important of the plasma inhibitors is antithrombin III, identified by Rosenberg (1975) as the heparin cofactor. This inhibitor has an arginine residue that seeks out active serine sites to form a stable complex. Thus, it inhibits not only thrombin but also other serine proteases, including Factors XIIa, XIa, IXa, and Xa. Its effect on Factor VIIa is relatively weak.

The combination of heparin with antithrombin III enhances its affinity for serine proteases by as much as several thousand times, converting a slow reaction to one that is almost immediate (Fig. 4–26). In the absence of antithrombin III, heparin has no effect on clot formation. Hence, the inhibitor is also known as heparin cofactor. Heparin binds to a specific lysine residue at a point on the molecule that is distant from its active arginine. The heparin complex induces a conformational change that makes the arginine much more available for binding to active serine sites on neighboring molecules. After the active serine is bound and inhibited in the stable complex, heparin is released and is available for recycling.

Endothelial surfaces are richly endowed with heparan, a heparin-like substance found on a variety of cell surfaces. In fact, parenterally administered heparin is concentrated on endothelial surfaces (Jaques, 1979). Thus, it ap-

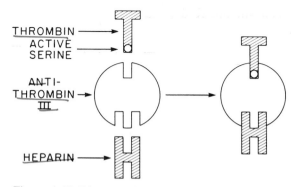

Figure 4–26 Diagram of the mechanism of action of antithrombin III. Thrombin and other serine proteases are inhibited at their active centers by complex formation at an arginyl residue on the antithrombin III molecule. The active serine is shown by an open circle. The affinity of antithrombin III for serine proteases becomes several thousand times greater as the result of binding of heparin to a distant lysine site on the molecule. (Adapted from Bussel, J. B.: Hosp. Pract., *18(2)*:171, 1983.)

Table 4–3 INHIBITORS OF PLASMA COAGULATION FACTORS

Factor	Molecular Weight (Daltons)	Action	Normal Plasma Concentration (μg./ml.)*	Deficiency State
Antithrombin III	50,000	Anti serine protease	240	Thrombosis
α_2-Antiplasmin	70,000	Antiplasmin	70	Bleeding
α_2-Macroglobulin	725,000	Antiprotease	2500	None known
Protein C	56,000	Anti-Factors V and VIII:C; vascular plasminogen activator release	5	Thrombosis

*Data from McKee, P. *In* Stanbury, J. B., et al. (Eds.): The Metabolic Basis of Inherited Disease. New York, McGraw-Hill Book Co., 1983, p. 1534, and Harpel, P. C. *In* Colman, R. W., et al. (Eds.): Hemostasis and Thrombosis. Philadelphia, J. B. Lippincott Co., 1982, p. 743.

pears likely that the anticoagulant effect of antithrombin III in complex with heparin or heparan is most active on the lining of the vascular tree (Fig. 4–27).

Heparin in plasma prolongs the prothrombin time by only a few seconds. Its action on the partial thromboplastin time and thrombin time is much more pronounced. Its clinical effect is immediate and is present in vitro as well as in vivo, in contrast to the coumarin anticoagulants, which are active only in vivo. Heparin is rapidly cleared from the circulation, demonstrating a half-life of 90 minutes, and its effect on plasma coagulation tests is dissipated within 6 hours. Although there is significant renal excretion, the metabolic fate of heparin is not well understood.

Another inhibitory system that depends on the vascular endothelium has been described more recently. The normal endothelium contains a substance called *thrombomodulin*. When thrombin binds to thrombomodulin, the complex activates *protein C* (Gardiner and Griffin, 1983). This anticoagulant protein is vitamin K–dependent and, like the procoagulant vitamin K–dependent factors, it contains a cluster of γ-carboxyglutamyl residues near its N terminus. Activated protein C has several anticoagulant effects. These include the release of plasminogen activator from the vessel wall and the inactivation of Factors Va and VIII:Ca. Protein S, another vitamin K–dependent plasma protein, acts as a cofactor for activated protein C. Deficiencies of antithrombin III, of protein C, or of protein S are associated with hypercoagulability.

At the other end of the reaction sequence, the forces of clot lysis are contained by α_2-antiplasmin, a plasma inhibitor of plasmin, with which it forms a complex to block the active center of the enzyme. It also reacts with the lysyl residues on fibrin and fibrinogen, blocking access of plasmin to its substrates at these sites. Deficiency of this inhibitor leads to hemorrhagic diathesis because of the lack of plasmin control.

The only other plasma inhibitor of significance is α_2-macroglobulin, a relatively weak nonspecific protease inhibitor. It is a large molecule with antithrombin and antiplasmin activities. Deficiency apparently leads to no clinical effects. It inhibits by engulfing its target, which retaliates by breaking peptide bonds in its attacker. This in turn promotes macrophage uptake of the complex. This inhibitor serves as a backup system. For example, the plasma contains only half as much α_2-antiplasmin as plasminogen. If plasminogen activation is so extensive that the capacity of α_2-antiplasmin is overwhelmed, α_2-macroglobulin steps in and fills the gap.

Synthesis and Turnover

Most of the coagulation factors are made in the liver, with only a few notable exceptions. Factor VIII:R is synthesized by endothelial cells and megakaryocytes, but the site of synthesis of Factor VIII:C is still unknown. Megakaryocytes also appear to be the source of one of the Factor XIII subunits. The other may be made in the liver.

Fibrinogen and Factor VIII are acute-phase

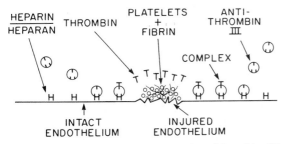

Figure 4–27 Schematic illustration of antithrombin III interactions with heparin or heparan or both on endothelial surfaces to control the local growth of the thrombus. (Adapted from Bussel, J. B.: Hosp. Pract., *18(2)*:181, 1983.)

reactants, and their levels rise in response to inflammatory states, surgery, and pregnancy. An epinephrine response is rapidly followed by a transient rise in both the platelet count and the plasma Factor VIII level. The platelets are presumably temporarily released from the splenic pool. The origin of the Factor VIII increase is still not clear. A similar increase in Factor VIII also occurs following administration of a synthetic derivative of vasopressin, which appears to stimulate release from endothelial cell stores (Mannucci et al., 1983).

The biologic half-lives of most of the clotting factors are relatively short (Table 4–2). Factor VII has the shortest, and fibrinogen and Factor XIII have the longest. The disappearance of a plasma protein from the intravascular space is a complex function determined not only by its catabolism but also by its passage into extravascular spaces. Thus the meaning of "half-life" is open to considerable discussion. Nonetheless, the value is useful in scheduling the frequency of replacement infusions in patients being treated for bleeding due to known factor deficiencies.

Coagulation Tests

Most of the tests of the clotting mechanism depend on the appearance of a fibrin clot in

Table 4–4 COAGULATION TESTS AND HEMOSTATIC PARAMETERS EVALUATED

Primary

Prothrombin time: extrinsic and common systems
Activated partial thromboplastin time: intrinsic and common systems
Clot retraction: clot size, clot lysis, platelet contractile function
Platelet count: platelet quantity
Bleeding time: platelet function

Secondary

Fibrinogen concentration: fibrinogen lack or excess
Thrombin time: direct conversion of fibrinogen to fibrin clot
Fibrinogen-fibrin degradation products: fibrinogen-related antigens in serum
Protamine sulfate paracoagulation test: soluble clottable fibrinogen derivatives in plasma (fibrin monomer, fragment X)
Substitution tests with normal plasma, fresh adsorbed plasma, fresh serum, and aged plasma: identification of factor deficiency
Factor assays: confirmation and quantitation of factor deficiency
Tests for pathologic inhibitors: detection of pathologic endogenous anticoagulants and of "lupus inhibitor"
Urea clot solubility: Factor XIII deficiency
Platelet aggregation reactions: qualitative platelet defects

the test tube (Table 4–4). The simplest of these is the whole-blood clotting time, which is a crude measure of the intrinsic system. A much more convenient, accurate, and reproducible method of measuring the clotting time in the laboratory rather than at the bedside is to collect citrated plasma and subsequently measure the plasma clotting time in the laboratory by adding excess calcium. The normal "recalcification time" is about 100 to 240 seconds, compared with 5 to 15 minutes for the whole-blood clotting time. The addition of various reagents to recalcified plasma gives considerable information about the coagulation mechanism. The addition of a substitute for platelet phospholipid (a "partial thromboplastin") shortens the time to about 60 to 90 seconds; this is the "partial thromboplastin time," which reflects the status of the intrinsic system. The activation of Factors XII and XI by surface-active materials, such as kaolin, celite, and ellagic acid, shortens the time to about 25 to 40 seconds and gives a more reproducible test ("activated partial thromboplastin time"). If tissue factor is added, the plasma clotting time is about 13 seconds, and the corresponding test, somewhat erroneously called the prothrombin time, is a measure of the extrinsic system. The addition of Russell's viper venom (Stypven time) activates Factor X directly and thus eliminates Factor VII as a variable in the assessment of the extrinsic system. The addition of thrombin (thrombin time) is a direct measure of the ability to form a fibrin clot in the test plasma and normally produces a clot so rapidly (about 6 seconds) that dilution of the thrombin is necessary in order to lengthen the time and thus to obtain more accurate and meaningful results. It is obvious that all tests that depend on the appearance of a fibrin clot require an adequate concentration of fibrinogen in the test plasma.

In summary, the initial clinical evaluation of a hemostatic disorder requires an activated partial thromboplastin time (APTT) and a prothrombin time (PT) to evaluate the intrinsic and extrinsic systems. Deficiencies of Factor X, V, II or of fibrinogen or the presence of heparin or "split products" prolong both the APTT and the PT. Factor VII lack prolongs the PT but not the APTT, whereas the reverse is true for deficiencies of Factor XII, XI, IX, or VIII. The thrombin time detects fibrinogen abnormalities, heparin, or "split products." Although the concentration of fibrinogen is readily measured, one may easily obtain a rough index of fibrinogen level by inspecting the bulk of a retracted clot in a test tube.

Rapid lysis of the incubated clot indicates pathologic fibrinolysis. In vivo fibrinolysis is revealed by an elevated level of fibrinogen-fibrin degradation products. The routine hemostasis evaluation is completed by a platelet count and sometimes by tests of platelet function, of which clot retraction and bleeding time are the most useful.

Tentative conclusions about the identity of a plasma factor deficiency are drawn from substitution tests in an "expanded" partial thromboplastin time. The reagents used for substitution are aged plasma (which lacks the labile Factors V and VIII), fresh adsorbed plasma (which lacks the vitamin K–dependent Factors II, VII, IX, and X), and fresh serum (which lacks the consumable Factors II, V, and VIII and fibrinogen). For example, the prolonged APTT in a patient with Factor VIII:C deficiency (hemophilia A) is corrected by substitution with normal fresh adsorbed plasma, but not aged plasma or serum. In Factor IX deficiency (hemophilia B), the abnormality is corrected by normal serum or aged plasma, but not adsorbed plasma. Final confirmation and quantitation is accomplished by specific factor assays using a test plasma of known deficiency mixed with patient plasma.

PATHOPHYSIOLOGY

The hereditary abnormalities of the coagulation factors are readily classified because they are definable in terms of a single inherited abnormality in either the amount or the structure of a single protein (Mammen, 1983). Acquired defects are more difficult to categorize in that they frequently affect many different aspects of the coagulation sequence as well as multiple coagulation factors (Table 4–5).

The general effects are those of bleeding or clotting or both. The clinical nature of the bleeding gives clues about its underlying cause. Intra-articular hemorrhage is highly characteristic of hemophilia and is seen only rarely in other disorders, whereas petechiae are strongly suggestive of thrombocytopenia. Ecchymoses and purpura are very nonspecific; deep hemorrhage into muscles or the retroperitoneum is more a feature of hemophilia or of adverse effects of anticoagulants. Intracranial hemorrhage, regardless of the underlying hemostatic defect, is the most dreaded complication. Bleeding from the umbilical stump or following circumcision may be the first sign of a hereditary disorder. Later in life, the onset of the

Table 4–5 CLASSIFICATION OF DISORDERS OF PLASMA COAGULATION

I. Disorders of fibrinogen and related factors
  A. Hereditary
    1. Afibrinogenemia
    2. Dysfibrinogenemia
    3. Factor XIII deficiency
  B. Acquired
    1. Disseminated intravascular coagulation
    2. Primary fibrinolysis
    3. Liver disease
II. Disorders of the intrinsic, extrinsic, and common systems
  A. Hereditary
    1. Hemophilia A
    2. Hemophilia B
    3. Deficiencies of surface active Factor XII or XI
    4. Other deficiencies: Factor VII, X, V, or II
    5. Von Willebrand's disease
  B. Acquired
    1. Vitamin K deficiency
    2. Liver disease
    3. Hemorrhagic diseases of the newborn
    4. Exogenous anticoagulants
    5. Endogenous anticoagulants (antibodies to Factor VIII and other Factors)

menses, dental extraction, and surgical procedures are natural tests of hemostasis. Delayed hemorrhage several days after completion of a procedure raises the index of suspicion that there is a disorder of plasma coagulation factors.

Disorders of Fibrinogen and Related Factors

A low level of circulating fibrinogen may be secondary to decreased production or more frequently to an increase in the rate of its degradation. The excess in fibrinogen consumption above its production rate is most often due to a process of intravascular coagulation. Rarely, it is caused by the presence of a high level of circulating plasmin.

Several different terms have been used to describe the process of *extensive intravascular clotting,* none of them entirely satisfactory (Merskey, 1982). "Consumption coagulopathy" emphasizes the depletion of the plasma coagulation factors, but not all the factors are consumed, and the "panel" of depressed factor levels is neither uniform nor predictable. "Disseminated intravascular coagulation" places major emphasis on the pathogenetic importance of the deposition of large quantities of fibrin throughout the microcirculation but does not fit those situations in which the fibrin deposition is extensive and yet mostly or entirely localized to the vascular beds of certain tissues.

If not fatal, the process may be acute and self-limited, subacute, or chronic, depending on the underlying cause. It may be set off by a pathologic activation of the extrinsic or the intrinsic clotting systems. In many circumstances, the triggering mechanism is not known. The activation of the extrinsic system is caused by the entry into the circulation of large amounts of tissue factor. Examples are the hypofibrinogenemic states associated with pregnancy: abruptio placentae, amniotic fluid embolism, toxemia, and retained dead fetus. Since fibrinogen concentration normally increases in pregnancy, the finding of a plasma concentration within the normal range may be indicative of significant consumption if found late in pregnancy in association with one of the aforementioned complications. Widespread carcinoma may incite intravascular clotting, also presumably on account of the tumor content of tissue factor that finds its way into the circulation. The intrinsic system may be activated by bacterial septicemia and certain rickettsial and viral infections (Rocky Mountain spotted fever, epidemic hemorrhagic fever) that lay bare the vascular endothelium and expose collagen. Antigen-antibody complexes trigger intrinsic clotting by an unknown mechanism in massive transfusion reactions (although the thromboplastic properties of red cell membranes may play some role) and in anaphylactic reactions. It has been suggested that an immunologic mechanism underlies purpura fulminans, a serious and often fatal disorder primarily of children that characteristically follows a minor viral infection (Spicer and Rau, 1976). Properly timed injections of endotoxin given to animals have been experimentally used to produce the so-called "generalized Shwartzman reaction," a disseminated intravascular coagulation syndrome, but in this model the precise initiating event also remains obscure. The classification of intravascular coagulation syndromes is given in Table 4–6.

Local factors may prepare the vascular bed of a certain organ or tissue for selective fibrin deposition. In pregnancy, the kidney is particularly vulnerable, and the syndrome that may ensue is bilateral renal cortical necrosis with oliguric renal failure. In cavernous hemangiomas, a large vascular bed with a high ratio of endothelial surface area to vascular cross-sectional area accommodates a large volume of blood with static flow. This may be sufficient to set up a chronic process of extensive but

Table 4–6 CLASSIFICATION OF DISSEMINATED INTRAVASCULAR COAGULATION SYNDROMES

I. Pregnancy
  A. Abruptio placentae
  B. Amniotic fluid embolism
  C. Toxemia
  D. Retained dead fetus
  E. Saline abortion
  F. Septic abortion with septicemia
  G. Hydatidiform mole
II. Malignant disease
  A. Metastatic carcinoma
  B. Acute leukemia (promyelocytic)
III. Infectious disease
  A. Bacterial septicemia (meningococcal, other gram-negative and gram-positive organisms)
  B. Rickettsial (Rocky Mountain spotted fever)
  C. Viral (epidemic hemorrhagic fever)
  D. Parasitic (malaria)
IV. Pediatric syndromes
  A. Neonatal (respiratory distress syndrome, retained dead twin fetus, septicemia, rubella, abruptio placentae)
  B. Purpura fulminans
  C. Hemolytic uremic syndrome
V. Antigen-antibody complexes
  A. Anaphylactic reaction
  B. Massive transfusion reaction
VI. Miscellaneous
  A. Liver disease
  B. Aneurysm
  C. Vasculitis
  D. Postoperative (open heart and other thoracic surgery, prostatic surgery)
  E. Massive trauma (including burns and severe head injury)
  F. Heat stroke
  G. Drowning
  H. Snake bite
  I. Giant hemangioma

localized fibrin deposition, with the endothelium contributing high plasminogen-activating activity and thus releasing fibrin degradation products into the circulation.

An adequate hepatic perfusion is necessary for rapid clearance of activated coagulation factors as well as fibrinogen-fibrin degradation products and their complexes from the circulation. Any impairment of this process will prolong and aggravate the severity of the coagulopathy. Clinical states of hypovolemia, whatever the underlying primary cause, lead to poor perfusion and may seriously increase the magnitude of the syndrome. Macrophage blockade with substances such as thorium dioxide (Thorotrast) contributes to the severity of intravascular coagulation syndromes experimentally in animals. A similar blockade may be of pathogenetic significance in septicemia or in massive hemolysis.

The ischemic consequences to local tissues

from the blockage of the microcirculation are fortunately usually self-limited owing to the local fibrinolytic efficiency, which rapidly removes the fibrin deposits. However, renal failure is one of the most dire of the ischemic effects. Cutaneous patches of gangrene and acrocyanosis are more externally visible signs seen in purpura fulminans and sometimes in septicemia. Erythrocyte fragmentation, occurring as red cells are forced through the obstructing fibrin meshwork, causes the morphologic appearance of microangiopathic hemolytic anemia on the peripheral blood film (Fig. 2–100). The picture may be accompanied by clinical signs of hemolysis. Intravascular coagulation causing oliguric renal failure and erythrocyte fragmentation is therefore one of the "hemolytic uremic" syndromes.

Laboratory tests reflect the paradoxic circumstance that excessive intravascular clotting brings forth a hemorrhagic diathesis. The consumption of coagulation factors in vivo resembles the process of conversion of plasma to serum in vitro. The most consistent changes are decreases in the platelet count and in the levels of fibrinogen and Factors II, V, and VIII. Plasminogen activation releases fibrinogen-fibrin degradation products into the circulation. These form complexes with fibrin monomer and interfere with the normal polymerization of fibrin monomer during clot formation. The widespread derangements in the coagulation mechanism are reflected by abnormalities in all the routine laboratory tests. These include prolongation of the prothrombin time, the activated partial thromboplastin time, and the thrombin time. The concentration of "split products" in the serum is elevated, and tests of paracoagulation, as described earlier, may be positive. The test tube clot is small and easily broken up. Serial measurements of the routine coagulation tests, platelet count, and fibrinogen concentration may help one make the clinical decision about the presence of and the course of a suspected case of extensive intravascular clotting. Measurement of the levels of other factors, although helpful, is generally unnecessary. Laboratory confirmation may be difficult in mild cases and especially in some of the more chronic varieties.

Treatment varies with the individual circumstances. In acute syndromes, the prompt and vigorous treatment of the primary underlying cause and the correction of hypovolemia are the most important measures. Heparin is sometimes used to arrest the deposition of fibrin, but not without fear of increasing the bleeding tendency. Repletion of coagulation factors with fresh frozen plasma or cryoprecipitate and platelets may be indicated. Replacement therapy is best combined with heparin if the process has not been arrested and fibrin deposition is continuing. Inhibitors of fibrinolysis such as epsilon aminocaproic acid usually are contraindicated, since they will delay the physiologic resolution of the fibrin clots within the vasculature.

Primary fibrinolysis is an acute severe bleeding state that resembles intravascular clotting but must be distinguished from it because the treatments differ. The high levels of circulating plasmin that set up this state are generated secondary to metastatic carcinoma of the prostate, after thoracic surgery or injury to the genitourinary tract with extravasation of urokinase-containing urine into tissues, or in association with cirrhosis or shock with impaired ability to clear plasminogen activators from the circulation. Plasmin attacks circulating fibrinogen and causes a decrease in its concentration along with the appearance of fibrinogen degradation products in the circulation. These unfortunately cannot be easily distinguished from the fibrinogen-fibrin degradation products of disseminated intravascular coagulation (although cross-linked derivatives of fibrin can be distinguished by a more cumbersome electrophoretic method from the non–cross-linked fragments that result exclusively from fibrinogen degradation). Other coagulation factor levels may also be depressed. However, in contrast to intravascular coagulation syndromes, the test-tube clot that initially forms dissolves completely within 1 or 2 hours, the platelet count is normal, the red cell morphology does not show fragmentation, and the bleeding improves with the therapeutic use of fibrinolytic inhibitors. Under certain circumstances, such as metastatic prostatic carcinoma, primary fibrinolysis occurs together with disseminated intravascular coagulation, and laboratory distinction of the two states is not possible.

Inherited disorders of fibrinogen are rare. Afibrinogenemia is a quantitative deficiency secondary to a profound lack of synthesis, whereas dysfibrinogenemia refers to a variation in the structure of the molecule. Only trace quantities of fibrinogen are detectable in hereditary afibrinogenemia, an autosomal recessive condition that is of clinical significance only in the homozygous form. Whole-blood and recalcified-plasma clotting times are indefinitely long and are not corrected with the addition of thrombin. Successful arrest of hemorrhage is achieved by replacement therapy sufficient to raise the fibrinogen level above 60 mg. per 100 ml. *Hereditary dysfibrinogenemia* is a mild or even asymptomatic disorder. Several different types have been described, presumably differing in the specific amino acid substitution in the molecule (Ebert and Bell, 1983). Plasma coagulation tests may be broadly deranged. Fibrinogen concentration measured by immunochemical or physical methods may be normal, but methods that depend on "clottable fibrinogen" give low values. The condition is autosomal, and affected heterozygotes therefore have normal fibrinogen along with the variant molecule. *Acquired dysfibrinogenemia*, due to an abnormality in oligosaccharide processing, occurs in patients with severe liver disease and also in association with hepatoma (Martinez and Palascak, 1982).

Hereditary deficiency of Factor XIII is properly included among disorders of fibrinogen, since Factor XIII also affects clot structure. Deficiency is detectable in the laboratory by virtue of the fibrin clot solubility in 5M urea. The defect, also autosomal recessive, is clinically severe and, as in hereditary afibrinogenemia, may first come to attention because of bleeding at the site of the sloughed umbilical cord. Wound healing is impaired because fibroblastic organization of the clot is not normal. Affected homozygotes have less than 1 percent of the normal concentration and respond particularly well to replacement therapy because Factor XIII has a relatively long half-life and only small quantities are required. Factor XIII is among the factors consumed in disseminated intravascular coagulation, another explanation for a lowered level. Consumption or decreased hepatic synthesis accounts for low levels in patients with liver disease.

Intrinsic and Extrinsic System Disorders

Hemophilia A and *hemophilia B* are hereditary deficiencies of Factor VIII and Factor IX, respectively. The two disorders are clinically indistiguishable except by laboratory test. Both are sex-linked and thus transmitted by asymptomatic carrier females to half their sons. Half their daughters will be carriers. Sons of hemophilic fathers are normal, whereas daughters are obligate carriers. Female homozygotes, offspring of affected fathers and carrier mothers, are extremely rare. Hemophilia A occurs with a frequency of 1 per 10,000, about four to five times the frequency of hemophilia B.

Severe hemophilia is characterized by repeated hemarthroses and ultimately by chronic arthritis and joint destruction. Ankles, knees, and elbows are most susceptible. The normal ineffectiveness of the extrinsic clotting system in the articular structures may explain the particular susceptibility of this tissue to hemorrhage in the face of severe deficiencies of the intrinsic system. Patients with hemophilia of moderate severity may have only occasional joint hemorrhages, whereas patients with mild cases usually have normal joints. Deep hematomas may dissect along fascial planes and cause nerve compression or compromise the vascular supply of an extremity. Pseudotumors may develop. Even with intensive treatment the surgical risk is great. Intracranial hemorrhage may be provoked by minor head trauma and culminate with a fatal outcome.

In severe hemophilia A, Factor VIII:C is less than 1 percent the normal level, in moderate cases 2 to 5 percent, and in mild cases 6 to 30 percent. The defect is limited to the procoagulant piece of the Factor VIII molecule, VIII:C, which either is missing or is present but not functioning. Factor VIII:R is unaffected. It has been possible to classify patients with hemophilia A into two groups, based on reactions of their plasma with certain neutralizing antibodies to VIII:C. Plasma from about 10 percent of patients with hemophilia A will neutralize these antibodies and is designated as cross-reacting material positive (CRM$^+$) or A$^+$. The remaining 90 percent are CRM$^-$ or A$^-$. The pathogenetic significance of this observation and its possible relationship to genetic polymorphism are still not clear.

In hemophilia B, the deficiency may similarly be due either to lack of production of Factor IX or to normal production of an immunologically measurable but functionally deficient molecule.

The accurate diagnosis and classification as to degree of severity of hemophilia A and B ultimately rest on the direct measurement of the levels of Factor VIII:C and Factor IX activity (Aledort, 1982). The treatment of major hemorrhagic episodes or the preparation of patients for surgery also requires the ability to measure the specific factor level to ensure that it remains in excess of 30 percent at all times. The partial thromboplastin time is sensitive to levels below 20 percent and thus is almost always prolonged in untreated patients of any degree of severity. The prothrombin time and the bleeding time are normal. Female carriers cannot be identified with certainty by simple measurement of their Factor VIII:C levels because their functional levels, 25 to 75 percent for hemophilia A heterozygotes and 9 to 90 percent for hemophilia B heterozygotes, overlap considerably, with the normal range of 50 and 150 per cent. Ratnoff and Jones report 94 percent accuracy in identifying female carriers of hemophilia A with the use of a method that compares the ratios between the levels of procoagulant (VIII:C) and antigenic activity (VIII:RAg). In hemophilia A heterozygotes, the ratio is about half the value expected in normals.

Replacement therapy with plasma or plasma derivatives is effective in both hemophilia A and hemophilia B (Fig. 4–28). Treatment must be specific, however. Cryoprecipitate and other Factor VIII-rich preparations lack Factor IX activity, whereas fractions containing Factor IX and the other vitamin K–dependent factors lack Factor VIII. Cryoprecipitate is a fraction prepared by thawing fresh frozen plasma at 4°C. Because it contains concentrated fibrinogen in addition to Factor VIII, it may also be used for replacement therapy of hypofibrinogenemic states when volume expansion from fresh frozen plasma would be excessive. Factor IX is relatively stable and is present in stored plasma, which is a poor source of Factor VIII. The longer biologic half-life of Factor IX (about 24 hours as compared with 12 for Factor VIII) is also important in that less frequent infusions of Factor IX are required to maintain its functional activity at the desired level. Factor VIII is predominantly intravascular, but about half of the total pool of Factor IX is extravascular. A relatively larger dose of Factor IX is therefore required to allow for loss into the extravascular space.

The availability of concentrates containing Factor VIII or Factor IX plus the growth of publicly supported centers for financing the cost of treatment has led to the common use of home treatment programs. Patients learn how to treat themselves with intravenous infusions at the earliest sign of hemorrhage or even occasionally on a routine prophylactic schedule. As a result, there has been a decrease in the incidence and severity of arthropathy and of hospital admissions and disability in general.

Von Willebrand's disease is also a disorder of Factor VIII that is usually inherited, although acquired forms have been reported (Zimmerman and Ruggeri, 1982). The VIII:R aspect of the molecule is primarily affected, usually but not invariably leading to an associated lack of VIII:C activity. Platelet adhesion to injured blood vessels is impaired, and the bleeding time is prolonged. Platelet adhesion to glass beads in vitro is reduced. Platelet aggregation reactions to ADP, epinephrine, collagen, and thrombin are all normal, but ristocetin-induced platelet aggregation is usually impaired. Factor VIII:C levels may be reduced below 50 percent to as low as 1 to 5 percent. The partial thromboplastin time is prolonged only in those with VIII:C levels below 20 percent. Other routine coagulation tests are normal. Factor VIII:C levels fluctuate in individual cases, in contrast to their constancy in hemophilia A. Pregnancy stimulates an increased VIII:C level, as in normal women, and thus may ameliorate hemorrhagic symptoms.

One of the difficulties in laboratory confirmation of the diagnosis is the lack of a method for directly measuring Factor VIII:R activity. The immunochemical determination of VIII:RAg and the measurement of ristoce-

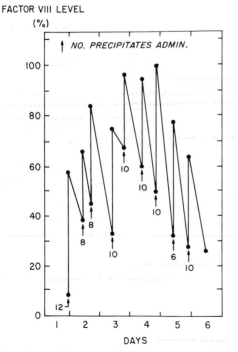

FACTOR VIII LEVEL
(%)

Figure 4–28 Plasma Factor VIII:C levels measured during treatment of a patient with hemophilia A by repeated infusions of cryoprecipitate. (Redrawn from Pool, J. G., and Shannon, A. E.: N. Engl. J. Med., *273*:143, 1968. Reprinted by permission.)

tin cofactor activity are VIII:R–associated properties that may correlate with VIII:R activity, but this is not always the case, as discussed subsequently.

The disorder is inherited as an autosomal dominant or recessive trait and is characterized by epistaxis, menorrhagia, and gastrointestinal hemorrhage. Joint hemorrhage is unusual. Some forms are clinically recessive and are asymptomatic in heterozygous carriers but cause severe bleeding in homozygotes. Other forms are dominant and cause mild to moderate hemorrhagic disease in heterozygotes. Because there are several different genetic types, double heterozygosity is also possible.

The most common genetic form is Type I, or "classic," von Willebrand's disease. In this variety, there is a concordant decrease in VIII:C activity and in VIII:R levels as measured by VIII:RAg or by ristocetin cofactor activity, both of which reflect the concentrations of VIII:R. The defect is a quantitative lack of VIII:R without qualitative abnormalities, leading secondarily to a parallel loss of VIII:C activity. In Type II variant, the changes are discordant, primarily related to the fact that there are qualitative abnormalities on the Factor VIII:R aspect of the molecule that cause defective association into the large multimers necessary for platelet binding. Factor VIII:C and VIII:RAg concentrations may be normal or only minimally reduced. Ristocetin cofactor activity is decreased in the Subtype IIA, but it is paradoxically increased in Subtype IIB. The paradox apparently is related in some way to the preservation of the large multimers of VIII:R within the platelet but not in the plasma.

Commercial Factor VIII concentrates possess VIII:C activity but are deficient in the high molecular weight components necessary for VIII:R activity. Therefore, they should not be used for the treatment of patients with von Willebrand's disease. Cryoprecipitate is the treatment of choice and should be used with the objective of normalizing the bleeding time.

One of the most intriguing differences between hemophilia A and von Willebrand's disease lies in their response to plasma or cryoprecipitate infusions. The increase in VIII:C level in hemophilia A is entirely accounted for by the amount of infused material; the maximum occurs immediately after infusion and the declining level thereafter follows the known biologic half-life of VIII:C, about 12 hours. Plasma infusions given to patients with von Willebrand's disease actually stimu-

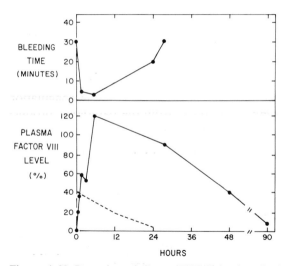

Figure 4–29 Response of Factor VIII:C level and of bleeding time in a patient with von Willebrand's disease after, given at time zero, a single infusion of a fraction prepared from normal plasma. The interrupted line represents the response in Factor VIII:C level to be expected in a patient with hemophilia A. (Modified from Williams, W. J. *In* Williams, W. J., et al. [Eds.]: Hematology. New York, McGraw-Hill Book Co., 1972, p. 1340.)

late the production of VIII:C. Levels, reaching a peak at 4 to 24 hours, are higher than those that could be explained on the basis of the amount of infused material. The subsequent decline to original pretreatment levels occurs slowly over several days (Fig. 4–29). Donor plasma taken from patients with hemophilia A indeed has more potent VIII:C–stimulating activity than normal plasma. The correction of the prolonged bleeding time, if it is corrected at all, is much more transient and may last only a few hours. The persistence in the circulation of VIII:R tends to be intermediate, less prolonged than the VIII:C elevation but more prolonged than the period of bleeding time correction. The only sure conclusion that can be drawn from these observations is that the metabolic behavior of Factor VIII is complex. The explanation for the relative inefficacy of infusions in favorably influencing the bleeding time may point to the significance of intraplatelet and/or endothelial cell depots of VIII:R that cannot be easily repleted by simple infusion of exogenous material. However, platelet transfusion does not correct the bleeding time defect as it does in hereditary or acquired defects of platelet aggregation.

Ristocetin-induced platelet aggregation is also deficient in the *Bernard-Soulier syndrome,* a hemorrhagic condition in which the intrinsically defective platelets are large, heavy, and decreased in number. In this disorder, there is a deficiency in the platelet receptor for VIII:R. There is no plasma deficiency of Factor VIII constituents.

Acquired defects in Factor VIII, other than those found in the intravascular coagulation syndromes, result from the pathologic production of autoantibodies directed against Factor VIII. Somewhat paradoxically, about 5 to 20 percent of patients with hemophilia A develop antibodies against Factor VIII after repeated replacement therapy. These greatly complicate successful therapy when they are present in high titer. Fortunately, the titer falls with time, and if the intervals between hemorrhagic episodes are sufficiently spaced, intensive replacement therapy may successfully arrest the bleeding before the anamnestic response to the infused Factor VIII raises the antibody titer to levels that would preclude successful treatment. Acquired antibodies to Factor VIII are also seen in association with such autoimmune disorders as lupus erythematosus, rheumatoid arthritis, ulcerative colitis, and regional enteritis. A third variant occurs days to weeks post partum. A fourth type is found without obvious relationship to other coexisting factors, especially in older people. The antibody behaves as a natural circulating anticoagulant, and its addition to normal plasma will delay its clotting time. Specific confirmation is made by measurement of the neutralization of the Factor VIII:C activity of normal plasma by plasma containing the antibody. Therapy may be difficult if spontaneous disappearance does not alleviate the problem. Immunosuppressive therapy has been successfully used in a few instances. Concentrates of vitamin K–dependent factors have been reported to be effective in the control of bleeding because of their content of Factor Xa, which bypasses Factor VIII (Lusher et al., 1980). They are not without adverse effects, including thrombosis and hepatitis. Autoantibodies to other plasma coagulation factors have also been discovered, but the great majority have been directed against Factor VIII.

Hereditary deficiencies of the remaining plasma coagulation factors are uncommon. Of the surface-active factors, Factor XII deficiency is not associated with any bleeding abnormality, and the hemorrhagic diathesis of Factor XI deficiency is mild. Deficiency of Factor X, V, or II will prolong prothrombin and partial thromboplastin times. In Factor VII deficiency, only the prothrombin time is long. All are associated with mild to moderate bleeding manifestations.

Inadequate supplies of vitamin K cause depletion of the vitamin K–dependent factors: II, VII, IX, and X. Absorptive impairment secondary to gastrointestinal disease or to obstruction of the biliary tract causes clotting factor depletion, which is correctable by parenterally administered vitamin K. Nutritional deficiency of vitamin K is an especially common plight of the critically ill hospitalized patient who cannot eat and at the same time receives broad-spectrum antibiotics.

The coumarin and indanedione derivatives are vitamin K antagonists that are therapeutically useful as orally administered anticoagulants (Walsh, 1983; Wessler and Gitel, 1984). A large number of medications interact with these anticoagulants by either increasing or decreasing their effects. Barbiturates, for example, cause relative coumarin resistance, whereas most nonsteroidal anti-inflammatory agents have the opposite effect (Koch-Weser and Sellers, 1971). The Factor VII level is the first to fall after administration of a coumarin anticoagulant because of its short biologic half-life. Factors II, IX, and X reach their nadir at about 5 to 10 days after anticoagulant therapy is begun. Vitamin K is occasionally required to arrest hemorrhage in patients treated with anticoagulant and will significantly increase the levels of the dependent factors within 6 hours. If more rapid correction is necessary, replacement therapy with plasma or with concentrates of the vitamin K–dependent factors can be given. Vitamin K therapy is ineffective if the low factor levels are the result of severe liver disease (Blanchard et al., 1981).

As summarized by Martinez and Palascak (1982), severe liver disease is plagued by a variety of hemostatic malfunctions. Of these, lack of the vitamin K–dependent factors and of other factors produced in the liver, such as Factor V and fibrinogen, are the most important. Add to these thrombocytopenia secondary to congestive splenomegaly, qualitative platelet abnormalities, a significant incidence of disseminated intravascular coagulation, and increased fibrinolysis, and the entire spectrum of bleeding dyscrasias is included. The presence of disseminated intravascular coagulation is difficult to distinguish from the primary coagulation factor deficiencies found in patients with severe liver disease. Because Factor VIII is not made in the liver, a lowered level in the patient with liver disease suggests a consumptive process.

The normal newborn infant has lower concentrations of the vitamin K–dependent factors than the adult, partially because of the immaturity of the fetal liver and partially because of low vitamin K stores. Prematurity exaggerates the phenomenon. Breast milk is a poor source of vitamin K, but cow's milk contains significant quantities. A hemorrhagic disease occurring 2 to 3 days after birth owing to low levels of the vitamin K–dependent factors has been associated with a sufficiently high mortality rate that prophylactic administration of a small quantity of vitamin K is considered warranted, even though only a partial correction of the coagulation abnormalities is achieved. The syndrome must be distinguished from other neonatal hemorrhagic syndromes, such as the thrombocytopenias, disseminated intravascular coagulation disorders, and hemophilia. The coumarin drugs cross the placental barrier and therefore are not given to pregnant women.

Hemorrhagic complications following heparin therapy are relatively infrequent, considering how extensively this drug is used (Wessler and Gitel, 1976). The duration of heparin action is limited to 4 to 6 hours, and thus the use of protamine, which neutralizes heparin, is rarely necessary in the management of hemorrhagic complications. Hemorrhagic complications may also occur following therapy with plasminogen activators, such as streptokinase or urokinase, but these agents also are rapidly removed if phagocytic clearing mechanisms are functioning normally.

Hypercoagulable States

Pathologic thrombosis in the coronary or cerebral circulation, in the deep veins of the legs, in the heart interior, or in other vascular sites is among the most important of public health problems. Yet, with some exceptions to be discussed, it has been impossible to predict which individuals will suffer this often devastating aberration of blood coagulation.

Table 4–7 lists some conditions that are known to be associated with a thrombotic tendency. These are classified as diseases of the vascular integrity, of stasis of blood flow, cellular abnormalities of the blood, and plasma abnormalities, but overlap between categories frequently occurs. In several of these conditions, the thrombotic tendency occurs concomitantly with a bleeding tendency.

Just as lack of procoagulant can bring on excessive bleeding, a deficiency of one of the natural plasma anticoagulants may be associated with a tendency to thrombosis, usually

Table 4–7 HYPERCOAGULABLE STATES

Altered intravascular surfaces
Atherosclerosis (and predisposing conditions such as diabetes mellitus, hypertension, the hyperlipidemias, etc.)
Prosthetic heart valves
Vasculitis
*Thrombotic thrombocytopenic purpura
Homocystinuria
*Pseudoxanthoma elasticum

Stasis of blood flow
Deep venous thrombosis (and predisposing causes, such as immobilization, venous compression, valve incompetence, etc.)
Valvular heart disease
Congestive heart failure
Cardiac arrhythmia

Cellular abnormalities of the blood
*Polycythemia vera
*Thrombocythemia
Sickle cell disease
Paroxysmal nocturnal hemoglobinuria
*Leukemia

Plasma abnormalities
*Disseminated intravascular coagulation (see Table 4–6)
Postoperative state
Pregnancy
Oral contraceptive use
Malignancy
Antithrombin III deficiency
*Dysfibrinogenemia
Plasminogen deficiency
Protein C deficiency
Protein S deficiency
Lupus anticoagulant

*Also often associated with pathologic bleeding.

venous in origin. *Hereditary deficiency of antithrombin III* is an autosomal dominant condition in which heterozygotes within affected families have an increased incidence of venous thromboembolism in early adult or middle life (Cosgriff et al., 1983). *Hereditary deficiency of protein C* is another autosomal dominant condition in which heterozygotes incur an increased incidence of venous thromboembolism, but homozygotes die in the neonatal period because of massive venous thrombosis (Seligsohn et al., 1984). It has been suggested that the rare complication of skin necrosis observed in patients being treated with coumarin anticoagulants is related to depression of this vitamin K–dependent factor. Heterozygosity for protein S deficiency is associated with a thrombophilic state similar to that seen in individuals with heterozygosity for protein C deficiency (Schwarz et al., 1984). *Hereditary deficiency of plasminogen* is also associated with thrombosis, as are some of the equally rare dysfibrinogenemias. It should be pointed out that lowered levels of antithrombin III, protein C, and plasminogen may also be seen in patients with liver disease or disseminated intravascular coagulation.

Antibodies directed against phospholipids occur in the plasma of 5 to 10 per cent of patients with systemic lupus erythematosus. These interfere with in vitro coagulation tests, which depend on the presence of phospholipid. Despite the laboratory abnormalities, in vivo hemostasis is usually normal. The term *lupus anticoagulant* is used to describe such antibodies, even though they are occasionally seen in other situations, such as in cases involving patients under treatment with certain medications, most notably chlorpromazine (Shapiro and Thiagarajan, 1982). The majority of the patients show false-positive reactions for syphilis, also related to the antiphospholipid antibody. The partial thromboplastin time is prolonged, and the prothrombin time is normal or only slightly prolonged. Paradoxically, these patients show a high incidence of thromboembolic disease (Elias and Eldor, 1984). How this might be related to the antiphospholipid antibody is unknown, although endothelial effects have been postulated. Pathologic bleeding is extremely rare in the absence of other defects, such as thrombocytopenia and hypoprothrombinemia.

References

Aledort, L. M.: Current concepts in diagnosis and management of hemophilia. Hosp. Pract., *17(10)*:77, 1982.

Blanchard, R. A., Furie, B. C., Jorgensen, M., et al.: Acquired vitamin K dependent carboxylation deficiency in liver disease. N. Engl. J. Med., *305*:242, 1981.

Bussel, J. B.: Circulating anticoagulants. Physiologic and pathophysiologic. Hosp. Pract., *18(2)*:169, 1983.

Colman, R. W.: Surface-mediated defense reactions. The plasma contact activation system. J. Clin. Invest., *73*:1249, 1984.

Cosgriff, T. M., Bishop, D. T., Hershgold, E. J., et al.: Familial antithrombin III deficiency: its natural history, genetics, diagnosis, and treatment. Medicine, *62*:209, 1983.

Doolittle, R. F.: Fibrinogen and fibrin. Sci. Am., *245(12)*:126, 1981.

Duckert, F.: Thrombolytic therapy. Semin. Thromb. Hemost., *10*:87, 1984.

Ebert, R. F., and Bell, W. R.: Fibrinogen Baltimore II. Congenital hypodysfibrinogenemia with delayed release of fibrinopeptide B and decreased rate of fibrinogen synthesis. Proc. Natl. Acad. Sci., *80*:7318, 1983.

Elias, M., and Eldor, A.: Thromboembolism in patients with "lupus" type circulating anticoagulant. Arch. Int. Med., *144*:510, 1984.

Gardiner, J. E., and Griffin, J. H.: Human protein C and thromboembolic disease. Prog. Hematol., *13*:265, 1983.

Gurevich, V.: Guidelines for the management of anticoagulant therapy. Semin. Thromb. Hemost., *2*:176, 1976.

Jaques, L. B.: Heparin: an old drug with a new paradigm. Science, *206*:528, 1979.

Koch-Weser, J., and Sellers, E. M.: Drug interactions with coumarin anticoagulants. New Engl. J. Med., *285*:487, 1971.

Laffel, G. L., and Braunwald, E.: Thrombolytic therapy. A new strategy for the treatment of myocardial infarction. New Engl. J. Med., *311*:710, 1984.

Lusher, J. M., Shapiro, S. S., Palascak, J. E., et al.: Efficacy of prothrombin-complex concentrates in hemophiliacs with antibodies to Factor VIII. A multicenter therapeutic trial. N. Engl. Med., *303*:421, 1980.

Mammen, E. F.: Congenital coagulation disorders. Semin. Thromb. Hemost., *9*:1, 1983.

Mannucci, P. M., Remuzzi, G., Pusineri, F., et al.: Deamino-8-D-arginine vasopressin shortens the bleeding time in uremia. N. Engl J. Med., *308*:8, 1983.

Martinez, J., and Palascak, J. E.: Hemostatic alterations in liver disease. *In* Zakin, D., and Boyer, T. D., (eds.): Hepatology. A Textbook of Liver Disease. Philadelphia, W. B. Saunders Co., 1982, p. 546.

Merskey, C.: DIC: Identification and management. Hosp. Pract., *17(12)*:83, 1982.

Nemerson, Y., and Bach, R.: Tissue factor revisited. Prog. Hemost. Thromb., *6*:237, 1982.

Ratnoff, O. D., and Jones, P. K.: The laboratory diagnosis of the carrier state for classic hemophilia. Ann. Intern. Med., *86*:521, 1977.

Rosenberg, R. D.: Actions and interactions of antithrombin and heparin. N. Engl. J. Med., *292*:146, 1975.

Rosenberg, R. D., and Rosenberg, J. S.: Natural anticoagulant mechanisms. J. Clin. Invest., *74*:1, 1984.

Russell, F. E.: Snake venom poisoning in the United States. Ann. Rev. Med., *31*:247, 1980.

Saito, H.: The "Contact system" in health and disease. Adv. Int. Med., *25*:217, 1980.

Schwarz, H. P., Fischer, M., Hopmeier, P., et al.: Plasma protein S deficiency in familial thrombotic disease. Blood, *64*:1297, 1984.

Seligsohn, U., Berger, A., et al.: Homozygous protein C deficiency manifested by massive venous thrombosis in the newborn. N. Engl. J. Med., *310*:559, 1984.

Shapiro, S. S., and Thiagarajan, P.: Lupus anticoagulants. Prog. Hemost. Thromb., *6*:263, 1982.

Spicer, T. E., and Rau, J. M.: Purpura fulminans. Am. J. Med., *61*:566, 1976.

Walsh, P. N.: Platelets and coagulation proteins. Fed. Proc., *40*:2086, 1981.

Walsh, P. N.: Oral anticoagulant therapy. Hosp. Pract., *18(1)*:101, 1983.

Wessler, S., and Gitel, S. N.: Warfarin. From bedside to bench. New Engl. J. Med., *311*:645, 1984.

Wessler, S., and Gitel, S.: Control of heparin therapy. Prog. Hemost. Thromb., *3*:311, 1976.

Zimmerman, T. S., and Ruggeri, Z. M.: Von Willebrand's disease. Prog. Hemost. Thromb., *6*:203, 1982.

Vascular Factors

STRUCTURE AND FUNCTION

Intact blood vessels provide an almost perfect nonleaking and nonactivating circuit for blood cells and plasma. The vascular diameter at its narrowest in capillaries is about 8 μ, which permits fairly free transit of red cells but demands considerable change in the shape of leukocytes. Because cells, regardless of their number, must pass capillaries in a single file, increased blood counts are sensed less by capillaries than by large vessels. All vessels are lined with a confluent monolayer of endothelial cells anchored to a basement membrane by an extracellular subendothelial matrix. In the capillaries, the junctions between endothelial cells may permit some fluid seepage and leukocyte migration, but most fluid and cellular transfer probably occurs via endocytotic vesicle formation. In large vessels, the intima, consisting of the endothelial cells and subendothelial matrix, is surrounded by the media with its concentric layers of smooth muscle cells and by the adventitia with its network of fibroblasts (Fig. 4–30).

The confluent endothelial cells provide a

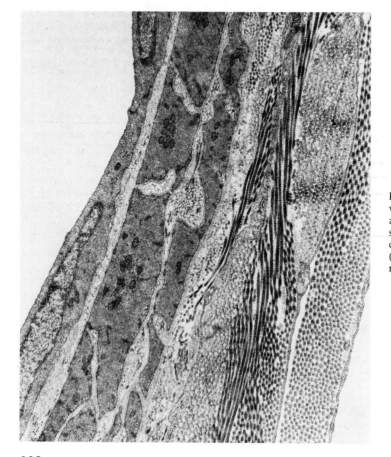

Figure 4–30 Cross section of a vessel wall with monolayer of fused endothelial cells, a basement membrane, subendothelial tissue and media with longitudinal and circular smooth muscle fibers. (×2500). (From Sedar, A. W., et al.: Arteriosclerosis, *30*:278, 1978.)

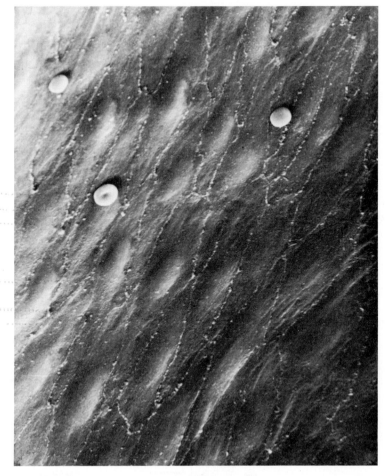

Figure 4–31 Electron microscopic scan of vascular surface showing the confluent monolayer of endothelial cells. Three red cells but no platelets are visible (×2500). (From Sedar, A. W., et al.: Arteriosclerosis, *30*:278, 1978.)

nearly perfect nonadhesive barrier for circulating platelets (Fig. 4–31), and aggregation occurs only at sites of injury with exposure of subendothelial tissue (Jaffe, 1983; Legrand et al., 1983). Such injury will lead to adhesion of platelets (Fig. 4–32) either directly to exposed collagen or indirectly via von Willebrand's factor and fibronectin, a ubiquitous sticky protein. Von Willebrand's factor is synthesized by the endothelial cells and deposited in the subendothelium, and, as suggested by the impaired platelet adhesion in von Willebrand's disease, it plays a major role in fastening the platelet to the subendothelium and initiating platelet aggregation and thrombus formation (Fig. 4–4) (Meyer and Baumgartner, 1983). In addition, platelet factor 4 released by activated platelets will inactivate heparin-like compounds secreted by mast cells in the subendothelial tissue. This sequence is inhibited, however, by prostacyclin, another factor synthesized by endothelial cells. In capillaries, with their relatively high density of endothelial

cells, prostacyclin plays an important role in retarding the effect of aggregating agents and permits platelets to seal endothelial injury without causing capillary obstruction.

In addition to denuding endothelial cells, tears in larger vessels will expose smooth muscle fibers, fibroblasts, and their intercellular collagenous matrix. The procoagulant effect of activated platelets will be augmented by activation of the extrinsic clotting pathway following release of tissue factor and activation of the intrinsic pathway by Hageman factor (Factor XII). Concomitantly, anticoagulant factors will be mobilized to limit the growth of the thrombus. Additional prostacyclin will be released from muscle fibers and counteract serotonin-induced vasoconstriction. Heparin-like compounds in the subendothelium will enhance the anticoagulant activity of antithrombin III, and thrombomodulin, a thrombin receptor in the endothelium, will activate protein C, a potent inhibitor of Factors V and VIII. Furthermore, tissue plasminogen activator will

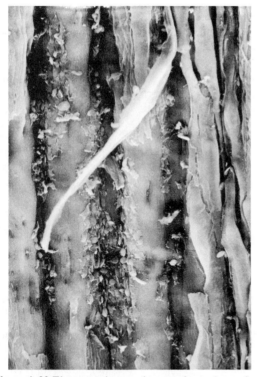

Figure 4–32 Electron microscopic scan of vascular surface after mechanical abrasion of endothelial cells. Numerous platelets adhere to the subendothelial tissues in the gaps between injured endothelial cells (×1000). (From Sedar, A. W., et al.: Arteriosclerosis, *30*:278, 1978.)

Table 4–8 VASCULAR HEMORRHAGIC DISORDERS

I. Hereditary
  A. Hereditary hemorrhagic telangiectasia (Rendu-Osler-Weber disease)
  B. Ehlers-Danlos syndrome
  C. Marfan's syndrome
II. Acquired
  A. Senile purpura
  B. Purpura simplex
  C. Scurvy
  D. Cushing's syndrome
  E. Amyloidosis
  F. Allergic purpura (Schönlein-Henoch syndrome)

cause the activation of plasmin, which will remodel the hemostatic plug. Finally, platelet-derived growth factor will stimulate proliferation and migration of smooth muscle cells and fibroblasts and adjacent intact endothelium will provide endothelial cells to cover the vascular tear completely.

PATHOPHYSIOLOGY

Table 4–8 lists a number of purpuric and bleeding disorders that occur in the absence of platelet or coagulation dysfunction. These vascular disorders, ranging from cosmetic blemishes to life-threatening illnesses, are caused by extravascular, vascular, or endothelial dysfunction. The most common of the extravascular dysfunctions result from age-related loss of elasticity and turgor of the supporting tissue around the vessels. This disorder, somewhat injudiciously called *senile purpura,* involves primarily the face, neck, and distal extremities. The purpuric spots are bluish-violet, have

sharply demarcated borders, resolve very slowly, and appear to be localized in the most superficial part of the dermis. They are not associated with overt bleeding and are primarily of cosmetic concern. A similar purpura, called purpura simplex, occurs frequently in women around their menstrual periods and in their postmenstrual years. However, the bleeding that occurs with purpura simplex is present in deeper dermal layers and resolves quickly. In diseases characterized by impaired collagen synthesis, such as in the hereditary disorders, Ehlers-Danlos and Marfan's syndromes, and in acquired scurvy and Cushing's disease, purpura is common. Purpuric lesions have little clinical significance in vascular hemorrhagic disorders, except scurvy, in which perifollicular hemorrhages are a valuable diagnostic clue. Infiltration of the vessel wall with immunoglobulin fragments, as in amyloidosis and other paraproteinemic disorders, can cause vascular wall weakness and purpura. Among vascular disorders, hereditary hemorrhagic telangiectasia (Rendu-Osler-Weber syndrome) is a striking and refractory illness. It is autosomal dominant and causes localized dilatations of small vessels. These commonly first appear as punctate vascular spots on the nose and fingertips and on the mucous membranes of the nose and mouth. As age progresses, these dilatations eventually can be found throughout the body, causing epistaxis, gastrointestinal bleeding, and arteriovenous fistulas.

Immunologic damage to endothelial cells is the most important endothelial disorder. The resulting purpuric lesions resemble those of thrombocytopenic purpura in that they have a predilection for the dependent parts of the body. However, the eruptions are frequently mixed with urticarial raised lesions and appear more violet and confluent than those of thrombocytopenic purpura. When these purpuric lesions are associated with gastrointestinal hemorrhages and joint swellings, the condition is designated *Schönlein-Henoch purpura.* In children, it often occurs following an upper respiratory infection and is of short duration. In adults, it may be associated with a variety of drug exposures and can be prolonged, lasting for years. However, the etiology and immunologic pathogenesis are still obscure. In either age group, the most severe complication is renal involvement, with renal failure only marginally responsive to corticosteroid or immunosuppressive therapy.

A previously rare endothelial disease causing local endothelial proliferation and purpura is Kaposi's hemorrhagic sarcoma. Dilated blood vessels with endothelial hyperplasia, local hemorrhage, and hemosiderin deposits provide substance and color to the dermal nodules. They may ulcerate and bleed, but in the past only sporadic cases involved internal organs. Since 1981, however, there has been an almost epidemic outbreak of this disease in young people with the acquired immunodeficiency syndrome (AIDS). Kaposi's sarcoma in these patients appears far more aggressive and potentially fatal than the disease observed previously in older individuals (Friedman-Kien et al., 1982). The cause is not known but obviously must be related to the impaired immune system.

DIAGNOSIS

The diagnosis of primary vascular purpuric syndromes rests primarily on clinical recognition. Laboratory confirmation is at present unsatisfactory. The bleeding time and the tourniquet test (in which the appearance of petechiae is observed after inflation of a blood pressure cuff to a level sufficient to occlude venous return but not arterial filling) are primarily tests of adequacy of platelet numbers and function and they are not of great assistance in establishing a diagnosis of primary vascular disorders. The fact that almost 10 percent of normal people have a positive tourniquet test also diminishes the diagnostic value of this procedure.

References

Friedman-Kien, A. E., et al.: Disseminated Kaposi's sarcoma in homosexual men. Ann. Intern. Med., 96:693, 1982.
Jaffe, E. A.: Vascular function in hemostasis. *In* Williams, W. J., et al. (eds.): Hematology. 3rd ed. McGraw-Hill Book Co., 1983, p. 1277.
Legrand, Y. J., et al.: The molecular interaction between platelet and vascular wall. Blood Cells, 9:263, 1983.
Meyer, D., and Baumgartner, H. R.: Role of von Willebrand factor in platelet adhesion to the subendothelium. Br. J. Haematol., 54:1, 1983.
Rosenberg, R. D., and Rosenberg, J. S.: Natural anticoagulant mechanisms. J. Clin. Invest., 74:1, 1984.

Appendix

NORMAL ADULT LABORATORY VALUES*

		Range	International Units
Red cell count	Men:	4.7–5.9 (5.1) $\times$ 10^6/mm.^{3}	$\times$ 10^{12}/L.
	Women:	4.0–5.2 (4.5) $\times$ 10^6/mm.^{3}	$\times$ 10^{12}/L.
Hemoglobin	Men:	14–17 gm./100 ml.	gm./dl.
	Women:	12–15 gm./100 ml.	gm./dl.
Packed cell volume	Men:	42–52%	.42–.52 L./L.
	Women:	37–47%	.37–.47 L./L.
Erythrocyte indices:			
Mean corpuscular volume		82–92 μ^3	fl.
Mean corpuscular hemoglobin		27–32 $\mu\mu$g.	pg.
Mean corpuscular hemoglobin conc.		32–36 gm./100 ml.	gm./dl.
White cell count		5000–10,000/mm.^{3}	5–10 $\times$ 10^9/L.
Differential:			
Neutrophils (segs)		54–62%	%
Neutrophils (bands)		5–10%	%
Neutrophils (total)		3500–7100/mm.^{3}	3.5–7.1 $\times$ 10^9/L.
Eosinophils		0–3%	%
Basophils		0–1%	%
Lymphocytes		18–35%	%
Monocytes		3–7%	%
Platelet count		175,000–375,000/mm.^{3}	175–375 $\times$ 10^9/L.
Reticulocyte count		0.5–2.5%	%
Absolute reticulocyte count		25,000–125,000/mm.^{3}	25–125 $\times$ 10^9/L.
†Prothrombin time		11–13 sec.	sec.
†Partial thromboplastin time		50–90 sec.	sec.
†Partial thromboplastin time, activated		20–35 sec.	sec.
†Thrombin time		20–26 sec.	sec.
Fibrinogen		150–400 mg./100 ml.	2.0–4.0 gm./L.
Bleeding time (Ivy method)		2–7 min.	min.
Euglobulin lysis time		More than 2 hrs.	hrs.
Fibrin degradation products		0–4 μg./ml.	mg./L.
Factor VIII and other coagulation factors		50–150% of normal	0.5–1.5 U./ml.
†Serum iron		70–140 μg./100 ml.	12–25 μmol./L.
†Total iron binding capacity		250–400 μg./100 ml.	45–72 μmol./L.
% saturation		20–50 (35) %	%
†Serum ferritin	Men:	20–200 ng./ml.	μg./L.
	Women:	10–200 ng./ml.	μg./L.
†Serum B$_{12}$		200–1000 pg./ml.	ng./L.
†Serum folate		3–20 ng./ml.	μg./L.
†Shilling test	Stage I	10–40 (18)% of dose	%
	Stage II	10–42 (18)% of dose	%
Haptoglobin (hemoglobin binding capacity)		50–150 mg./100 ml.	.5–1.5 gm./L.
Bilirubin (total)		0.1–1.2 mg./100 ml.	1–12 mg./L.
Bilirubin (direct)		0–0.3 ng./100 ml.	0–3 mg./L.
†Serum lactic dehydrogenase		100–225 mU./ml.	0–90 I.U./L. 30° C.
Hemoglobin A$_2$		1.8–3.3%	%
Hemoglobin F		<2.0%	%
Erythropoietin (plasma)		3–20 mU./ml.	mU./ml.
Erythropoietin (urinary excretion)		2–5 U./24 hr.	U./24 hr.

*Ranges given in terms of ± 2 standard deviations. Mean values in parentheses.
†Normal values vary with technique used.

INDEX

Note: Page numbers in *italics* indicate illustrations; those followed by (t) indicate tables.